THE ONE YEAR® BOOK OF HEALING

THE ONE YEAR® BOOK *of* HEALING

Daily Appointments with God for Physical, Spiritual, and Emotional Wholeness

DR. REGGIE ANDERSON
with JENNIFER SCHUCHMANN

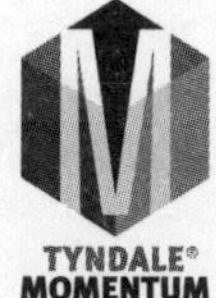

An Imprint of
Tyndale House Publishers, Inc.

Visit Tyndale online at www.tyndale.com.

Visit Tyndale Momentum online at www.tyndalemomentum.com.

Tyndale Momentum, the Tyndale Momentum logo, *The One Year*, and *One Year* are registered trademarks of Tyndale House Publishers, Inc. The One Year logo is a trademark of Tyndale House Publishers, Inc. Tyndale Momentum is an imprint of Tyndale House Publishers, Inc., Carol Stream, Illinois.

The One Year Book of Healing: Daily Appointments with God for Physical, Spiritual, and Emotional Wholeness

Designed by Alyssa Force

Published in association with the literary agency of Creative Trust, Inc., 210 Jamestown Park Drive, Suite 200, Brentwood, TN 37027.

Printed in the United States

22 21 20 19 18 17 16
7 6 5 4 3 2 1

Introduction

As a primary care physician practicing rural medicine in a small town outside of Nashville, Tennessee, I have witnessed a lot of healing. Some of it has been through the work of medical professionals, whom God uses to carry out his good work, and some has happened supernaturally—the result of God's direct intervention.

The devotions in this book are meant to encourage you to pursue a closer relationship with our Lord and Savior, Jesus Christ. I want you to see the many ways that he intervenes in the lives of the sick and the hurting—and the many ways that he heals—so that you will be inspired to have hope; the faith to know that he can bring healing to your life, as well; and the patience to wait for him to act on your behalf. I want you to see what I see every day—that God is alive and that he is active in our lives. I want you to know how much he cares for you. I have written these brief daily offerings to help you meditate on his healing promises.

Because we live in a broken, sinful world, we are all sick or hurting in some way. Some of us need to be healed of things that can easily be fixed, like a sprained ankle or a treatable illness. Others of us need to be healed from things that aren't as easy to see—like abuse suffered in the past or emotional wounds from a broken relationship. Perhaps you have a chronic, debilitating disease that won't go away without miraculous intervention. Or maybe it's a temporary condition that will get better with time. Whatever your sickness, whatever your hurt, I want you to know that God loves you and wants to heal you. Whether you're seeking relief from pain or want your energy to return or your cancer to go into remission or to have control over your spiraling negative thoughts, you need your Father's healing hand to reach out and free you from the bondage of your physical body. One thing we all have in common as human beings is that we need healing—God's healing.

But sometimes we're not able to see how God is at work, and we wonder if he's even there or if he cares. That's why I've chosen to tell these stories about my patients—stories about God's faithfulness that I've seen with my own eyes and sensed in my own spirit. *How* God's healing work will be accomplished cannot be predicted—only that it *will* happen.

Sometimes, God heals us partially by removing our disease or fixing our wounds. Sometimes, he heals us completely by taking us to our forever home in heaven. Often, he uses modern medicine—lab results, high-tech treatments, doctors, and nurses—to accomplish his healing. Less frequently, he does it miraculously and instantaneously, without intervention from the medical community.

From my thirty years of practicing medicine, I've learned that we can't explain why one person gets sick and another one doesn't. With our society's focus on fairness, this can be hard to understand. We feel as if there must be a plausible reason why we got cancer or why our child has autism. But whether we have played a part in our illness through lifestyle choices we've made, or it has happened through no fault of our own, God's desire for us to be healed, healthy, and whole remains the same.

Over the years, I have discovered several common truths in the lives of my patients when it comes to healing.

1. God is the one who heals. Medical professionals can treat, cure, recommend, advise, prescribe, and preserve, but no matter how talented the physician, he or she alone cannot heal the human mind, body, and soul. Only God can do that. God often uses doctors and other health practitioners in the healing process, but ultimately only God can restore us fully and completely. This is especially true when it comes to spiritual healing and healing from emotional issues or abuse. A physician can prescribe a mood elevator, but if we want to be fully healed, God must ultimately renew our minds. As you read and meditate on the devotions in this book, look for stories of miraculous healing. I have also included stories of times when God healed someone by nudging me toward a diagnosis or treatment option I would not have chosen based on medical science alone.

2. Sometimes emotional healing must come first. Because we don't always recognize the symptoms of emotional injury or illness, we're often slow or reluctant to seek treatment. However, emotional or spiritual wounds can affect our physical health. Look for stories in this book about people who realized that they had to heal emotionally before they could become physically healthy.

3. Healing comes in many forms. In medicine, nothing is 100 percent. There is always an exception to the rule. What should work doesn't always work. So, when someone recovers, I know that God played a part in it. This book is filled with these stories. Some are miraculous—that is, there is no medical explanation for what happened. Others will seem like they are simply the natural outcome of a course of treatment. God doesn't always heal in the same way or within a predictable time frame. But just as a bird watcher uses a guidebook to recognize rarely seen birds in the field, I hope this book becomes a field manual to help you recognize the different ways that God heals ordinary people living ordinary lives.

4. Our hope for healing is only in Jesus Christ. In conversations about chronic or deadly diseases, it's common to hear people say, "I hope they find a cure." We all hope for scientific breakthroughs in prevention, diagnosis, and treatment of disease. But our real hope isn't in a scientist developing a new drug or treatment. Our real hope is in the God who saves us. As Psalm 25:5 reminds us, "All day long I put my hope in you." And our hope extends beyond our days on earth. As the apostle Paul says, "If our hope in Christ is only for this life, we are more to be pitied than anyone in the world" (1 Corinthians 15:19). As you read the devotions, the verses and stories will remind you that unless our hope is in Christ, our hope is in vain.

5. Prayer is an important part of the healing process. Whether we are praying for ourselves, or someone else is praying for us, prayer is more powerful than any medicine a doctor can prescribe. That's why I take time to pray with my patients who are willing. I know that nothing pleases God more than when we turn our worries and fears over to him, trusting him to work. Look for devotions about the power of prayer, intercessory prayer, anointing the sick with oil, and how prayer can change us.

6. Healthy living leads to healthy lives. If I didn't address the subject of healthy living, the book would be incomplete. Too many people become concerned about their health only after it's gone. I've used stories of my patients to remind you that healing begins before we get sick. We must intentionally take care of our bodies, our minds, our emotions, and our relationship with God in order to prevent, postpone, or lessen the impact of illness.

7. Sometimes we must overcome obstacles to healing. Despite our desire to get well and God's desire to heal us, we may encounter obstacles to our healing. Look for stories of people whose fear, anxiety, unbelief, or unwillingness to ask for help or follow a treatment plan held them back from recovering their well-being.

As you meditate on these devotions, my prayer is that God will give you hope, peace, and patience to trust, believe, and wait for him to do what only he can do—heal you from the inside out.

How to Use This Devotional

This book is divided into twelve months, with a devotion for each day of the month.

Each month begins with a checkup—an overview of common experiences or what you may expect that month to bring physically or emotionally. In those monthly introductions, I suggest a spiritual challenge, something you can do for the next thirty days to enhance your relationship with God. Feel free to adapt or replace my suggestion if it doesn't work for you. My objective is to help you see God through fresh eyes each month.

Just as many of your childhood visits to the doctor may have ended with a shot, I finish each monthly checkup here with a Booster Shot, intended to encourage you to greater health and wellness during the month that follows.

At the beginning of each devotion, I have included a verse or two of Scripture. But I encourage you to have your Bible handy so you can look up the verses in context to gain a more complete understanding.

Following the Scripture verse, each devotion has a story of healing. Sometimes the story is directly related to the verse; others are stories that came to mind after I prayed about the verse. My hope is that the combination of these verses and stories will show you that our sovereign God is still very much in the healing business. I want to assure you that he loves you and desires for you to be whole and healthy—though sometimes we won't experience complete healing until we join him in our forever home. Even when healing doesn't happen as quickly or completely as we may desire, I hope these stories demonstrate that God is always present in your pain and suffering. My patients continue to amaze me with stories of how their faith has grown, even when their prayers weren't answered the way they hoped they would be.

At the end of each devotion, I offer a suggestion (Today's Rx) for something specific that you can do or consider that will make you feel better, grow stronger, or draw closer to our Father. Then I close in prayer.

The personal stories from my own life and medical practice are all true. But to protect the privacy of my patients, I have changed their names, circumstances, and other identifying information. After three decades of practicing medicine, I have seen many similar cases dozens of times, so some of the stories are composites of details from different cases. Conversations have been reconstructed based on my best recollections.

The medical information provided in this book is specific to the patients I saw in my office or in the emergency room. The treatments prescribed are not intended to diagnose, cure, or treat anyone else's medical or health condition. It is not medical advice and should not replace the advice of your physician. Please consult your doctor to determine what is right for you and your situation.

And while I am adding disclaimers, it would be wise for you to consult with your pastor before following my spiritual advice, as well. After all, I'm not a theologian; I'm just a country doctor.

I hope the stories in this devotional will convince you that the healing hand of God isn't limited to the pages of the Bible. Our Lord continues to heal the sick and hurting today.

How do I know?

I've seen his extraordinary work in my own life and in the lives of my patients. My prayer is that you will see God work in your own life, as well.

Dr. Reggie Anderson

JANUARY CHECKUP

January is a month when new life can seem distant and unreachable. The days are short, and the sky is often gray. In many parts of the country, the weather isn't conducive to going outside, and when we look out the window, we see a barren landscape and naked trees.

As winter takes hold, the excitement we felt during the holidays is gone, and we're left with nothing but the bills. Along with family and friends, we have resumed the daily grind, and spring cannot come soon enough.

During these often gloomy days, I think of a seed buried in the dark, cold, and lonely ground and how necessary the winter season is in the cycle of life. You see, that seed needs the time underground in order for the plant inside to burst through its shell and sprout new life. We won't see evidence of the growth until spring, but the seed is already in the process of transforming into a blossoming flower.

January can feel a bit like the Saturday after Jesus' death on the cross. It seems as if all hope is lost. But take heart; just as Sunday came and Jesus was resurrected, so too, spring is coming and everything will feel fresh and new.

During this first month of the year, learn the lesson of the seed, and concentrate on your interior life. Make a special effort to set aside time each morning or evening to pray. Pick a new topic each week—finances, relationships, health, family, friends, or whatever you think will most affect your year—and concentrate on praying about that topic for seven days. During your prayer time, take time to listen to what God is telling you. Align your goals with his. Just as a seed prepares to send out green shoots of new life during this cold, dark month, you can prepare for new growth in your spiritual life.

In addition to preparing your heart for renewal, take this time of hibernation to rest and relax from the busy holidays so you will have the strength to blossom in a few short weeks. Make your New Year's resolution something that will not only improve your health, but will also improve your wellness.

January Booster Shot: Depression is one of the most common maladies health-care providers see during the winter. It's often referred to as *seasonal affective disorder* (SAD). If you find yourself feeling sad, sluggish, depressed, or tearful, get as much sunlight as possible. If the symptoms persist, seek medical advice.

THE BEST TIME TO START IS NOW

My child, pay attention to what I say. Listen carefully to my words. Don't lose sight of them. Let them penetrate deep into your heart, for they bring life to those who find them, and healing to their whole body. PROVERBS 4:20-22

Do you remember the last time you visited a doctor or a counselor? After discussing your ailments, the practitioner likely gave you a set of instructions to help you feel better.

When you left the office, you were committed to implement the recommended plan. But maybe that's as far as it went. Maybe life got in the way, and before you knew it, the doctor's advice had been shuffled to the bottom of your to-do list. A week later, you had forgotten you even had a plan. The advice that had once seemed important enough to consult with and pay a professional for had somehow slipped away.

The all-too-common pattern of wanting answers to our problems but never implementing them can also happen with God's Word. We go to him looking for wisdom and guidance, but even when we receive his instructions, we file them away for a day when applying them seems more convenient. But the right time never seems to come. We all have good intentions, but we're lacking on the follow-through. We keep putting off until later what we should do right now. When we procrastinate, it often means we never get around to what is important.

If we really want the life and healing that God promises, we can't let his wise words slip away. If we lose sight of God's wisdom, it's worse than if we had never received it. We need to abide in God's Word, allow it to penetrate our hearts deeply, and put into action the things we've heard God say. Write down what God has said, and place reminders where you won't lose sight of them. That is how they will penetrate deeply into your heart.

TODAY'S RX

Has God asked you to forgive someone? Call that person now. Has God asked you to give something? Give it now. Has God asked you to show love to someone? Love that person now.

Lord, thank you for giving me wisdom and counsel through your Word. Help me to draw from it daily, impressing your instructions upon my heart and applying your words to the problems I face.

THE POWER OF PRAYER

Are any of you sick? You should call for the elders of the church to come and pray over you, anointing you with oil in the name of the Lord. JAMES 5:14

We've all had times when we've been sick. Whether we had a minor cold or something more serious, we learned how miserable we can feel when we're under the weather. With proper care and rest, we typically recover fairly quickly, and even those with chronic or debilitating illnesses would say they have good days along with the bad. But there's one thing that is always true: When we're sick, we want to feel better.

In today's key verse, James describes the importance of praying for healing when we're sick. Many Christian churches have a formal time for these kinds of prayers. Other churches may be less structured and more spontaneous as needs arise, but they are nonetheless committed to this practice. Having people pray for us when we're sick helps us to feel better. It's a sign that people love us when they will intercede with the Great Physician for our well-being. But prayers don't only help us to *feel* better; they can also help us *get* better.

In medical literature, there is scientific evidence that patients who have people surrounding them with love and prayer generally fare better than those who don't. Patients who have been prayed for recover faster, report less pain, require less medication, and have fewer complications.

As a doctor, I've been at the bedside of many patients when elders from their church have come to pray for their healing. And I've personally seen many patients with severe illnesses recover and return home to their families and continue living fruitful lives.

I've also been at the bedside of many patients when prayers for healing were not answered as hoped, and we had to trust God for his higher purposes. But even when those illnesses ended in death, the process of praying brought emotional healing and comfort to those who were present. It's as if we were able to catch a glimpse of the patient's soul completely healed on the other side of heaven's veil.

TODAY'S RX

Whatever kind of healing you need—spiritual, emotional, or physical—ask others to join you in prayer today for your healing.

God, thank you for the comfort of bringing my requests to you and knowing that you hear me and love me. Where I am weary, please bring healing and strength, and help me to fully trust in you.

TURNING BACK TO SEE WHO IS THERE

O Lord, you alone are my hope. I've trusted you, O Lord, from childhood. Yes, you have been with me from birth; from my mother's womb you have cared for me. No wonder I am always praising you! Psalm 71:5-6

I grew up in a churchgoing family in Plantersville, Alabama. From the day I was born, any time the church doors were open, my family was there. But even as a young child, I knew that I didn't have to go to a special building to be with God. I felt his presence each time I lay on my back in the lush, green grass and watched the puffy marshmallow clouds float by in the silky blue sky.

When I was four and a half, my favorite cartoon show advertised a contest to win a free pony. One night, I dreamed that God wanted me to have that pony, so I talked to my mom, and she helped me mail the entry. A few days later, I found out I had won! Because God had given me this gift, I promised that I would share that pony with all the children who came to visit.

And as I grew older, the coral colors of the sunset and the twinkling stars in the heavens were all the proof I needed that God was real and always with me.

But when I was in high school, my beliefs changed when some close friends of mine and members of their family were brutally murdered in a senseless massacre. It was hard for me to believe that the God of twinkling stars and marshmallow clouds could allow this to happen. So I turned my back on the God of my childhood and ran as far as I could from him.

Professing to be an atheist, I searched for answers about life but only found more questions. When I finally wore myself out, I turned back and surrendered to the God I'd left behind in Plantersville—only to find that he'd been running alongside me all along, even when I didn't care to admit that he existed. He was patiently waiting for me to run back into his arms. Because of his unwavering faithfulness, I will praise him all the remaining days of my life.

TODAY'S RX

If you are running from God, stop and turn back. He has always cared for you—and he always will.

Father, I confess I turn my back on you all too often, doubting your goodness in my life. Thank you for always chasing after me and welcoming me with open arms.

HIDDEN DEVILS

Jesus went around doing good and healing all who were oppressed by the devil, for God was with him. Acts 10:38

As a third-year resident in family medicine, I had the opportunity to serve as the medical director of a mental health hospital in Jackson, Tennessee. The duties, for the most part, were routine. It was my job to make sure that the patients were medically healthy. If we had to admit someone, it was typically because his or her outpatient treatment plan had failed.

Larry was an exception. He was sent to the hospital by a court order because he thought he was possessed by Satan. An unusually large man with a massive forehead, Larry had had periodic outbursts toward his family, and the police had been called to his house on several occasions for domestic violence.

As I examined him, he seemed to look right through me—peering off into a world that the rest of us couldn't see. He had been diagnosed with schizophrenia, but his medical history was unusual. His symptoms had appeared much later in life than was typical for schizophrenia. Larry also suffered from migraines, and there was something unusual about the size of his hands and feet.

When his lab work came back, I could see that he had diabetes mellitus and renal failure. There were now more questions in his chart than answers. I spoke with the psychiatrist who was treating Larry's mental illness and requested a CT scan of Larry's head. When the results came back, we were able to see for the first time what was going on. It turned out that Larry had a pituitary tumor that was causing acromegaly—a hormonal disease that causes growth hormones to be released long after the body should have stopped growing. This explained the unusual size of his face, feet, and hands. They had continued to grow well into adulthood.

We began treatment on the tumor immediately, and within three weeks, his "schizophrenia" symptoms improved. God had removed "the devil" that had tormented this man for so many years.

TODAY'S RX

Regardless of your affliction, whether spiritual or physical, God wants to heal you. Sometimes he uses a pastor, and other times he uses a physician.

God, only you can see my innermost parts. Please detect in me where I need healing, both in body and spirit. I give myself to you.

GOD WANTS YOU TO BLOSSOM

The LORD said to me, "Look, Jeremiah! What do you see?" And I replied, "I see a branch from an almond tree." And the LORD said, "That's right, and it means that I am watching, and I will certainly carry out all my plans." JEREMIAH 1:11-12

After the holidays, the long, dark days of winter can begin to take a toll on our moods. Many doctors and counselors find that their patients are in a funk during this time of year. But for some people, it could be even worse. They could be suffering from depression. Twenty percent of the world's population will struggle with depression at some point in their lives. In fact, it's so common that it's often referred to as the "common cold" of mental illness.

The brain chemistry involved in depression is both simple and mysteriously complex. Three main chemical engines—serotonin, norepinephrine, and dopamine—make us feel happy and hopeful. God designed these neurotransmitters to work in concert to help us maintain a hopeful outlook. But when one or more of the systems isn't working properly, depression can set in.

I have counseled many patients with depression. Often they mention, "No one cares whether I live or die." If this statement resonates with you, reread today's verse, which contains a promise from God that he is watching over you and actively involved in your life.

Almond trees are native to the Mediterranean climate and are known for being one of the first plants to blossom. The white and pale pink flowers sometimes bloom as early as January or February. Because of their early blossoming, almond trees are mentioned several times in the Bible—often as a symbol of God's vigilance and faithfulness.

Do you ever wonder whether God is looking out for you or if he even cares what happens in your life? Wonder no more. The almond tree is a reminder that God wants you to blossom under his care. You are not alone in the battle. God wants you to enjoy the world he has created, and he wants you to hope for even better things to come—in the next world, our forever home.

TODAY'S RX

Depression often happens when we focus on the past. Focus on the future, and God's promises will help to brighten your day.

Jesus, I ask that you breathe life into this dreary season—that you lift my head and help me focus on you. Thank you for never leaving me in the dark and always sending me reminders of your faithfulness and love.

MODERN MIRACLES

"Now put your hand back into your cloak," the LORD *said. So Moses put his hand back in, and when he took it out again, it was as healthy as the rest of his body.*
EXODUS 4:7

In today's verse, God reveals his power over sickness and health. If we witnessed today what God did for Moses, we'd certainly call it a miracle.

I believe that miracles still happen. Just because we use medical science to treat people doesn't mean that God is any less involved or that the cure is any less miraculous—like the night when medical science saved a woman's life early in my career.

On a slow evening in the ER, I was relaxing in the doctor's lounge when I received an urgent summons. Before I could even get to the exam room, I heard a woman named Allison pleading for help.

"I'm itching all over. My skin feels like it's on fire! Please help me!"

Allison was in anaphylactic shock, on the verge of total collapse and cardiac arrest. This was a true life-and-death emergency.

I followed the standard protocol: putting her on 100 percent oxygen and starting an IV of epinephrine, Benadryl, and steroids.

"I can barely breathe," she said in a panic. She looked terrified. "Are you sure this will work? I feel like I'm about to pass out."

"Your blood pressure is low, and your heart rate is pretty high. That's why you're feeling this way," I said. "Give the medication a few minutes to kick in, and you'll start feeling better."

Soon her shortness of breath began to subside. I saw the fear in her eyes abate as her blood pressure and heart rate returned to normal. It turned out she'd had an allergic reaction to shellfish. If she had gotten to the ER five minutes later, she probably would have been in full cardiac arrest.

Though we used modern medicine to treat her, I have no doubt that it was God who saved Allison's life. The efficacy of the drugs is really no less miraculous than when God healed Moses of leprosy by telling him to put his hand inside his cloak.

God knows the dangers we face, and it's a miracle of his grace that we can be saved through modern medicine.

TODAY'S RX

Don't overlook or dismiss everyday miracles just because they don't happen the same way they did in the Bible.

Lord, your power is beyond my imagination. Help me to recognize your hand at work throughout my day. I praise you for how intimately you know my needs.

MY SECRET

Don't worry about anything; instead, pray about everything. Tell God what you need, and thank him for all he has done. Then you will experience God's peace, which exceeds anything we can understand. His peace will guard your hearts and minds as you live in Christ Jesus. PHILIPPIANS 4:6-7

Over the years, I've had more than one person ask me, "Dr. Anderson, why are you so cheerful all the time? I always see you with the sickest of patients, yet you never get sick. You're surrounded by people who are dying, and yet you always seem happy. What's your secret?"

My secret is contained in today's verses.

When I started medical school, I was an atheist. One night, I had a date with a pretty blonde woman who told me she was a Christian. When she found out that I didn't believe in God, she wasn't interested in pursuing a relationship.

At the university we both attended, she co-led a Bible study. As a part of her preparation, she had to memorize the book of Philippians. The only way she would spend time with me was if I helped her memorize those verses. Night after night, I'd go to her apartment and quiz her on verses, then chapters, and finally the entire book of Philippians. As I helped her study, I memorized the verses too.

Months later, I read a book by C. S. Lewis that she gave me. Then I started reading the Gospel of John. When Jesus revealed himself to me in a dream and I gave my life to him, it took a while for Karen to believe that the changes in me were real. But eventually, that pretty blonde woman became my wife.

At the time, I had no idea how precious the book of Philippians would become to me as a doctor. During the darkest moments, when delivering the worst news—an unfavorable diagnosis or telling parents about an untimely death of a child—today's verses in particular would come to mind. When I share these verses with patients, they often find peace, knowing that God is with them.

What the patients don't know, unless I tell them, is that the very same verses once healed my heart and refreshed my broken life.

TODAY'S RX

Memorizing Scripture has a lot of health benefits. Start today by memorizing today's verses from Philippians.

Help me to keep your Word hidden in my heart, Lord. May I store up your commands, draw from your well of knowledge, sing your praises, and remember Jesus' parables to help me through every season. Thank you for allowing me to know you better through the Bible.

HEALING POWER OF TEARS

You keep track of all my sorrows. You have collected all my tears in your bottle. You have recorded each one in your book. PSALM 56:8

As a young man growing up on a farm, I had no idea what the phrase "I just need a good cry to feel better" meant. It wasn't until I got married and had three daughters that I understood the importance of that statement.

Men are sometimes reluctant to show their emotions. We think of shedding tears as being weak. We'll often just buck up and swallow our emotions, internalizing the things that need to be brought up and dealt with.

Generally, women are much better communicators—especially when it comes to feelings. They're much less reserved about pouring out their hearts and souls. Over the years of being in a predominantly female house, I have seen, up close and personal, the positive effects of crying at the right time for the right reasons.

God created us to have emotions, and tears can be very therapeutic. In fact, even Jesus wept at the death of Lazarus.

In addition to the spiritual benefits, tears have documented healing properties. For example, our tears are similar in composition to the saline solution we use to resuscitate people when they are about to code. And biologically, the release of tears is accompanied by chemical changes in the brain.

There are times when we need to cry and times when we need to cry out to God and ask him to intercede for our needs. Healing tears can be used to reset our emotional center toward all that is good and godly.

And perhaps you'll learn what I learned: understanding our own tears can help us to understand the tears of others.

TODAY'S RX

Know that it is healing to release your fears with tears.

Thank you, Father, for hearing my cry when I am feeling sad. I take comfort in knowing that you're alongside me during my time of need and that none of my sorrow is ever in vain.

BABY BLUE MIRACLE

I love the L*ORD because he hears my voice and my prayer for mercy. Because he bends down to listen, I will pray as long as I have breath!* PSALM 116:1-2

The mother burst through the doors of the trauma center and ran toward the nurse's desk.

"My baby! My baby! Please help my baby!"

In her arms was a little boy, probably nine or ten months old. He was blue. She handed the child to a nurse, who in turn handed him to me—a limp and lifeless body.

"Tell me what happened," I said, trying to calm the mother.

"I was feeding him breakfast, and I turned around to grab his cereal. When I turned back, he was choking! Please, you have to save him!"

I tried not to panic as I placed the baby on a cot and listened for any sign of breathing. None. I swept his throat with my finger. Nothing.

I wasn't sure we even had time to wait for the code team to assemble, and I was out of my league. What else could I do? I began to pray, "God, please help me save this baby."

Instantly, I felt God's presence, and it gave me confidence beyond my training.

I grabbed the laryngoscope, stuck it in the baby's throat, and looked around. Nothing. I knew by now that he'd been without air for too long. As I called for the nurse to prepare a tracheotomy tray, I sensed God saying, *You won't need it.*

Then something caught my eye—like a ball bobbing back and forth. The hard back of the laryngoscope dislodged it, and the baby took one quick breath.

"Hemostat," I said to the nurse.

When she handed me the clamp-like device, I reached into the baby's throat and pulled out a small square of plastic with a notch on one side. A clip from a bread bag.

The little boy took a deep breath and started crying. It was an exhilarating experience to hand him back to his mother, healthy and howling.

Later, I thought about how little control I'd had over the fate of that young boy. But God did. I had felt his hand guiding me throughout the entire event—and I was so thankful he had![1]

TODAY'S RX

Pray for a miracle today, and give credit to God, the miracle maker.

God, give me ears to hear your voice today. Speak your instruction to me as I make decisions and interact with others. Thank you for guiding me every step of the way.

TWO MIRACLES IN ONE

Jesus led him away from the crowd so they could be alone. He put his fingers into the man's ears. Then, spitting on his own fingers, he touched the man's tongue. MARK 7:33

As Jesus was traveling from Tyre to Sidon, he encountered a deaf man with a speech impediment. The man's friends begged Jesus to heal him. After Jesus led the man away from the crowd to where they could be alone, he put his fingers into the man's ears and then spit on his own fingers and touched the man's tongue. Looking up to heaven, Jesus said an Aramaic word that means, "Be opened." Instantly, the man could hear and speak plainly.

In that moment, Jesus demonstrated his power over disabilities that most people would consider permanent and irreversible—conditions such as deafness. In the same moment, Jesus also demonstrated his power over time.

Even after the man was able to hear, one would expect that it would take some time for him to learn to speak properly. After all, speech is developed over years of repetition, with lots of trial and error. Yet this man spoke immediately and plainly. Jesus compressed years of learning into an instant.

This miracle demonstrates that our Lord not only has power over the physical realm, but he also has power over time. This should give us hope that no matter how long we've suffered, Jesus can heal us of even our most chronic disabilities, according to his will.

TODAY'S RX

No matter what the diagnosis is or how long you've suffered, Jesus has the power to heal you immediately, if he so chooses. Trust his wisdom and timing.

Jesus, just as you have opened this man's ears and mouth,
I ask for your healing touch—not just for my physical
ailments, but also for the sin that lurks in my heart.

EXPERIENCING HEAVEN ON EARTH

Since you have been raised to new life with Christ, set your sights on the realities of heaven, where Christ sits in the place of honor at God's right hand. Think about the things of heaven, not the things of earth. COLOSSIANS 3:1-2

On July 4, 1980, I had a dream of heaven that changed my life. In that dream, I experienced the sights, sounds, and smells of heaven. That one experience changed me from an atheist to a believer in God.

Ever since that night, I have searched the world for signs of the heaven to come. I truly believe it is closer than we think—perhaps just on the other side of the veil between life and death. I know this because, as I've paid attention, God has given me glimpses of heaven.

In fact, I believe God marks the pathway for all of us to our eternal home, drawing us onward toward heaven. But we must be spiritually awake and aware of those bread crumbs to experience them in this world.

Often, while walking around my farm, I will get a whiff of a tantalizing aroma or see a majestic butterfly, and I'll again experience that sense of heaven. Those moments take me back to what I experienced in my dream.

C. S. Lewis said, "If I find in myself a desire that nothing in this world can satisfy, the most probable explanation is that I was made for another world."[2]

Standing at the bedside of a believer who is ready to cross the threshold into eternal life is like standing on holy ground. It is an opportunity to witness the veil blowing open momentarily to welcome a new saint into heaven. I have treasured every chance I've had to be a part of these transitions. Each experience is slightly different—yet, at the same time, familiar.

We must be fully awake and spiritually aware of the bread crumbs that lead us ever so gently toward home. Who knows? We may just get the opportunity to escort a loved one to heaven's foyer. If that happens to you, inhale deeply and fully experience the moment. You might just be breathing in heaven's air.

TODAY'S RX

You don't need to run toward heaven; heaven is walking alongside you.

Father, I long for a glimpse of what awaits me—to shed the weight and pain of this life and to experience the majesty of your Kingdom. Until that day, send me reminders of your glory so that I may remember that I was made for more than just this world.

SET ASIDE YOUR ANSWERS TO HEAR HIS

Harden the hearts of these people. Plug their ears and shut their eyes. That way, they will not see with their eyes, nor hear with their ears, nor understand with their hearts and turn to me for healing. ISAIAH 6:10

Early one morning, Mike called my office. He was having stomach pains and was convinced he had a rare form of cancer. He insisted on seeing me that day.

When he arrived that afternoon, he had a stack of printouts listing diseases and symptoms that matched his experience. He told me about the research he'd done online and the diagnoses he'd considered. He firmly believed that he had a particularly nasty—and rare—cancer, and he was understandably stressed.

When I asked about his symptoms, Mike listed several things that had been bothering him. Though some of his symptoms were consistent with the cancer he had discovered on the Internet, I was able to quickly rule it out. Ultimately, it was something much easier to diagnose and treat—irritable bowel syndrome—but it had worsened as a result of his worrying. After we discussed a treatment plan, Mike went home with a relieved smile on his face.

Coming up with our own answers to physical or spiritual problems can often make us anxious. That's why I love the opening line of Psalm 46:10: "Be still, and know that I am God!" Even with my years of medical training and experience, I still rely on God to guide me and to give me insight into the diseases or injuries that cause my patients' symptoms.

When we go to God with our own list of answers, telling him what we think is wrong, we miss an opportunity to hear his wise diagnosis. Instead, we should present him with our spiritual symptoms—whether we're experiencing fear, anger, or anxiety—and allow his Word to diagnose our spiritual diseases. No matter if our pain is physical or emotional, God is the one who can heal us. Sometimes he uses doctors—or even an article on the Internet—but if we want to be blessed by his wisdom, we must go to him prepared to listen.

TODAY'S RX

When you hear hoofbeats, you're more likely to see a horse than a zebra, so take a deep breath before diagnosing yourself with something you read about on the Internet.

Thank you, God, that you have the answers to all my needs. Help me to be still before you, listening for your wisdom as I go through times of worry.

STRIKING A TUMOR SO IT NEVER RISES AGAIN

Hit their enemies where it hurts the most; strike down their foes so they never rise again. DEUTERONOMY 33:11

As I listened to Brad's chest, things didn't sound right. "How long have you been coughing up blood?"

"Maybe two or three months, off and on." He didn't sound very confident. "I thought it would just go away, but now the right side of my chest hurts."

"This could be serious. I'm going to call the X-ray department and order a CT scan as soon as possible."

Later that afternoon, I gave Brad the sobering results. "I'm sorry to report that you have a spot on your right lung."

Brad had been a smoker for years, and he knew the risks.

"Is it cancer?"

"I don't know yet. We'll need to do more tests. I'm going to order a fine needle aspiration for tomorrow at the interventional radiology department in downtown Nashville. We'll probably have the results back in a week or so."

Brad looked worried when he left. I'm sure he was thinking about what his family would do if he wasn't there to take care of them.

Four days later, a pathologist called me with the results: adenocarcinoma of the lungs. The workup was otherwise negative. I called Brad. "It's a primary tumor of the lung, but there is no metastasis. We can have it removed with a CyberKnife treatment."

Brad's response was assuring: "You know, you've been telling me to quit smoking for years. I think you've finally convinced me."

After the surgery, I thought about today's Scripture verse. Because of the size and location of the tumor, the CyberKnife was able to hit it directly, strike it down, and completely eradicate it, so it wouldn't grow again.

Five years later, Brad is still cancer free. He sees me regularly for checkups, and each time he praises God for guiding his treatment and for the tools we had available. If this had happened before the invention of the CyberKnife, the diagnosis would have been an almost certain death sentence.

Only God knows the number of days we have here on earth. Brad and his family are thankful that God granted him healing and allowed him more time on earth.

TODAY'S RX

The best way to quit smoking is to never start; but if you've already started, the best advice is to stop before it stops you.

Lord, I realize I have some unhealthy habits. Please provide me with strength and determination to break free of them, especially in weaker moments.

STRONG AND COURAGEOUS FOR THE FIGHT

Be strong and courageous, all you who put your hope in the LORD! PSALM 31:24

"He just doesn't seem as strong as before. He says it hurts to run and that he doesn't feel well. He used to want to play outside all the time, but now he wants to stay in."

Tommy's mom was concerned. Tommy was only five, and he'd started losing weight and having night sweats.

"It's the middle of winter, and he's burning up every night. Last year he had strep. The year before that, both ears were clogged, and you sent him to get tubes in his ears. Do you think it could be one of those problems again?"

Tommy looked pale, and he was thinner than I remembered. When we weighed him, he'd lost five pounds—a significant amount in a child that young.

"Hmm. Let's look and see." I got my light out. "His throat looks good. Ears look good—the tubes have fallen out, and his tympanic membranes are normal." I felt his neck and could tell that his lymph nodes were enlarged. They were also enlarged in his armpits. "Let's get some lab work done and see if that will tell us anything."

When the blood work came back, it gave us a definitive answer—but one we had all hoped and prayed against. Tommy had acute lymphoblastic leukemia (ALL), cancer of the blood and bone marrow. I joined hands with Tommy and his mother, and we prayed, "Lord, this diagnosis is not what we'd hoped for, but now that we know the answer, help us to fight this battle. Give us courage and strength, Lord, for our hope is in you."

The next year was a difficult battle for both Tommy and his mother. The treatments seemed to last a lifetime, but he made it through. Tommy is now in remission with about an 85 percent chance of a cure.

In the midst of adversity, the Lord answered our prayers and gave both Tommy and his mom the strength and courage they needed during his fight.

TODAY'S RX

We all have areas in our lives where we must fight. Place your hope in the Lord, and ask him to provide you with the strength and courage you need to make it through.

Lord, sometimes the road ahead is daunting, and I'm overcome by the challenges I face. Help me to trust in you for courage and strength during these times of trial.

DOUBLE BLESSINGS

Isaac pleaded with the LORD on behalf of his wife, because she was unable to have children. The LORD answered Isaac's prayer, and Rebekah became pregnant with twins. GENESIS 25:21

"Ohhh!" The petite Chinese woman doubled over in pain.

I froze. As a medical student, I had shadowed a resident who showed me how a typical labor and delivery should progress. But now I couldn't remember anything. The woman didn't speak much English, and it was probably a good thing. If she had, it would have been obvious that we shared the same fear about what was going to happen. Fortunately, the labor and delivery nurse had been coaching new moms and new doctors for more than twenty years.

When the mom was fully dilated, I made an exaggerated pushing motion with my hands and said, "You push." Then, pointing to myself and rounding my hands like a football receiver, I said, "I'll catch." I'm sure the nurse thought I was a complete fool.

Fortunately, she stepped up to the patient's bedside and took control of the situation. Looking the woman in the eye, she began to model the proper breathing. Soon the mom was following her lead.

Before long, a patch of dark hair appeared as the baby crowned, and it took only another minute before the infant's head emerged. I reached in to guide the shoulders, and out came a healthy baby boy. I clamped and cut the cord and handed the baby to the nurse. He was crying, which was a good sign. I wasn't crying, which was also a good sign.

When I pushed down on the mother's abdomen, expecting to feel a postpartum uterus, it felt larger than I expected. What could I have missed? It was my first solo delivery, and I didn't want to make a mistake. Grabbing the fetoscope, I listened to the woman's abdomen.

A second heartbeat!

Pointing to the woman's stomach, I held up two fingers. Her eyes grew large. A few minutes later, baby boy number two came kicking and screaming into the world.

Although every delivery has a sense of wonder, this one—my first—was extra special. No one—not even the woman herself—knew she was having twins. But God knew. And he chose me to be a part of it.[3]

TODAY'S RX

When we ask God to bless us, sometimes he unexpectedly gives us a double blessing.

Thank you for blessing me, Father, with many good gifts. Help me to always be in wonder of you.

STANDING BETWEEN TWO WORLDS

As I looked, I saw a door standing open in heaven, and the same voice I had heard before spoke to me like a trumpet blast. The voice said, "Come up here, and I will show you what must happen after this." And instantly I was in the Spirit, and I saw a throne in heaven and someone sitting on it. The one sitting on the throne was as brilliant as gemstones—like jasper and carnelian. And the glow of an emerald circled his throne like a rainbow. REVELATION 4:1-3

As the medical director of a nursing home, I've learned that sometimes those who need the most help aren't my patients—but the children of my patients.

One day, as I was making my rounds, the senior nurse asked if I would stop in and see the Browns.

Making my way to Mrs. Brown's room, I stepped in and asked how their mother was doing. The eldest son, Alex, said, "I'm not sure."

"Sometimes, Momma talks to us, and sometimes she seems to be talking to Daddy," his sister Amy said. "But Daddy went to be with Jesus more than twenty years ago."

"Does she seem to be in any pain?" I asked.

"Not really. She's groaning, but she seems calm and relaxed, almost like she did when we were younger and we'd catch her praying."

Over the years, when I've had the honor of being with people on their deathbeds, I've encouraged their family members to hold their loved ones' hands, pray with them, and sing to them. But mostly I just want them to be present and aware that they're standing on sacred ground.

"When I examined your mother a few days ago, I saw no evidence of pain or distress. It's my opinion that she's close to leaving this world, but only the Lord knows the hour. Her responses make me believe that, right now, she's standing between two worlds—heaven and earth."

Alex blinked back tears. Amy let them flow. I had just confirmed what they had already been thinking.

"Though she's lying in bed, she's resting on holy ground. I know it will be hard for your family to say good-bye, but I believe she is already making plans for the reunion you'll have with her in your forever home."

TODAY'S RX

Earthly words cannot adequately describe heaven or explain God's glory. Sometimes, groaning is the best we can do.

God, I cannot begin to grasp how beautiful heaven must be. Thank you for making a place for us there. Help me not to lose sight of your glory in my daily life, but to always remember what awaits me.

SLIPPERY ICE

Give your burdens to the LORD, and he will take care of you. He will not permit the godly to slip and fall. PSALM 55:22

When the ice storm hit, we expected to see a lot of broken bones in the ER. Typically, the patients would be growing boys with too much energy to stay inside. Broken arms or legs from sledding or a slip on the ice were par for the course.

So when the EMS radioed that an eighty-five-year-old woman had been found in her front yard, my heart sank. A broken bone on a teenage boy would heal just fine, but a bad fall on the ice could be deadly to an elderly person.

When they brought Florence in, I learned she had gone outside to clear her walk. After she fell, she had lain on the icy ground for nearly an hour before someone noticed and called for help. Her core temperature was 94 degrees—a little low, but nothing a warming blanket couldn't fix.

The X-rays revealed that Florence had an intertrochanteric fracture of the left hip, which prevented her from getting up. "It only hurt when I tried to stand," she said. "So I just lay there hoping someone would come by."

When I asked Florence if she knew how blessed she was to still be alive, she answered with a question of her own: "I don't want to be a burden to anyone. Can I get this fixed and go home as soon as you're done?"

"Florence, your hip fracture will take some time to fix. Then you'll need to stay in rehab for a few more weeks while you heal. After that, I pray you can return home with the help of home health care and physical therapy."

A shadow crossed her face as she absorbed the news.

"Florence, know that when we slip and fall, God is right there to catch us. He will pick us up and help us walk again. He was there for you while you were lying in the yard, and he'll be there as you heal from this break. Don't worry. Just give your burdens to God."

Florence smiled. "I always have, and I always will. I may have slipped on the ice, but I have never slipped in my faith."

TODAY'S RX

Be mindful of your neighbors and elderly friends during the winter season. Offer to help them with their needs.

Lord, only you know how many slips and falls I've had—both physically and spiritually. Thank you for not leaving me on my own, and for tenderly caring for me through each one.

BETTER LIVING THROUGH GOD'S CHEMISTRY

Be strong and courageous! Do not be afraid and do not panic before them. For the LORD *your God will personally go ahead of you. He will neither fail you nor abandon you.* DEUTERONOMY 31:6

"It's so bad, I'm afraid to leave the house," Eloise said. "Now my husband has left me because I won't go out. I lost my job, and I can't find another one because I miss too much work. I'm swimming in anxiety, and when it gets to be too much and I feel as if I'm going to drown, I start to panic."

Eloise wrung her hands and bit her bottom lip. "Everything in front of me seems like a much bigger deal than it used to be. I feel as if I can't be fully present because I'm obsessing about the future. I don't know what to do."

"Panic and anxiety are usually related to making the future too big," I said. "When we look at how normal thought patterns operate, the past, present, and future typically have equal focus. When one is out of proportion with the others, we see the consequences. If you're worried about the past, then depression usually follows. If you're worried about the future, then anxiety follows. Our goal is to try to restore balance to your thought life."

I reminded Eloise that God is sovereign over the past, present, and future. He lives beyond the constraints of time, and he protects us even when we don't realize we need his protection.

"When you start to worry, Eloise, I want you to realize that God is in control. He's got this. You can turn all your cares over to him. I recommend that you start with therapy to help restore balance in your thought life. But I can also prescribe medication if you need more help."

"I understand how God could use a Christian counselor to help me with this," she said. "But what about medication?"

"God created our bodies with a certain chemistry, and we can use medicine to reestablish a chemical balance. But either way, with therapy or medication, you can be assured that God goes with and before you."

TODAY'S RX

If you're suffering from anxiety or depression, don't be a prisoner to it. Get help. Your quality of life may improve through Christian therapy or God-given chemistry.

God, thank you that time is in your hands. When I become overwhelmed with worry about the future, help me to reflect on your past faithfulness—how you have always seen me through times of difficulty and have drawn me closer to you.

WRESTLING WITH GOD

But you have made me as strong as a wild ox. You have anointed me with the finest oil. PSALM 92:10

Entering the exam room, I encountered a mountain of a man. He was massive even for our local farming community, in which physical strength was a ticket to prosperity.

Charlie looked to be about seventy-five years old but with the build of a much younger man. I could see that his arms had new scars on top of old scars—no doubt a story to go along with each one of them. With that many scars, it was odd that I hadn't stitched him up once or twice before.

"After twenty-five years in practice, I thought I'd met everyone in town. Are you from around here?" I asked.

"I was born and raised here, but I left when I was nineteen. I just moved back after retiring from being on the road."

"Are you a musician?"

"No," he said with a chuckle, "I'm a professional wrestler—well, I was."

"I guess that explains the scars."

"When I was a young man, I always pushed the limits of my God-given strength whenever I was in the ring. I won a lot of trophies, and I made some good money. But as you can tell, it wasn't an easy way to make a living."

"It looks like you've been in a few battles," I responded.

"Yeah, but none was worse than the spiritual toll of being on tour. When I was no longer top billing on the circuit, I lost my way. I went broke and life seemed meaningless. That's when I turned to Jesus, and he anointed me. He gave me a fire in my belly to teach his Word to the same crowd who used to watch me wrestle. Except now, instead of beating my chest, I proclaimed the Bible to anyone who would listen."

Charlie was the real deal. Until the day he died, he sought to reach as many people as he could. He would stop people on the street, at the mall, or at wrestling events to talk about his faith. (I know that if a man his size asked me to listen, I would!)

Charlie was a mighty man, and God used him mightily.

TODAY'S RX

God can use everyone for his glory . . . no matter their line of work.

Father, however it may unfold—in my job, in my relationships, in my community—I pray that you will use me for your good works today and in the days to come.

THE WISDOM DIET

Don't be impressed with your own wisdom. Instead, fear the LORD *and turn away from evil. Then you will have healing for your body and strength for your bones.*
PROVERBS 3:7-8

Betsy had been a patient of mine for years. And for as long as I'd known her, she had struggled with her weight, trying diet after diet. Most of them didn't work at all. But the only thing worse for her than a diet that failed was one that succeeded—because once she hit her goal, she would return to her normal way of living and gain back everything she'd lost, plus more. Still, it didn't surprise me when she showed up in my office excited about yet another diet plan.

"Dr. Anderson, I lost fifteen pounds the first week! And ten pounds this week! That's twenty-five pounds in two weeks!"

I could tell she was excited. But that was a lot of weight to lose so quickly, and I was concerned.

"Tell me about your new diet."

Betsy described the latest fad diet that was currently getting a lot of attention thanks to a few well-known people who claimed to have lost weight from it. "I think you should recommend it to all your patients!" Betsy said.

Unfortunately, I knew what Betsy didn't, and I had some well-founded reservations. The plan wasn't well balanced, nor was it sustainable over the long term. In fact, I had recently admitted a patient to the hospital who was in renal failure. When we narrowed down what was causing her kidneys to fail, we linked it to the same diet that Betsy was talking about.

Though Betsy was happy with her results so far, I knew that the diet could do a lot of harm if taken to the extreme. I spent the next few minutes debunking the "wisdom" of what appeared to be such a great thing.

Sometimes we're like that with God, aren't we? We forsake his wisdom in favor of what we think will be a faster, better, or less demanding way to get what we want. But God knows what we don't, and he is the source of all wisdom. That includes nutritional wisdom. If my patients would follow God's dietary wisdom, they would be much healthier.

TODAY'S RX

Eat healthier by choosing fruits and vegetables over processed foods. That one change today will improve your health tomorrow.

Help me to choose healthy ways of living, Lord, that will benefit both my body and my spirit for the long run. Steer me in your direction, and keep me grounded in your Word.

A TALE OF TWO SISTERS

The tongue can bring death or life; those who love to talk will reap the consequences.
Proverbs 18:21

"My sister is always putting me down. She tells me I can never do anything right," Justine complained. "She tells me my perfume stinks, that blonde hair is 'out,' that I don't earn enough money at my job, and that I should go back to school so I can get a better job and make more money."

I had asked Justine if she had any stress in her life, and her answer was a lot more than I expected.

"She even picks on my husband. She says he's a bum and that he's ugly. Why does she have to constantly run me down in every area of my life?"

Justine obviously looked up to her sister, and their contentious relationship was wearing on her. She wanted to have a more loving relationship, but her older sister's cutting remarks made that impossible. "Tell me about your sister and your relationship while you were growing up," I suggested, hoping to get a handle on what was happening.

"She's two years older, and she won every award there was to win in high school. Most beautiful, most intelligent, most likely to succeed . . ."

As Justine continued to list the accolades her sister had received when they were younger, I didn't sense any jealousy or bitterness; she was simply stating the facts.

"When we were younger, we got along great. After high school, she met her husband, they got married, had three kids, and moved away. Then something happened. I don't know the details, but her husband left her and moved in with another woman. After that, my sister just grew bitter, and now that she's moved back, she's so hard to be around!"

"Justine, you have a great life with a terrific job and loving children. Your sister's bitterness is aimed at you because you're a safe target for her."

"I never thought of it that way, but I think you're right. If she said these things to her kids, it would destroy them. Justine resolved to pray that her sister's heart would heal quickly so that they could have a warm relationship again.

TODAY'S RX

Sometimes, people say mean things that aren't intended to hurt us. Instead, these words reveal the condition of the speaker's heart and help us to know how to pray for them.

God, I pray that my words will be uplifting to those around me today. Let me be quick to listen and slow to speak, bringing light to those in need.

ALL IN ONE BOX

Whenever someone turns to the Lord, the veil is taken away. For the Lord is the Spirit, and wherever the Spirit of the Lord is, there is freedom. So all of us who have had that veil removed can see and reflect the glory of the Lord. And the Lord—who is the Spirit—makes us more and more like him as we are changed into his glorious image. 2 Corinthians 3:16-18

In my medical practice and my personal life, God has allowed me to see some marvelous things. He has offered me glimpses of heaven that most people haven't had, as well as the privilege of walking with many people at the beginning or end of their lives. As a result, I don't view death the way many others do.

I don't dread my own death or that of anyone who belongs to Jesus. I envision death as a joyful homecoming for those who know Christ. When an opportunity arises to escort someone home, I want to be there beside them. Those opportunities energize me and make me want to be a part of the miracle. Death is not a failure of medical science; it is a victory of the soul.

When I tell other physicians about the things I've seen, they often try to compartmentalize them, to fit them into a box formed by their own understanding—especially those who don't have faith in Jesus. It's as if they're saying, "Your scientific training is the only thing that can be used in your medical practice. Your experiences should stay in a religious box." In other words, they don't think my appointments with heaven should have any bearing on how I practice medicine.

I understand their point of view, but when I practice medicine, I can't separate my faith from my training. To me, it all comes from the same source; it's all in one box.

If you've separated your faith from your job or your relationships, or if a hurt in your life has separated you from God, don't wait for a future event to upend your boxes. Ask God to reconcile and restore everything into one integrated box—*his* box.

TODAY'S RX

Whatever your circumstances, keep your heart and mind centered on God. Only he can give you peace and joy in every aspect of life. And only he gives us the promise of heaven.

God, whether my day is filled with busyness or boredom, keep my heart and mind centered on you, that I might have access to the peace and joy that only you can give in every circumstance. Thank you for the promise of heaven.

WHEN THERE ARE NO WORDS

Instantly Zechariah could speak again, and he began praising God. LUKE 1:64

"After having two kids, my tubes were tied twenty years ago," Martha said. "I'm too old to be pregnant, but that's exactly how I feel."

Martha was right. At fifty-eight, she was too old to be pregnant again. The oldest new mom I'd ever diagnosed was forty-four, and even that was a surprise.

"I think my belly has been growing since last fall. I remember feeling pressure, but the size increase was so gradual that I didn't realize how big I'd gotten—until the kids mentioned it."

When Martha removed her outer clothing, I could see why she thought pregnancy was a possibility. But my training and years of experience told me there was a different story. When I laid my hands on her abdomen and felt the mass in her belly, I knew what it was. For a woman her age with a tumor that size that had grown that quickly, it was usually ovarian cancer.

"Martha, you're not pregnant, but we're going to have to admit you to the hospital for some tests."

The next morning, after receiving word that the CT scan and blood tests pointed toward cancer, I quietly approached Martha on my rounds. When I took a deep breath and hesitated before speaking, she knew it wasn't a good sign.

"Why are you speechless?"

"It doesn't look good, Martha. I've consulted with a gynecological oncologist to help us figure this out. Based on the tests, he thinks it's cancer, but I'm praying that those preliminary tests are wrong."

After discussing her treatment options, Martha and I prayed together for a miracle.

The day after Martha's surgery, the oncologist caught me on rounds. "The pathology came back clean. I really don't understand why. Perhaps this is a benign cyst pretending to be cancer. It was a very large mass, but it all came out okay, and she shouldn't have any problems."

When I delivered the good news to Martha, once again I was speechless. But when I finally got the words out, neither one of us could contain our joy. We simply praised God for all he had done.

TODAY'S RX

Does trying to explain what God has done in your life leave you speechless? Words aren't necessary. You can still praise God in your heart.

Jesus, I'm often speechless when I think of your great love for me. You are the ultimate physician, having healed me of my physical needs and the sin in my heart. Thank you for continuing to work miracles in the lives of your people to this day.

SOUL PROVIDER

At that time you won't need to ask me for anything. I tell you the truth, you will ask the Father directly, and he will grant your request because you use my name.
JOHN 16:23

"Sorry to bother you again," Victor said. "But since you're the guy who holds the keys to helping me get well, I need another referral—this time to see a specialist for my back pain."

Victor had struggled with back trouble for several weeks. It had started with mild pain but grew worse until it radiated down his right leg. He was unable to work his factory job, and I had to write an explanatory note so he would be excused without being fired. Next, I wrote a referral for an MRI. Now he was back in my office a third time for authorization to see a neurosurgeon.

Have you ever found yourself in a similar dilemma, having to ask your doctor or insurance provider for permission to treat your basic health-care needs? It's not easy for patients to do this—or for doctors to stay on top of all of the requests.

With all the changes in health care, "Mother, may I" situations are becoming more common. One doctor must determine whether the patient is sick enough to consult with a specialist, who then decides if more diagnostic tests are needed. But to schedule the tests, the patient must get permission from the first doctor. This creates obstacles that can delay the desired outcome of restored good health.

It's easy to see how ridiculous this is in medicine. But how often do we do something similar in our spiritual lives? For example, have you ever asked a friend for advice rather than asking God?

Historically, many people have gone to a priest or pastor for guidance or to request permission to ask God for grace and forgiveness—rather than going to God directly. But Jesus, the Great Physician, is our mediator in heaven. We can go directly to him. He holds the keys to our spiritual health and growth. There is no need for a referral. All our healing comes from his hands.

God's diagnostic and treatment plans have already been written and completed, before we even ask. God is our soul provider.

TODAY'S RX

The Father holds the keys to your healing. Seek him first.

Father, I confess that I often seek advice and counsel from family and friends before coming to you with what's on my mind. Help me to turn to you first when I have important decisions to make, knowing that you've prepared the way for me to go.

THE BLIND SHALL SEE

When Jesus heard them, he stopped and called, "What do you want me to do for you?" "Lord," they said, "we want to see!" Jesus felt sorry for them and touched their eyes. Instantly they could see! Then they followed him. MATTHEW 20:32-34

Too often, we think we see clearly when we really can't see much at all. For one of my patients, it was the exact opposite. He was completely blind, but he had much better vision than most.

Looking at my list of rounds that morning, I saw that Herb was my first patient for the day. At 104, he was also one of my oldest and most resilient patients. I saw him every month, but he couldn't see me. Macular degeneration had stolen his eyesight nearly twenty years earlier. He had no visual response to even the brightest of exam lights.

When I walked into his room that day, the air immediately seemed lighter and fresher, as if spring had arrived there before it reached the rest of the town. As I drew closer to Herb's bedside, I noticed that he gripped a photo in each hand—one was of his wife, who had died ten years earlier, and the other was a group photo of his children.

The nurse was having trouble getting a systolic blood pressure reading above 90, and she asked me to listen to Herb's heart. As I bent forward, I heard him exhale. Three heartbeats later, I heard him draw his final breath on earth. Immediately, I was aware that I stood on holy ground, and I was awed by the sacredness of the occasion.

As I thought of Herb's final moments, I had to pause to catch my own breath. He had clung to two photos he could no longer see, while before his very eyes a world of immense clarity and color suddenly unfurled. The last things to pass through his hands were pictures of those he loved most dearly—those who had gone before him, and those who would come after him.

I immediately knew that the scents of lilac and citrus I had smelled upon entering his room were the aroma of heaven. And now Herb could see the heavens, the earth, and those he loved in all their glory.

TODAY'S RX

Pray that God would grant you to see the world through his eyes.

God, you've given me many gifts on this earth. Help me not to take them for granted but to see them as precious, and to make the most of my time with family and friends.

THE GREAT GOODNESS

How great is the goodness you have stored up for those who fear you. You lavish it on those who come to you for protection, blessing them before the watching world.
PSALM 31:19

In college, I bent to the peer pressure of my friends. I wanted to be liked and to be like everyone else.

Day in and day out, it was the same routine. We went to class and then went out drinking. Down the Hatch was the name of our favorite bar—and it was aptly named. When we were through, if we had any time left, we'd grab a little sleep before heading off to class again. In medical school, I more or less kept up the same routine. Classes, drinks, and a few hours of shut-eye.

Then I met Karen and asked her out. When she saw the routines of my life and learned that I was an atheist, she questioned the trajectory I was on. One day, she gave me a copy of C. S. Lewis's *Mere Christianity* and asked me to read it.

I read the book while camping, and it made a tremendous impression on me. As a young man, Lewis had wrestled with many of the same issues I had, including questions about God. Eventually, he came to realize that God truly *was*, *is*, and *forever will be.*

That night, through a dream, my transformation from being an atheist to a believer occurred instantly. I was thrown off my high horse, and my eyes were opened to the new person that God wanted me to become.

Your transformation may have been more gradual, but the end result is the same. God renews our minds as he makes us into new creatures. The way we think about this world changes as we realize how temporary it is. As today's verse says, God has stored up goodness for us, and he will lavish it upon us when we fear him and come to him for protection. I felt his goodness that day—and have every day since.

Since college, my routines have certainly changed, but the biggest change is this: I used to run from God, but now I run *to* him.

TODAY'S RX

If you're dissatisfied in this world, perhaps it's because you were created for another world, as C. S. Lewis suggests. Today, reflect on the goodness of God that awaits us in heaven.

Lord, as I look back on my past, I see how you have faithfully been working in my life, molding me day-by-day into the person you desire me to be. Continue to renew my mind, Lord, as I live out each day so that I may see with brighter clarity the treasure that awaits me.

THE POWER OF PRAYER TO BRING A SMILE

Have compassion on me, LORD, for I am weak. Heal me, LORD, for my bones are in agony. PSALM 6:2

"Thank you for keeping your appointment today, Helen," I said. "I know how the cold and dampness make your rheumatism feel worse."

Helen nodded. In addition to rheumatoid arthritis, she also had lupus. I knew she had to be in a lot of pain.

"Mom's had most of her joints replaced, but she still has so much pain," her daughter said. "I don't understand how that can be."

She was right. Over the years, Helen had had a hip and both knees replaced, and her wrists were permanently fused in a neutral position. In the years before current treatments were available, the arthritis had done tremendous damage.

"I know," I said as sympathetically as I could. "The problem is that the pain gets worse with movement, but if she doesn't move, her muscles will weaken and atrophy, which will cause even more pain. We can try giving her more pain medicine."

Helen sat there and never said a word. It was as if we weren't even talking about her.

"The problem is that she's limited by the medications she can tolerate," her daughter added, "so I don't know if we can do that."

"I see. What do you think helps her most?"

"She seems her best on the days we go to church and when she sees other people. She prays for them and has prayers offered for her.

Helen smiled. It was the first time I'd seen her smile.

I learned something that day. Though Helen didn't say a word, she reminded me how important it is for us to pray for ourselves *and* pray for others. We may never see the results firsthand, but our prayers may be the only thing that eases someone else's pain.

TODAY'S RX

Prayer is like a soothing balm to both body and soul. Apply it liberally.

Lord, put on my heart today people who need prayer. Help me to be aware of their needs and to lift them up to you.

BACK IN THE LAND OF THE LIVING

I am confident I will see the LORD's goodness while I am here in the land of the living.
PSALM 27:13

"Everything in this world seems broken," Harvey said, "like it's all upside down from what it should be."

I'd known Harvey and various members of his family for years. But I had never heard him sound so despondent, and I was concerned.

"Tell me what's going on."

"In the last two years, I've lost ten of my closest family members. It's like God doesn't even care."

Harvey wasn't exaggerating. Most of the deaths had been expected—several were of relatives in their seventies and eighties. But at least one death had happened unexpectedly: a beloved niece who had died in a car accident on a rainy night.

"I'm guessing you feel as if God isn't listening to your prayers right now," I said.

Harvey started to cry.

"I understand your pain because I've felt that way too."

I told Harvey about the personal loss I had experienced when my close friends were murdered. "From what I went through, I know that grief isn't always a short journey. It's hard to navigate, and it can be difficult to find a spiritual oasis where you can reconnect with God."

Harvey nodded. I could see he was relieved that someone understood what he was going through. I encouraged him and prayed with him. But as his doctor, I also recognized that depression had set in, and he would need medication to restore his brain chemistry. "I'm going to prescribe something to help you, but you'll need to come back frequently so I can monitor your progress."

For weeks, nothing seemed to change. Harvey was as despondent as ever. But as time went on, I noticed that the doom and gloom weren't quite as prevalent as before. A few months later, when I walked into the exam room, he had a smile on his face—the first I had seen from him in a long time.

"I've been trying to get back into the swing of things, Doc. And you know what? It's not so bad out there."

That's when I knew for sure that Harvey had rejoined us in the land of the living.

TODAY'S RX

If your glass is half empty and you can't lift it on your own, see a doctor for help.

God, so often the darkness of this world overshadows the light. I pray that you make yourself present to me today and to those around me who are hurting. Bring healing to us, God, and help us to recognize your light.

MEDICINE CHANGES, GOD DOES NOT

Whatever is good and perfect is a gift coming down to us from God our Father, who created all the lights in the heavens. He never changes or casts a shifting shadow.
James 1:17

I have practiced medicine for more than thirty years. Occasionally, I've reflected on the exponential growth and changes that have occurred in medicine during that time.

Recently, while cleaning out an old filing cabinet, I found some notes I'd taken while in medical school. For the better part of an hour, I sat on the floor and read through them. I laughed out loud about some of the things I'd written down. At the time, the gold standard advice and treatment we were told to give our patients seemed rock solid. But with new discoveries, many of those solid rocks had crumbled under the weight of new evidence.

For example, my notes contained information on an antibiotic that was the recommended first line of treatment for a certain infection. We now know that this treatment is totally ineffective. It used to be thought that peptic ulcer disease was caused by stress. We now know that it is often caused by the Helicobacter pylori bacteria, and it's treatable with antibiotics. Back then, MRIs were still on the drawing board; we had never seen one. Now we use them daily to diagnose problems that weren't detectable even a few years ago.

As our knowledge of medicine grows, it seems that the ground we once stood on continues to shift. The one and only constant in healing is God himself.

The same prayers of hope and healing prayed for patients thirty years ago, fifty years ago, one hundred years ago, even one thousand years ago, are still heard at the bedside here and now. God never changes. Even in our evidence-based world of medicine, he is, has been, and always will be the gold standard in healing.

TODAY'S RX

God heals, and God never changes; but with the advancement of human discovery, he may change the tools he uses to heal us.

God, in this ever-changing world, thank you for remaining constant from the beginning of time. You are and always have been a loving, gracious Father who hears and answers prayers.

GOD'S UNFAILING LOVE

I am always aware of your unfailing love, and I have lived according to your truth.
PSALM 26:3

In today's verse, the psalmist reminds us that when we live according to God's truth, we can always be aware of his unfailing love.

Growing up in Plantersville, Alabama, I felt that love. My parents were schoolteachers. They were also active in the small Baptist church in town. Dad was a deacon and the treasurer, and Mom taught Sunday school. To this day, when I recall the story of baby Jesus in the manger, I hear it in my mother's sweet Southern drawl. Other family members were teachers, preachers, and farmers.

Our family life was inextricably woven and intertwined with the God of the universe. From an early age, I knew that he had sent his Son to die for me and to pay the debt of my sin. There was no question in my mind how much God unconditionally loved all of us.

Though I was young, I was always aware of God's omnipotence. I would chuckle thinking about how he must smile watching my siblings and me play and enjoy the world around us. To me, God was as real as the air I breathed. He filled not only my lungs, but the world around me. I would romp through the woods, marveling at his creation and how much he loved us all. At the deepest level, I knew that God's love for me was as solid as the red clay beneath my feet.

Though later in life I wandered far from those powerful truths, I never forgot what it was like to experience those feelings of God's unfailing love in my youth.

TODAY'S RX

The things of this world are temporary, but God's unfailing love is not. He will continually draw us back to our forever home in heaven.

Father, I take such comfort in knowing that you have provided all that this world has to offer. Thank you for creating the beautiful mountains, rivers, cities, and fields that make up this world.

HE KNOWS US BY NAME

The L*ORD replied to Moses, "I will indeed do what you have asked, for I look favorably on you, and I know you by name."* EXODUS 33:17

Grace's appointment was scheduled for ten o'clock, but I was running late—as usual. I knocked on the exam room door and walked in gingerly, fully expecting an earful for how long she'd had to wait.

"I'm so sorry that I'm running late this morning, Grace."

"That's okay, Dr. Anderson. I've waited a lot longer for other doctors. And when I come here, you always take your time with me. I've known you for so long that I don't think of you as our family doctor."

"You don't?" I asked, puzzled.

"Nope, I just think of you as family."

I was humbled to be invited into the inner circle of so many of my patients' lives, and I was honored to share their journeys with them. Unfortunately, I didn't have good news for Grace that day.

"Your tests came back, and they're not good. You're going to need surgery, probably followed by rehab. Your hip has walked its last mile."

"That's okay. I know I haven't walked it alone."

Grace's surgery went well, and I came to see her in the rehab unit. She was smiling, though I could tell she was in great pain.

"I haven't worked this hard in a long, long time," she said. "But I will do this so I can get back on my feet for my family."

Like all of my patients, Grace wasn't just a number. She was a person whom the entire staff knew by name, and she knew our names, as well. To be considered family by her was something we never took for granted.

In today's verse, when the Lord replies to Moses, he doesn't treat Moses' prayer as just one in a long line of requests; instead, God acknowledges Moses' request and assures Moses that he will look on it favorably. If that wasn't enough, God reminds Moses that he knows his name.

What a marvelous thing to consider. The God of the universe knows our names, and he hears every one of our requests. More important, he looks favorably on us.

TODAY'S RX

Today, when you meet new people, look favorably on them, and remember their names. It will remind you of what God does for us.

God, it's reassuring to know that I'm not just a face in the crowd to you, but rather your child whom you know by name, care about, and desire to hear from. I lift up to you all that is on my heart today.

FEBRUARY CHECKUP

In South Georgia, where my family is from, February is the month when farmers start their tractors and break ground for the new crops. Some casual gardeners plant seeds indoors so they can later transfer them outside. It seems crazy; it's the dead of winter. The ground is still hard and frozen. But this is the best time to start the cycle of new growth again.

Maybe your life has been frozen in time—waiting, watching, and anticipating a new beginning. The ground around you feels cold and hard, but it's time to start anticipating the little things you can do to help your own growth this year. Maybe it's time to join a book club, start a blog, or begin a new exercise program.

February is a great time to start a new Bible study. Find a couple of friends and meet for coffee. Read through a book of the Bible together and discuss it. You don't have to be an expert to learn from God's Word and the lives of other believers—you only have to be willing. If you prayed each day last month, congratulations! You've now started a new habit. Keep on praying! If you haven't been as consistent as you wanted, it's not too late. Start now with a short morning prayer or a head-on-your-pillow prayer each night, thanking God for your many blessings.

For many people, February 14 is a special day. Valentine's Day can signal new courtships and promises of new or renewed love. For some who have lost a loved one or who are longing for a relationship, the days leading up to Valentine's Day can seem particularly cruel. It can also be a difficult day for spouses in struggling marriages, where one or both partners feel let down by unmet expectations.

Don't let your disappointment derail you. February can be a month to use your feelings constructively. Many people need love. What if you used this month to find others who need some love and gave them encouragement and appreciation? Whether it is a child, an elderly neighbor, or a single person at work, you might find great satisfaction and fulfillment in meeting the needs of others. Remember, Jesus told us to love others as we love ourselves. How can you put this principle into practice this month?

February is also a great month for falling deeper in love with Jesus. Take a moment to write a list of all the reasons he deserves your love. Make a second list of all the reasons you love him. Then pray over both lists, asking him to reveal himself to you in fresh and exciting ways so you can grow in your love for him.

Intentionally plant love in your heart and mind. The seeds of love that you plant this month will become the relationship flowers that blossom in future seasons.

February Booster Shot: Take time during one of the coldest months of the year to break the ice in your relationships. Just as a farmer prepares the soil, prepare your soul for a springtime of renewed and refreshed relationships.

A PRAYER FOR OTHERS MAY BE AN ANSWER TO YOURS

The LORD listened to Hezekiah's prayer and healed the people. 2 CHRONICLES 30:20

The Israelites were a month late celebrating Passover, and many people were ceremonially unclean—meaning they should have been excluded from the Passover celebration. Hezekiah interceded on their behalf, asking God to overlook those details and see only their hearts as they began to turn back to him. God extended his grace, allowing the people to enjoy the festival with him. Hezekiah's prayer made a difference.

One of the great traditions of the body of Christ is to intercede in prayer for others. We serve a merciful and gracious God who hears our prayers and grants our requests. But sometimes those prayers aren't answered in the way we expect.

Gerard had struggled with post-traumatic stress syndrome (PTSS) ever since returning from Iraq. Though this wasn't unusual—many soldiers returned with those symptoms—the memories of war were particularly vivid for Gerard because he had lost both legs and had seen his best friend die when their military vehicle hit a roadside bomb.

His family brought him to see me because he needed a primary care physician. Though he was a big guy, he seemed to shrink into himself as he sat in his wheelchair. His eyes were vacant and despondent. I spoke mostly with his family during that initial visit and heard firsthand how much they valued the prayers of others. They attributed Gerard's survival to the prayers of many, many people they'd never even met.

Week after week, I watched as Gerard gained physical strength and seemed to reengage mentally and emotionally with the world around him. One day, when he came for an appointment, he walked into my office on brand-new prosthetic legs. And that wasn't all that was new. On his arm was an attractive young woman.

He introduced me to his fiancée, Emily, and said, "A lot of people prayed for me over the past two years, and Emily was one of them. When she began praying for my healing, she didn't know that one day my heart would belong to her."

A few months later, Gerard walked down the aisle with his new wife, accompanied by many prayers for their new life together.

TODAY'S RX

Pray for others. Though it may take months—or years—to see an answer, what a blessing it is when it happens!

Father, I ask that you place on my heart the names of those who need prayer. May I be steadfast in lifting them up to you, and may you be with these people, comforting them and giving them wisdom in their times of need.

HEART DISEASE AND DISEASE OF THE HEART

"O LORD," I prayed, "have mercy on me. Heal me, for I have sinned against you."
PSALM 41:4

Sickness has many causes. Unsanitary conditions, genetics, poor diet, lack of exercise, and lack of proper medical care can all cause disease or worsen the outcome of an illness. When sin entered the world, it not only separated us from God, but it also caused or contributed to many of the conditions that foster disease and illness.

Today, with our knowledge of biology, we put up a good fight against many of these disease contributors, but we often don't consider another cause to our pain that modern medicine can't treat.

When a patient complains of heart pain, sometimes it's not a physical problem—it might be better described as a heartfelt pain. The heart is suffering, but it isn't sick from a disease; it's sick from a lack of repentance or reconciliation. Whether the cause of the pain is a broken relationship with a loved one, private anger aimed at a coworker, or unmet dreams and desires, the illness isn't seated in the body; it's in the soul.

This kind of sickness can create legitimate medical symptoms such as stress, high blood pressure, increased cortisol levels, or chest pain. Though these sins of the spiritual heart can lead to real physical disease, the root of the problem is that the patient's sin is interfering with the person's healthy relationship with God.

If you recognize these soul symptoms in your life, the first step to a healthy relationship with your Creator is to ask for forgiveness. It's a simple step in his treatment plan, but it's a hard one for many people to take. When you ask for forgiveness, you can know that God's forgiveness is complete and his healing starts immediately. His treatment brings peace and hope for the future. That's where the journey to both spiritual and physical health begins.

TODAY'S RX

A doctor can perform a checkup on your body, but you have to perform a spiritual checkup on the condition of your heart and soul.

Lord, forgive me for the anger and resentment I harbor in my heart. Help me release this weight I've been carrying, and wash me clean with your Word.

A GIFT OF LIGHT

We know how much God loves us, and we have put our trust in his love. 1 JOHN 4:16

"They just told us that Rhonda's bone marrow transplant wasn't as successful as they initially thought." Rhonda's husband, Phil, had just stopped me in the hallway during my rounds.

"What happened?" Rhonda was my patient, and I was concerned.

"Apparently, she had a virus that was dormant since childhood, but it was awakened when they introduced the new bone marrow cells."

"I'm sorry to hear that," I said.

Over the next few days, I stopped by Rhonda's room during rounds. I watched as her strength dissipated and she began to develop fevers. In Rhonda's circle of friends, she had always been known as the one to call when things were down—she always brightened a bad day. Now as those friends stopped by to express their love for Rhonda, I watched as she received the gift of friendship she had been giving out her entire life.

When faced with the prospect of her impending death, it was easy to find examples to reassure Rhonda of the love of God that surrounded her. She was in love with Jesus and faithfully placed her trust in him. I knew that her only hesitation about running into his arms was concern for her family to find that love as well.

On Tuesday morning when I arrived, Rhonda's room was quiet. The sun hadn't yet come up; the eastern-facing window was still dark. I could see her lying in the bed with three people sitting beside her—Phil and their two children. We all sensed that her time was near.

I asked Rhonda if we could pray for her. When she nodded, I invited Phil to join us. Something about that prayer reassured Rhonda that her kids would be left in her husband's capable hands to continue her legacy of love. She smiled as her heartbeat and respiration slowed. Over the next two hours, she didn't say another word, but her face glowed as her body slowly released her soul into eternity.

When Rhonda left us that day, she left the world a better and brighter place because of the love of God she had showered on all who knew her.

TODAY'S RX

God's love surrounds us and protects us from all fear and pain—even in our darkest moments.

Father, I pray that my life will reflect your love and that my actions and words will make this world a better, brighter place.

LOVING SAUL TO UNCOVER PAUL

Ananias went and found Saul. He laid his hands on him and said, "Brother Saul, the Lord Jesus, who appeared to you on the road, has sent me so that you might regain your sight and be filled with the Holy Spirit." Instantly something like scales fell from Saul's eyes, and he regained his sight. Then he got up and was baptized. ACTS 9:17-19

When the Christians in Damascus heard that Saul had been struck blind, they may have thought that the Lord had answered their prayers by taking down their worst enemy. Finally they could sleep at night, no longer worried that Saul would make them his next victims.

But imagine how Ananias felt when God sent him to heal Paul. What if Jesus asked you to help an evil person? Would you do it?

I had the opportunity to find out for myself one night while working in the ER when a prisoner was brought from jail for treatment. Before I went in to see him, an officer pulled me aside.

"You need to know that this guy was arrested for first-degree murder. And not only does the evidence point to his guilt, but he also confessed. I need to warn you that he may be violent, so if you can't see him, we'll take him somewhere else."

This presented a conflict for me. When I was in high school, some very close friends of mine were murdered in a savage attack. After that incident, I had walked away from my faith for many years, returning only after a dream in which God showed me that my friends were safe and whole in heaven. Now God was asking me to treat a prisoner who had taken the lives of someone else's loved ones.

After saying a quick prayer, I cautiously approached the patient. What I found was a man just like me—fallen and broken. Though I'd never murdered anyone, I knew I was capable of evil if I strayed from the Lord. As I finished bandaging his wounds, I found myself thinking, *There but for the grace of God go I.*

Are you willing to be used by God as an instrument of grace to those who need it most? Who knows? You might be witness to a modern-day Saul-to-Paul conversion.

TODAY'S RX

Ask God to help you love the broken people in your life.

God, it's easy for me to forget that those who've committed evil in this world are your children too. Help me not to cast judgment on them, but to pray for them to see their need for you. Use me to be a light in their world.

CRUSHED WITHOUT A SCRATCH

He will order his angels to protect you wherever you go. They will hold you up with their hands so you won't even hurt your foot on a stone. PSALM 91:11-12

"The only thing I remember," Susan said, "was seeing everything go by in slow motion. I heard the tires screeching, and I smelled smoke. Pretty soon, there was so much smoke that I couldn't breathe. The stench of diesel fuel and burning rubber filled my nostrils."

The pictures of the car that Susan showed me on her phone were astounding. The entire front end of the car was demolished. Very little of the vehicle was even recognizable. The roof was gone, as well as both front tires.

"A semi jackknifed in front of us, and the only place to go was underneath it. I should have been killed or at least mangled as much as the car. I still don't understand why there isn't a scratch on me. I thought that little red car was going to be my coffin."

"Good thing you were the only one in the car," I said.

"But I wasn't. The whole family was headed to a revival when this happened. My husband and two children were also in the car. Satan wanted to destroy what we were doing."

"How in the world did four occupants survive that crash?" I said. The entire car was crushed and compressed—there didn't seem to be any room in there for four people to survive, let alone not be hurt.

"God intervened in a mighty way," Susan said. "He not only spared my life, but my family's lives as well."

I was shocked and amazed. It was nothing short of a miracle that Susan and her family were able to continue their journey after the detour they took under the carriage of that semitrailer. God was definitely with them that day. It was obvious that only he and his angels could have protected them in such a catastrophic situation.

TODAY'S RX

God is sovereign, and he performs miracles of healing and protection.

Lord, I praise you for how you work miracles. Thank you for taking me under your wing and protecting me this day. Please watch over my loved ones and keep them safe as well.

LEARNING TO WALK

The LORD directs the steps of the godly. He delights in every detail of their lives. Though they stumble, they will never fall, for the LORD holds them by the hand.
PSALM 37:23-24

When I read today's verse about how the Lord directs the steps of the godly and keeps them from falling, it reminded me of Ron, a local farmer who raised hogs, tobacco, and six children—his favorite crop. When the kids were learning to walk, Ron would hold out a thick finger for them to grip as they careened along. When Ron's kids had kids of their own, he offered the same "support service" as his grandchildren—his new pride and joy—found their footing.

Over the years, as their family physician, I'd walked with Ron's family through every laceration, broken bone, cough, and flu. But when Ron's wife passed away, it was the hardest thing the family had ever dealt with.

One night, while I was working a late shift in the ER, the EMS called and said that a sixty-eight-year-old man had been found lying facedown in a field. The EMTs said they thought it was a stroke. From the location they gave, I knew it was Ron. I thought about how the family had grieved when Ron's wife had died. To lose Ron, too, would be a major blow.

Ron's children arrived at the hospital before the ambulance did, and each had the same question: "Dad was always the strong one. He never wavered. What do we do now?"

"Once he gets here, we'll stabilize his vital signs and have neurology evaluate him," I said. "Then we'll go from there. If it's a stroke, it might take weeks or even months for him to recover, or—" I didn't say anymore. By now the ambulance had pulled in, and I started my exam and treatment.

Four months later, Ron walked into my office with a big lopsided grin. As he offered his left hand to shake, he said, "The Lord helped me stand back up on my own two feet. With his help, I know I'm going to have a long and productive life."

I assured him that I agreed. I knew that God was holding Ron's hand and helping him walk, just as Ron had done for his children and grandchildren.

TODAY'S RX

When you're holding the Lord's hand, even if you stumble, you won't fall.

Father, you have been with me every step of the way. You've shown me where to walk when the path seemed unclear and have guided me through important decisions. Thank you for caring about me so deeply and for walking with me each day of my life.

OVERFLOWING LOVE

I am giving you a new commandment: Love each other. Just as I have loved you, you should love each other. John 13:34

When I stop to think about how much Jesus loves all of us, it is overwhelming. The Son of God came to earth to invite us back into a relationship with him after we messed it up the first time.

Jesus loves us so much that he was willing to sacrifice his life for us. Are we willing to do the same for others?

That kind of love may seem incomprehensible. Perhaps we might see that kind of reckless, selfless love in the eyes of a mother who is willing to jump in front of a car to save her child, but even that is a rare occurrence. Yet, Christ did all of that—and more—for us.

Even when I ran away from him, even despite my sin, he patiently, kindly, and gently pursued me until I dared to turn and accept the love he had always shown me.

In today's verse, Jesus tells us to love others as he has loved us. But this only reveals the inadequacy in our own strength and will. We all know people who make this command seem nearly impossible to fulfill. Yet, Jesus must believe it is possible for us to love others as he did—or he never would have told us to do it. In those moments when I feel weakest, I stop to remember the quality of God's love for me. I remember his patience and kindness and how he was willing to show me his love, even when I wasn't ready to receive it.

So, in those moments when I am irritated, angry, or just forgetful, when I think more of myself than I think of the people around me, I stop and reflect on how much God loves me. Like a coffee mug that is filled to the brim and then overflows onto the table, I try to take the abundant love that God pours into me and allow it to spill out of my cup and pour onto others. If I can do that, I'll never fail to love other people because God constantly loves me more than I can contain.

TODAY'S RX

As you meditate on God's love for you, look for opportunities to show that love to other people, as well.

Heavenly Father, teach me how to love others from the abundance of love you have already poured out on me.

TUNING IN TO THE NEWS MAKER

Now, dear brothers and sisters, one final thing. Fix your thoughts on what is true, and honorable, and right, and pure, and lovely, and admirable. Think about things that are excellent and worthy of praise. PHILIPPIANS 4:8

In today's world, it is easy to be distracted from things that are true, honorable, right, pure, lovely, and admirable. All you have to do is turn on the news!

The news seems to be the antithesis of everything described in today's verse. Whether it is the local report, a network broadcast, or the twenty-four-hour nonstop news channel, it seems the stories that grab the headlines are always full of tragedy, heartache, terror, and brokenness. The more we listen to the news and the more we dwell on the ugliness of the world, the more likely it is that those dark thoughts will push us away from God.

On the other hand, time spent praying for God to intercede draws us closer to him. It's an opportunity for us to recognize that while we don't have all the answers, God does.

Karen and I have found that by limiting how much time we spend watching the news, we can use that time to pray for God to intervene in the hard situations that happen in the world every day.

I'm not saying that we should withdraw from society or put our heads into the sand. Far from it! But we must focus our attention on the one who can solve all these unsolvable problems, not on the problems themselves. When we focus on the overwhelming problems in the world, we lose our perspective on the blessings that God has granted us. He alone has the power to change the things that overwhelm our abilities, but we always have the ability to change *ourselves* through prayer.

If you find yourself dwelling on bad news, make time to dwell on the good news that comes from our good God. Only he is true, honorable, right, pure, lovely, admirable, excellent, and worthy of our praise. All the time.

TODAY'S RX

Instead of allowing tragic news to turn your head, step away from the news and bow your head in intercessory prayer.

Lord, in this dark world, thank you that your attributes are attractive and comforting. I praise you for being true, honorable, right, pure, lovely, and admirable. Whenever I am disheartened, help me to pray and remember that this world is in your hands.

GET A LITTLE R&R, NOT A TOMBSTONE WITH RIP

Why am I discouraged? Why is my heart so sad? I will put my hope in God! I will praise him again—my Savior and my God! Now I am deeply discouraged, but I will remember you. Psalm 42:5-6

Three chemical systems in the human brain—serotonin, norepinephrine, and dopamine—help us stay balanced emotionally. God created our bodies to have checks and balances, as well as backup systems to keep us healthy emotionally and physically. However, we were not created for a broken world. We were made to live in paradise. So there are times when our environment seems to overwhelm even our backup systems.

At times it can seem as if the world is spinning out of control. The days rush by, and the more we do, the more we feel we must do. We never seem to get enough rest. I think the rat race is especially bad in the United States, where the American Dream has become more of a nightmare. Depression affects more than one-third of the population to the degree that they will need outside help at some point.

There is no shame in needing help. And there is no shame in stepping aside to take care of yourself. I tell my patients the same thing I tell myself: Make time to recover from the battle. We all need to get some R&R (rest and relaxation), or we'll end up with an RIP sign over our resting place.

God knows we occasionally need a break from the world. That's why he wants us to rest in him. He wants us to sing songs from happy and hopeful hearts. The writer of Psalm 42 asks many of the same questions we ask; but ultimately he knows that his hope is in God. At night when he is discouraged, he sings songs of prayer and praise. This ancient practice is the same thing that will help us live happy, balanced lives even when we have a chemical imbalance.

Commit to getting out of life's rut and seek others to hold you accountable. Restoring your soul might be as easy as sitting quietly and enjoying the simple things in life.

TODAY'S RX

Sadness is commonplace, but you don't have to live there. You are not alone. Help is available. Step outside yourself to find someone who can help.

God, reveal to me moments in my day when I can take time to be quiet and rest in you. Place on my heart a desire to be in your Word, and help me to find my hope and joy in you.

SING TO THE LORD YOUR SONG

There I will go to the altar of God, to God—the source of all my joy. I will praise you with my harp, O God, my God! PSALM 43:4

Since the beginning of time, music has been a part of God's creation. I have heard that in the original Hebrew language of the Bible, it says that God sang us into existence. Can you imagine that? On earth, we occasionally refer to an accomplished singer as someone who has "a heavenly voice." But what must the voice of heaven itself sound like?

If it was through music that we were created, it makes sense that music would also sustain us and heal us. As a doctor, I recognize the importance of music in the healing process. The medical literature is full of studies of how music can help us to heal. Healers who want to specialize in this area can get a degree in music therapy.

We were created in God's image, so it is no surprise that we also create through music. From a mother's simple lullaby as she sings her baby to sleep to a symphony of musicians playing their parts to create something bigger than themselves, music reminds us that we are creators too.

I've been blessed with children, and now children-in-law, who are gifted in the art of music. It's hard to imagine our lives without music. One of my good friends, professional musician Steven Curtis Chapman, continues to write some of the most uplifting songs this world has ever heard. The highest praise a musician can receive is that his or her song has touched someone else's soul. I imagine that's also why God loves it when we sing to him—because our souls reach out to him.

As a doctor, I know there won't be a need for my services in heaven. So rather than risk unemployment, I am practicing my singing in the hopes that one day I can get a job in the heavenly choir.

TODAY'S RX

Worship the Creator through music. Sing a song today that heals your heart, and it just may heal your body, too.

God, thank you for the gift of music and how it is uplifting to so many. May I always sing songs of praise and worship to you.

THE SOURCE OF ALL COMFORT

All praise to God, the Father of our Lord Jesus Christ. God is our merciful Father and the source of all comfort. He comforts us in all our troubles so that we can comfort others. When they are troubled, we will be able to give them the same comfort God has given us. 2 CORINTHIANS 1:3-4

When our son, David, was born, he had a double cleft lip and palate. We grieved for the pain and surgeries we knew he would have to endure. But we also knew that God had given him to us for a special reason—even though at the time we didn't know what it was.

David's first two years of life were full of doctors' visits, hospitals, IVs, and surgeries. During that time, Karen and David bonded in a deep and meaningful way. Not only was Karen his mother, but she was also his protector, nurse, and voice when he had none.

After the last major surgery for his palate, the plastic surgeon mentioned that he often met with young parents who would soon be going through the same things we'd just finished. He asked Karen if she would be willing to meet with them and share her experiences. Being the giving soul that she is, she emphatically said, "Yes, of course!"

When the plastic surgeon called occasionally with the details of a new patient, Karen would arrange to meet with the young parents and their baby. Whenever she went on those visits, she took David with her as a living sign of hope for the parents to see that, in a few years, their babies would be healed as well.

Usually during these visits, Karen shared David's story and comforted and reassured the parents. Most visits ended with prayer for the parents and their baby—that God would give them all strength and courage to face the battle ahead.

I marveled at how Karen was able to comfort others, but I also knew the reason why—God had first comforted her. Because of her experience, she knew what others in the same situation needed. She was a willing vessel ready to pass on God's comfort to those who needed it most.

TODAY'S RX

If you need comfort, seek God, the source of all comfort. If you see others who are struggling, share your struggles. Empathy can be a great source of comfort.

Father, you've shown me your faithfulness time and again by comforting me during tough times. Help me to live out your example and be a comfort my friends and family.

COUNTING YOUR BLESSINGS

Be sure to fear the Lord and faithfully serve him. Think of all the wonderful things he has done for you. 1 SAMUEL 12:24

"How do I love thee? Let me count the ways." Poet Elizabeth Barrett Browning had it right when she wrote those lines. When we're in love, we count all the little things we love about the other person.

Maybe you can remember the earliest days of a courtship when every glance, hug, or kiss seemed thrilling. You never tired of the other person. You thought about him or her when you were alone, and you only wanted more of the same as you grew more deeply in love

This is the kind of enthusiasm we should have for our Lord. We need to stop and count all the blessings he has given us. If we can count all the cute smiles on our lover's face, why can't we count the times the Lord has done something to make us smile? If we can gaze longingly into our lover's eyes, why can't we gaze lovingly at nature and appreciate the tiniest details of our Father's creation?

Too often, we don't even notice the things that God has done for us or the blessings he has placed in our path. But even on those rare occasions when we do, we're more likely to attribute them to luck or coincidence.

Why is it that we interpret every positive signal from our love interest as an expression of his or her love, but we assume that every signal from our Lord is merely an accident of timing?

When we care enough to count the blessings God has bestowed on us, we learn to see with new eyes all the little things he's done for us. Over time, I have taught myself to recognize his subtle nudges just as well as when I recognize the ways that Karen looks at me and I know what she's thinking.

We may refer to our partner as our soul mate, but there is only one for whom our souls truly cry out—Jesus, our Lord and Savior, who created us, blessed us, and loves us unconditionally.

TODAY'S RX

Today, stop long enough to thank the one who created you, and ask him to help you perceive his other blessings as well.

Jesus, thank you for lavishing your love on me and blessing me with your beautiful creation. I am in awe of all you've done. Help me to have a grateful heart throughout my day.

UNFAILING LOVE MAKES THE DIFFERENCE

Each day the LORD pours his unfailing love upon me, and through each night I sing his songs, praying to God who gives me life. PSALM 42:8

On the night when Lisa entered the detox unit, she looked like all the other heroin addicts we took in—track marks on her arms and clothes that hung loosely from her anorexic frame. One of the most addictive substances on earth, heroin is a strong demon that takes its toll.

"How many times have you been in rehab?" I asked as I filled out her intake form.

"I've been in five or six times to get straightened out . . . but this time it's going to be different."

I could have told her that we heard this line several times a night, every night, but she seemed convinced. And then she told me why.

"Last week I walked into a little church down the street, and the preacher told me that Jesus loves me and would forgive me—no matter what I've done, no matter how bad my sin has been. The preacher said that all I had to do was ask for forgiveness and believe that Jesus is the Son of God, and Jesus would wash me white as snow."

Being white as snow probably seemed like an impossible dream to someone so filthy from living on the streets, but her face lit up, and her eyes sparkled as she spoke.

When she said, "Jesus is going to set me free from these drugs. I just know it," I, too, became convinced that this time would be different for Lisa. The nurses who witnessed Lisa's declaration later agreed that it was the most powerful and real testimony we'd ever heard.

Before entering the unit, Lisa asked for a Bible and a hymnal. For the next few days, and especially when her cravings were the strongest, we heard Lisa reading out loud from the Bible or singing from the hymnal.

By the time she went home, Lisa had been healed by the unfailing love of God. As she waved good-bye with a giant grin on her face, she almost seemed to glow.

To all of us, and in the eyes of God, she truly was white as snow.

TODAY'S RX

When you want things to be different in your life, ask God for forgiveness, and ask him to cleanse you of your sin.

Jesus, I am clean only because of your perfect sacrifice, so I ask that you please forgive me and wash away all that keeps me from drawing close to you. Thank you for loving me so deeply.

GENERATIONS OF ANSWERED PRAYERS

He will listen to the prayers of the destitute. He will not reject their pleas. Let this be recorded for future generations, so that a people not yet born will praise the LORD. PSALM 102:17-18

On February 14, 1908, my grandfather was the seventh child born into a south Alabama dirt farmer's family. He was the first boy, with six older sisters. In other words, he grew up with seven "mothers" fussing over him. With that many women in his life, he couldn't help but grow into a gregarious, fun-loving young lad.

The incessant demands of the farm required another worker just as soon as my grandfather was able, so before he had even finished second grade, he was taken out of school and put to work in the fields. There was no time to waste learning skills that didn't directly apply to crop production. During planting season, his bare feet barely hit the floor in the morning before he was called to start plowing the hard red clay to prepare the fields for seed.

Grandpa grew up, got married, and eventually took over the farm from his father. He and his wife had two boys, and he was grateful for both. With two boys, he could keep two mule teams busy.

But my grandfather wanted more for his sons than the life he'd had on the farm. During the long days working in the fields, he prayed that God would show him a way to break the cycle of poverty that had cursed the family for generations. Though he couldn't read or write, and his wife had made it only through the eighth grade herself, they knew that the boys needed to get an education in order to have a better life. So, when the boys were still babies, my grandmother began reading to them from the Bible, the only book they owned.

The elder son, James (my father), finished high school and college and became a teacher. In the next generation, I, of course, went all the way to medical school. The reason I am a doctor and a man of faith today is because of my grandfather's prayers, which began with my father and included me before I was even born.

TODAY'S RX

Is there anything more powerful than our prayers for our children and grandchildren? Write down your prayers so they will see the fruit of your faith.

God, I thank you for all the generations of family you've blessed me with. Help me to see your hand at work in their lives, and remind me to pray for them always.

JESUS, SHOW US HOW TO HAVE CONFIDENT COURAGE

The LORD is my light and my salvation—so why should I be afraid? The LORD is my fortress, protecting me from danger, so why should I tremble? When evil people come to devour me, when my enemies and foes attack me, they will stumble and fall. Though a mighty army surrounds me, my heart will not be afraid. Even if I am attacked, I will remain confident. PSALM 27:1-3

Twenty-one Egyptian Coptic Christian men knelt on the beach awaiting their fate. Dressed in orange jumpsuits, they faced away from their captors, who were all dressed in black. A few minutes later, the ocean tide ran red with the blood of the martyrs. These men of the Cross, these followers of Jesus, met their maker as silently as lambs.

It wasn't the first time, nor will it be the last, that Christian men have bravely faced their own deaths.

When Jesus calmed the storm on the Sea of Galilee, he revealed the scope and magnitude of his power over the elements. He showed us that we needn't be afraid of the storms of this world, whether physical, emotional, or spiritual. He was, and is, in control.

When he was mocked, beaten, and left hanging on the cross, he showed us how to face persecution and adversity with courage. His resurrection demonstrated that he had overcome death itself.

How will we respond when our lives are threatened? Will we face our mortality with courage and hope? Will we acknowledge that God is in control, regardless of the circumstances or the enemies that surround us?

I pray that God will give you the courage and strength to stand firm for him and that you will embrace the love and grace he has extended to you, even when the time comes for you to take your final breath.

Whether we are called as soldiers or martyrs, whether our foe is cancer or foreign terrorists, we must follow in the footsteps of Jesus. In the garden of Gethsemane, he prayed that his Father would take this cup of suffering from him. But regardless, he promised to do his Father's will.

May we do the same.

TODAY'S RX

Do not be intimidated. Engage your adversaries with the confidence that Jesus has shown you how to fearlessly face your foes and overcome death in his name.

Lord, may I always stand firm in my faith. Give me the courage and confidence to proclaim your name above whatever difficulties I face. Thank you for being with me wherever I am.

BREATHTAKING NEWS

We hoped for peace, but no peace came. We hoped for a time of healing, but found only terror. JEREMIAH 8:15

The Israelites had heard God's warnings through the prophet Jeremiah, yet they failed to heed his commands. Neither did they seek forgiveness for their sins. Thus, they sealed their fate—and instead of healing, they found only terror.

In our day and age, it seems we haven't changed much. There are still many who don't heed God's warnings, and they miss their chance to be healed.

Dylan was diagnosed with asthma at an early age, requiring daily breathing treatments. Both of his parents smoked, which made a difficult situation worse.

Then, during his teen years, Dylan himself started smoking. By his twenties, he was a three-pack-a-day smoker. Eventually, his asthma morphed into chronic obstructive pulmonary disease (COPD), and as a result, he was hospitalized two or three times a year.

Each time Dylan saw a doctor, he received an urgent warning. Both his pulmonologist and I told him there could be severe consequences from his smoking.

"I know, I know. I've got to quit," he said each time he was confronted. "But it's so hard when everyone around me is smoking."

"You're right," I said. "It is hard. But you're in control of your own destiny—and the only way to improve your health is to quit smoking."

Into his thirties, I heard the same song and dance. "I know, I know, I need to quit." Until one day when Dylan's complaint changed.

"I coughed up blood this morning. Is that bad?"

When the results came back from a CT scan and a bronchoscopy, I had the sad duty of informing Dylan that he had lung cancer, which had metastasized to his liver.

"We'll do everything we can," I said, "but this type of cancer is very aggressive. We'll try to keep you comfortable and pain-free on your journey, and we'll pray for you daily."

As the harsh reality set in, Dylan's face registered shock and horror. He was not prepared for his life to come down to this. Sadly, the time was past for him to change course for the better. Now he could only face the consequences of his lifelong choices.

TODAY'S RX

If you've been ignoring God's warnings in your life, repent now and seek healing and forgiveness before it's too late.

Lord, I am weak in so many ways. I give in to temptation, only to be met with regret. Please give me the strength to rise above temptation and to rely on you for complete fulfillment in my life.

HEALTHY PEOPLE DON'T NEED A DOCTOR

As Jesus left the town, he saw a tax collector named Levi sitting at his tax collector's booth. "Follow me and be my disciple," Jesus said to him. So Levi got up, left everything, and followed him. Later, Levi held a banquet in his home with Jesus as the guest of honor. Many of Levi's fellow tax collectors and other guests also ate with them. But the Pharisees and their teachers of religious law complained bitterly to Jesus' disciples, "Why do you eat and drink with such scum?" Jesus answered them, "Healthy people don't need a doctor—sick people do. I have come to call not those who think they are righteous, but those who know they are sinners and need to repent." LUKE 5:27-32

As a family care physician, I often do annual physical exams on my healthy patients. Sometimes they just want to make sure everything is okay. Other times, they need a physical for sports, school, a new job, or to qualify for insurance. If I declare them free of illness, they walk away happy—and I'm happy for them; but I find these encounters to be less fulfilling than working with patients who are sick or dying. My job, training, and experience are all about helping the sick and suffering. The more time I spend with my well patients or my worried-they-might-not-be-well patients, the less time I have to spend with those who truly need to see a doctor.

Before we can determine a treatment in modern medicine, we must first diagnose the underlying illness. Likewise, when we seek treatment for our souls, we must first understand that we have a spiritual sickness. We need to know that we are sinners in need of a Savior. If we self-righteously think that we have it all together, in effect we're saying that we don't need Jesus. But if we know we're sick and dying, and we want treatment, then we will come to Jesus to be healed.

Jesus didn't come to celebrate the righteous; he came to bring healing and redemption to sinners in need of forgiveness. That includes all of us. We need Jesus to cure our sin problem.

TODAY'S RX

If you recognize your soul's sickness, spend time today in the presence of the Healer.

Jesus, thank you for leaving your perfect place in heaven to dwell among the sinful and the sick. Thank you for bringing healing to this world and for showing me my need for you. Help me to learn from my past mistakes and follow you.

WHY DOES GOD ALLOW TRAGEDY?

The LORD is close to the brokenhearted; he rescues those whose spirits are crushed.
PSALM 34:18

During the first fourteen years of my life, my faith in God was innocent. It wasn't built on struggle or hardship, and it had never been tested. My life was pretty sheltered, and I was happy. I believed God was all-powerful and ever present. The role models in my life all demonstrated grace and kindness, which further reinforced my belief that God was good.

And then, one horrible day, my close friends (and distant cousins) Jimmy and Jerry Alday were senselessly murdered, along with several of their family members. Jimmy, Jerry, and I had worked summers together selling watermelons at the Atlanta State Farmers Market, and those two hardworking, God-fearing men had a tremendous influence on my life and faith. And in an instant they were gone.

For a long time after that, I accused God of turning his back on his people and not being powerful enough to take care of them. *Where were you when the Aldays were murdered?* I silently raged. *Why didn't you protect them?*

During the summer following their deaths, I spent hours at the market sitting alone with my memories, frightened by the prospect of evil. Heaven, which had once seemed as close to me as the wind in the trees, now seemed unapproachable. Sin had new depths, depravity had new meaning, and I felt vulnerable to the darkness.

My big brothers and earthly protectors were gone, and I was no longer certain that my heavenly Protector could be trusted. In fact, God seemed useless to me now.

It took years for God to woo me back to himself. Only as the Lord began to soften my heart did I recognize that he had been with me all along. Why hadn't I seen or heard him? Could it be that I had been the one to turn away from God just when I needed him most?

Over the course of my life and practice, I've learned that God does not willingly harm his people; rather, he is a God of infinite compassion. In times of grief, I encourage you to turn *toward* God instead of away from him.

TODAY'S RX

Ask God to help you see and celebrate his glory where it shows up—in the midst of pain as well as in joy.

Father, thank you for being a God of infinite compassion.
Help me to keep my eyes focused on eternity and to celebrate
your glory in the midst of pain as well as joy.

BLUE EYES SHINING

I will lead blind Israel down a new path, guiding them along an unfamiliar way. I will brighten the darkness before them and smooth out the road ahead of them. Yes, I will indeed do these things; I will not forsake them. ISAIAH 42:16

"My dad seems to be stumbling a lot more," Maggie said. "Can I set up an appointment for him to come in, so we can figure out what's going on?"

I had known Thomas and his family for more than twenty-five years. He and his children and grandchildren had one distinctive trait in common: the most beautiful deep-blue eyes I've ever seen. Thomas's eyes reflected sparkles of light and yet were as calm as the sea. I would recognize his kin anywhere because of those distinctive blue eyes.

"So, Thomas," I said, one afternoon when he came into my office "What seems to be the problem? Maggie seems worried about you."

"I think I'm going blind."

"Hmm, let me see." I pulled out my light and looked into his eyes. "They don't seem to be as bright and clear as they used to be. Have you noticed changes in your vision?"

"It seems like I'm stumbling over things more often. Especially when I go out at night."

When I had him look at my eye charts. I could see a noticeable drop in his visual acuity. As it happened, his vision was hindered by the yellow-green reflection of cataracts that had ripened rather quickly.

"Thomas, I'm going to refer you to a good ophthalmologist whose office is not too far from here. I'll see if he can fit you in this week to check things out a little more closely."

Thomas ended up needing two cataract surgeries, and he stayed with his daughter while he recovered. A month later, when Maggie brought him in for a follow-up appointment, Thomas was walking faster and had more pep in his step.

"The cataract surgeon fixed my vision!" he said. " It's great to be able to see all of God's creation again."

He winked at Maggie, and I could see that both father and daughter once again had that sparkle in their deep-blue eyes.

TODAY'S RX

Go for regular checkups and take good care of your eyes. Not only are they the window to your soul, but they are also the doorway to your good health.

God, thank you for guiding me through my struggles. I pray that you open my spiritual eyes today, giving me clarity for the decisions I must make.

TORN BETWEEN TWO WORLDS

To me, living means living for Christ, and dying is even better. But if I live, I can do more fruitful work for Christ. So I really don't know which is better. I'm torn between two desires: I long to go and be with Christ, which would be far better for me. But for your sakes, it is better that I continue to live. Knowing this, I am convinced that I will remain alive so I can continue to help all of you grow and experience the joy of your faith. PHILIPPIANS 1:21-25

When Karen and I first met, she was memorizing the entire book of Philippians for a Bible study. I was still walking away from God at the time, and the only way that Karen would spend any time with me was if I helped her with her memorization. As often as she would allow it, I'd go to her place and quiz her on long passages from Paul's letter.

Today's verse was one of the first Bible verses that really spoke to me when I came back to faith in God. As I've mentioned, the reason I had become an atheist was because two of my friends and several of their family members had been murdered, and I didn't believe that a good God would allow that to happen. But then I had a dream in which I saw my friends restored to wholeness and happiness in heaven, and they told me not to blame God.

That little glimpse of eternity made me never want to leave, but God let me know very clearly that I had work yet to do on earth. Ever since that day, I haven't feared death because I know what's on the other side of the veil. Even now, decades after I had that dream, the tranquility and beauty of that moment remains with me. That's why I can relate to Paul when he writes, "Living means living for Christ, and dying is even better."

Every day I wake up and ask God to help me share his love and joy for as long as I remain here on earth. I also thank him at the end of the day because I'm one day closer to returning to my forever home.

TODAY'S RX

God's heavenly banquet table has an open invitation. We're encouraged to invite as many people as we can to join us there someday.

Lord, I long to sit at your table and see you face to face. Thank you for the gift of salvation and the promise of heaven.

A CONFIDENT HEART

My heart is confident in you, O God; my heart is confident. No wonder I can sing your praises! PSALM 57:7

I love today's verse because it reminds me of one of my patients. Keith is a singer/songwriter with a history of heartbreak in his family—literally. He told me about it recently when he came in for an appointment.

"How are you doing?" I asked.

"Not so well. I'm worried that I might have what my dad and uncle had."

At first, I thought he was talking about being exposed to the flu or another airborne illness, but then he explained it was something much more serious.

"My dad and my uncle were both fifty-two years old when they had massive heart attacks and died. I'm fifty-three, and I'm finding it hard to walk up a flight of stairs without getting short of breath. I don't have much confidence that I am going to last a lot longer. I'm afraid I may have a broken ticker too."

I arranged for Keith to see a cardiologist the next morning. They put him on the heart catheterization table and quickly determined that his genetic makeup had caught up with him. Keith had a 99 percent blockage in one artery and significant blockages in three others—a common convergence of symptoms often referred to as a widowmaker.

The cardiovascular surgeon agreed that immediate bypass surgery was indicated, and the procedure was set up for the next day. I was thankful that Keith had come to see me when he did.

The surgery and postoperative recovery went well. Keith regained confidence in his heart and now had a new sense of hope about the future.

TODAY'S RX

Put your confidence in God. He can fix all kinds of broken hearts. And be certain to see your physician if you have a family history of heart problems.

Father, replace my worried heart with a heart of confidence. Help me to trust in you always, knowing you have the best in store for me.

RESCUED FROM DEATH

Jesus told her, "I am the resurrection and the life. Anyone who believes in me will live, even after dying. Everyone who lives in me and believes in me will never ever die. Do you believe this, Martha?" JOHN 11:25-26

All of medicine is dedicated to taking away our pain and sustaining life. Yet no matter how hard medical professionals try—no matter how many new drugs, treatments, or surgeries we invent—we cannot stop death.

We have found ways to sustain life through organ replacement, cloning of new parts, and regeneration through stem cells, yet those can also fail, and inevitably our bodies will give way. It seems that in the end, death wins. We are mortal. There is nothing we can do to change that.

But can there be victory over the grave? Can we triumph over death? Is there a life preserver that can rescue us from death's swirling waters?

The answer, of course, is a resounding yes, yes, yes! Jesus is our Savior. He did and will continue to conquer death.

Jesus undid Lazarus's physical death and gave him an extended life on earth. Though eventually, even Lazarus died a second physical death. But this time he died without fear because he joined Jesus in heaven.

Jesus conquered the grave with his own physical death and resurrection. We, too, will experience a physical death through which we will discard our earthly bodies. But once we reunite with Jesus, death will be no more.

I have had the privilege of sitting beside the deathbeds of hundreds of believers who have made this journey. I have watched them go without fear. They enter the next world at peace and with joy on their faces.

I do not fear the death of my body because I know that with death comes the freedom of everlasting life. Jesus asked Martha if she believed that. Do you?

TODAY'S RX

To have everlasting life, you must believe that Jesus is the Savior who came to rescue you.

Jesus, knowing that you have conquered the grave, I do not have to worry about dying. Thank you for the promise of everlasting life with you.

THE POWER IS HIS

I also pray that you will understand the incredible greatness of God's power for us who believe him. This is the same mighty power that raised Christ from the dead and seated him in the place of honor at God's right hand in the heavenly realms. EPHESIANS 1:19-20

"Tell me what's going on," I said to Erin. It had been a while since her last appointment.

"Oh, I'm not having any problems. I just haven't had a checkup in a while, and I thought I should probably get one."

"Great, I'm glad you're feeling well." As I glanced at her paperwork, something caught my eye. "Looks like you marked "yes" to both abdominal pain and recent weight loss. Tell me more about that."

"Oh, I just marked it because it asked, but I'm not really having any problems," she said.

I asked Erin more specific questions about her pain and the amount of her weight loss, but she assured me it was nothing.

"There are a couple of things that concern me," I said. "I think we should have them checked out just to make sure."

The following week, I sat at my desk staring in disbelief at Erin's test results. They showed a metastatic renal cell carcinoma—cancer of the kidneys that had spread to other organs.

When I gave Erin the diagnosis, her eyes filled with tears as she tried to understand how she could go from feeling good to being diagnosed with an incurable illness.

I took her hand and said, "Only the Lord knows our time on earth and the journey he has ordained for us to travel. As your doctor, I promise to do everything I can to make your journey as pain-free and comfortable as possible. As your friend and brother in Christ, I will continue to pray for God's healing hand and mercy upon you."

Though I look forward expectantly to one day crossing from this world to the next, I know that many people are not prepared to face the end of their time here on earth—certainly not before they might expect it. My best advice is to prepare your heart and soul for eternity before you are confronted with the reality of your mortality. Above all, trust God. Only he knows when your day will arrive.

TODAY'S RX

God holds the power of life and death. Entrust him with your destiny.

Plant a desire for heaven deeper in my heart, Lord. Help me to realize how temporary my time on earth is, and allow me to use the days I have left in a way that brings you glory.

THE JOY OF LIFE AND DEATH

This is a sacred day before our Lord. Don't be dejected and sad, for the joy of the LORD *is your strength!* NEHEMIAH 8:10

When I was young, funerals were sad events. It was hard for me to say good-bye to a loved one. Whether it was my friends who were murdered or beloved grandparents who had died, I missed those who had gone on before me.

As a doctor, I have grieved with parents who lost children much too early. When a child dies, the whole world seems out of order and upside down. Those events are forever seared into the parents' hearts and memories. They lose their ability to think rationally. Their joy in life is lost in a torrential, enveloping storm of grief.

But if we believe in Jesus, we know that what awaits us on the other side of that threshold is the Savior who died to forgive us of all our sins—past, present, and future. He is standing there with outstretched arms awaiting our arrival. On heaven's side of the veil, there is no sickness, sadness, or dejection. That is truly something to look forward to and celebrate.

When I was asked to speak at my father's funeral, what came to mind were all the memories I had of a great man who had lived a good life. Of course, I was going to miss him, but I rejoiced in the fact that he was now in heaven.

It's easy to focus on death. But life isn't about when we will die; it's about how well we will spend the time that God has given us here and now. We may celebrate the fact that we temporarily cheated death by surviving an accident or recovering from a terrible disease, but the only way to experience the pure joy of heaven is to step across the threshold of death.

My father fought the good fight. As I spoke of his life, it brought encouragement and hope to all of us who were there to celebrate him. We want to make the most of our time here on earth, but we also look forward to the joy of one day being reunited with those who have gone before us.

TODAY'S RX

Find joy in life today, and make every moment count.

Father, help me to fight the good fight and live wholeheartedly for you. May my words and actions reflect you and be life-giving to those around me.

SENSING ANOTHER WORLD

I give them eternal life, and they will never perish. No one can snatch them away from me. John 10:28

One of my favorite geriatric patients was a sweet lady who was petite but had the manners and voice of royalty. She was very precise in everything she said and did. When Annemarie arrived for her appointment, she took a seat in the exam room and smoothed her skirt so there wasn't a wrinkle across her lap. She seemed more regal than country.

"I'm ninety-two years old, Dr. Anderson. My body is wearing out. I can't hear very well—just a little ringing, a bit like tiny church bells. And I can't see much these days. Everything is hazy with a rainbow around it."

"How are you getting around?" I asked.

"The gravity of this world seems heavier to me these days, as if it is pulling me down. I find it hard to walk without a cane or a crutch in the purest sense of the word. But with all this, I know that God is with me, and I will not perish."

"I'm tracking with you, Annemarie. I clearly understand what you're saying."

As she became increasingly blind and deaf to the things of this world, she attuned her spirit to see, hear, and begin living in eternity.

"I'm here today to tell you that when my heart stops, I do not—repeat, I do not—want anyone to try to restart it. If I wake up from being dead, I will be quite upset."

"Don't worry, Annemarie. I think that when we finally get a glimpse of heaven, that is all we want. If God is calling us forward, nothing on this side of eternity can pull us back. But we will make sure that you have a do-not-resuscitate order in your chart. And we will honor your wishes."

TODAY'S RX

The very young and the very old seem to have more clarity of heaven than those of us in the middle.

God, help me to draw closer to you every day of my life. Keep me in tune with your Word so that I may live according to your will. Grow my love for you as I experience more of your blessings.

LET GO TO MOVE ON

When you are praying, first forgive anyone you are holding a grudge against, so that your Father in heaven will forgive your sins, too. MARK 11:25

Ricky was a new patient in my practice, so I asked him to tell me a little bit about himself.

"I ain't been to a doctor in years, ever since my wife, Kathy Sue, died. I still blame her doctor for not treating her cancer."

Ricky told me a little more about his wife and the kind of cancer she'd had. "They did surgery on her, but it had already spread all over. They just closed her up, and she only lived a few months after that."

It was evident that Ricky's bitterness still occupied his thoughts—and ate up a lot of his time.

"What brought you in to see me?" I asked.

"Well, I can't sleep. My head hurts, and I've lost so much weight my pants are fallin' off." He paused for a moment and then raised his eyes to look at me. "Am I gonna die now too?"

Looking at him, I could tell he was depressed, but I needed to rule out other possible causes of his symptoms. I ordered blood work, a CT scan of his head, and other tests. They all came back negative. At his next appointment, I told him the good news.

"Then what's wrong with me, Doc?" he asked.

"You've been mourning the loss of your wife, and you've been mad at her doctor for years," I said. "You're clinically depressed."

I explained how stress and anxiety created a serotonin deficiency in his brain. I recommended that he start on medication.

"But most important, I want you to know that Kathy Sue's death wasn't anyone's fault. You can't blame her doctor, you can't blame her, and you can't blame yourself. If you want to heal, you're going to have to let go of your grudge."

A doctor can prescribe medication to stabilize brain chemistry, but only we can let go of our pasts in order to move forward.

TODAY'S RX

Is there someone, or something, in your past that needs to be forgiven before you can move forward? To improve your health and happiness, do it today.

Jesus, whenever I am too stubborn to forgive, help me to remember your sacrifice and the ultimate model of forgiveness you displayed by dying on the cross. Let me be quick to forgive, knowing all you've done for me.

TOUCHING THE ROBE OF JESUS

[The woman] had heard about Jesus, so she came up behind him through the crowd and touched his robe. For she thought to herself, "If I can just touch his robe, I will be healed." Immediately the bleeding stopped, and she could feel in her body that she had been healed of her terrible condition. Jesus realized at once that healing power had gone out from him, so he turned around in the crowd and asked, "Who touched my robe?" His disciples said to him, "Look at this crowd pressing around you. How can you ask, 'Who touched me?'" But he kept on looking around to see who had done it. Then the frightened woman, trembling at the realization of what had happened to her, came and fell to her knees in front of him and told him what she had done. And he said to her, "Daughter, your faith has made you well. Go in peace. Your suffering is over." MARK 5:27-34

Imagine the crush of people jostling to get to Jesus as he walked with his disciples. A woman who had been bleeding for twelve years wanted what many others wanted—a healing miracle. But unlike many, she had the faith to believe that if she could just get close enough to touch Jesus' robe, she would be healed.

She pressed her way through the multitudes, and for a split second, when Jesus passed by, she reached out and touched his robe. Instantly, she felt his healing power surge through her. But then he stopped and spoke.

"Who touched my robe?"

Her instant reaction had to be one of fear. What would happen if she identified herself? Would Jesus, the healer, be angry? Would he take back the miracle?

The disciples were equally perplexed. How in this teeming mass of humanity could anyone know who had touched Jesus' robe?

But the woman chose to identify herself, and Jesus made it clear that God had used her belief in him to heal her.

How close do we try to get to Jesus when we feel unclean? Do we press our way through the crowd? Or do we give up, afraid that others will see how sick we are? I know that when my patients are willing to push forward, their outcomes are always better—maybe not always physically better, but always emotionally and spiritually better.

TODAY'S RX

Reach out to Jesus today. As you seek him, he will give you renewed life.

Lord, often my shame gets the best of me, and I draw away from you when I feel unclean. Help me, instead, to draw near to you, like the woman in this story, and trust you for deliverance from my sin.

OLD PATTERNS BECOME NEW

God is working in you, giving you the desire and the power to do what pleases him.
PHILIPPIANS 2:13

One cold February day, Ernie sat on the exam table and stared at the tile floor. Though he didn't seem to have any specific symptoms, his shoulders slumped.

"I just don't feel well. Every day, my job is the same monotonous grind. It pays all right, but it's not very exciting. I've got a great family, but I feel like we're stuck in a rut."

Ernie's circumstances weren't much different from those of countless others who put in an honest day's work and punched out at quitting time. But I heard something different in his voice, and it worried me.

"I don't know; I just feel like nothing is going to change or get better until I die. Some days, I think maybe everything would be better if I died."

I asked Ernie a few more questions and found out that he had not been sleeping well for months, and he didn't have much of an appetite. Here was a man who had lost his direction.

"Ernie, I think you're suffering from depression. But I can help."

We did the necessary medical work, and I helped him identify some positive things in his life that he could use as stepping-stones to a renewed life.

Over the next several months, Ernie quit drinking and began exercising, taking long walks in the neighborhood with his wife. He started attending church with his family regularly and began to foster his relationship with God.

The next time I saw Ernie in my office, he was not the same man I'd seen during the winter. Instead of looking down at all his circumstances, he was now looking up to God in worship. The changes hadn't happened overnight, but they took root and transformed his life.

In our darkest days, we search for the light. When we come to the end of ourselves, we become open to seeing the hand of God who faithfully walks alongside us even when we are unaware.

TODAY'S RX

If you're depressed, talk to a doctor or someone you can trust. Then change the old patterns in your life, and open your heart to God and his healing touch.

God, when I feel overwhelmed and life seems to be spinning out of control, pull me close to you. Help me to recognize how you have blessed me, and give me a renewed appreciation for your faithfulness.

MARCH CHECKUP

Our farm has a half-acre patch of buttercups that break through every March and blossom into a silky blanket of bright yellow on a carpet of green. This puts us on notice that spring is right around the corner.

As each day passes, there are more hints of renewed life—budding trees and green shoots bursting from the dark earth where they napped through the winter. We also smell the first scents of grass, flowers, and the waft of barbecue from the neighbor's grill.

By now, our New Year's resolutions may have fallen by the wayside and been replaced by a touch of guilt. But with the newness of the season, we can have a fresh start. It's not too late to rekindle our promises and renew our resolve. The apostle Paul says that we can be transformed by the renewing of our minds (see Romans 12:2, NIV). What better time than the month of March to start anew?

Consider renewing your mind through an online course or Bible study. Check to see if your church offers classes that can help you grow in your faith and in your ability to share it with others. Stop by a Christian bookstore, and ask the person behind the counter to recommend a good book that will expand your thinking and help nurture your faith.

This month, the warmth of the sun will cause cracks in the icy cold of winter. If you've been indoors hiding from the cold, this is a great time to carefully step out and start a new walking or exercise regime. Throughout the month of March, as you burst forth from your winter hibernation, pay special attention to the emerging sights and sounds of your environment. As you renew your mind, you will renew your energy as well.

March Booster Shot: Blossoming flowers, sprouting grasses, and spring cleaning send bits of pollen, dust, and mold into the air. This month begins the spring allergy season, and it's the perfect time to clean out the medicine cabinet. Properly dispose of the old to make room for the new.

HEALING HANDS

Be strong and immovable. Always work enthusiastically for the Lord, for you know that nothing you do for the Lord is ever useless. 1 Corinthians 15:58

In medical school, we were taught that if we listened to our patients, they would give us their diagnosis. When a doctor touches a patient, I believe he or she receives confirmation of what the patient has expressed in words. I often find myself "listening" with my hands so I can feel what my patient feels. I believe that God gave me a gift, similar to a mother's sensitivity to her child's pain or illness, which has been sharpened through my medical training and practice.

When I am examining a patient with my hands and come across sudden warmth, I know something may be awry. When that happens, I start my search for a diagnosis where my hands felt the warmest. Often, it leads me to diseases I might not otherwise have considered. Patients seem to appreciate my high-touch diagnostic skills, and the more I use them, the more I recognize them as a God-given gift.

God has given you certain gifts and talents as well. Maybe it's an ear for music, a heart for hospitality, or a special ability to relate to children or teenagers. Whatever it is, know that it is not merely a gift from God to you. It is a gift from God *through* you to those around you—a way for you to serve and bless others and use your talent for God's glory.

When we get to heaven, we will be exactly who God created us to be, minus the burden of sin and worldly concerns. We will freely do, to the fullest extent, what God created us to do. Here in this life, the deep joy and satisfaction we feel whenever we are faithful stewards of God's gifts is just a tiny foretaste of what awaits us in our heavenly home.

TODAY'S RX

Ask God what he wants you to do with the talents he has given you. If you feel as if you're not using your gifts to the fullest extent, what is holding you back?

God, thank you for the gifts you have given me. I know that any talents or abilities I have are not from my own doing, but are from you. Help me to use these gifts well so that I may point others to you.

BECOMING COMPLETE AGAIN

May you experience the love of Christ, though it is too great to understand fully. Then you will be made complete with all the fullness of life and power that comes from God.
Ephesians 3:19

"When Geoff died, I didn't know where to turn," Karla said. "I changed jobs, but that only brought a new set of stressors. I couldn't afford the house payment, so I had to sell and downsize. It was the worst summer ever. I've never felt so alone."

In the span of six months, Karla had endured three major events that had changed her life for the worse. No wonder she felt the way she did.

"Do you have anyone you can talk to?" I asked.

"I talk to my pastor. But I'm exhausted, and all I do is cry."

"I'm glad you're continuing to go to church and to meet with your pastor. Having a church family to rely on can be an important lifeline. What did your pastor suggest?"

"He said, 'Lean into God and read his Word every day, even if you don't feel like it.'"

"As your medical doctor, I couldn't agree more," I said. Even when Karla was exhausted and didn't fully understand the passages she was reading, God would meet her there, lift her up, and let her experience his love. She seemed to be doing the right things for her spiritual health, but her symptoms suggested she might also need treatment for depression.

"Here's a prescription," I said, "but I want you to continue to meet with your pastor as often as you need to and meet with God daily."

A few months later, during one of her regular appointments, Karla mentioned that she had met a man at church.

"First, he asked if he could help me in any way. Later, he started asking me out to dinner. I'm not sure. Is it too soon?"

"Karla, our timing isn't the same as God's. But if God is in this, then all will be good."

The next time I saw Karla, the transformation in her outlook—from darkness to a new lightness of being—was incredible to witness and something only God could have accomplished. We stopped her medication because God had cured her depression, and she was planning her wedding. She was truly a new creation.

TODAY'S RX

Lean into God and read his Word every day, even if you don't feel like it.

Father, thank you for faithfully showing me the way when I'm lost. Though I do not always know the direction to go, you guide me and comfort me through your Word, showing me examples of your love. Continue to show me the way.

I WILL RETURN

"I will return to you about this time next year, and your wife, Sarah, will have a son!" Sarah was listening to this conversation from the tent. GENESIS 18:10

"Doc, I'm afraid my life hasn't always been on the straight and narrow," Sean said. It was his first visit, and we were going over his past medical history. "When I was younger, I was an IV drug user, and I contracted hepatitis C."

Looking Sean in the eye, I could instantly see his anguish. He had repented of his old ways but was left with the consequences of those former sins. "Hepatitis C is a virus that attacks the liver, and in some cases, it can cause cirrhosis and liver failure," I said.

"Yeah. That's exactly what I'm afraid of. My cousin just died of liver failure. I was there with him, and he suffered tremendously. Can you make sure I don't suffer?"

I thought about how hard it must be to live with such severe consequences. "There are some new treatments in the final stages of testing by the FDA. The results look promising. Let's see if you qualify for one of those studies. But I don't want to get your hopes up."

"I'm willing to try," Sean said. "Even if I'm in the control group and get the placebo, maybe they will learn something that can help someone else."

In today's verse, the verb "I will return" in Hebrew means "to intervene in someone's life to change his or her destiny." Certainly, if Sarah had a baby, it would forever change her life. At the time, though, she had a lot of doubts about whether that would happen.

Often, my patients face the same kinds of doubts about their treatments, and so do I. Until they return to my office, we can't be sure whether the treatment is working. When Sean qualified for the new treatment in a double-blind trial, we didn't know which drug he had received. When I saw him several weeks after he started the trial, he seemed somewhat improved, but we still didn't know for sure.

When Sean returned to my office a year later, it was evident that he had been cured. His destiny had been changed because God had intervened, and his life was starting anew.

TODAY'S RX

Be alert to new ways in which God may want to intervene and change your destiny.

God, I praise you for providing for my needs. When I have doubts, you have answers, and I know my life is in good hands. Thank you for setting my path straight and leading the way.

THE JOY OF SERVING

Oh, the joys of those who are kind to the poor! The Lord rescues them when they are in trouble. The LORD protects them and keeps them alive. He gives them prosperity in the land and rescues them from their enemies. PSALM 41:1-2

Though my family was poor when I was growing up, I didn't know it until another ten-year-old, who was supposedly of a higher position in the pecking order, pecked me down to size.

"You're poor!"

"No, I'm not!"

Then he counted on his fingers all the material assets he had that I didn't. It was a revelation to me that he was so focused on possessions. My family may not have had his family's wealth, but we certainly weren't poor in spirit.

Growing up on the "wrong side of the tracks" gave me a unique vantage point on life. When I went to medical school, my scholarship came with an obligation that I would spend several years practicing medicine in a poor area of the country.

But I didn't consider that an obligation. That's what I had always wanted to do, anyway. My wife and I were excited when I found a job in Cheatham County, Tennessee. These were my people, and I wanted to live alongside them and serve them.

I was only the third doctor in a county of twenty-five thousand people, many of whom had great health needs. Good portions of the population, at the time, were living below the poverty line, and more walked that line like a tightrope.

Shortly after I arrived, the state of Tennessee developed plans to build a new hospital in our area—the first new hospital in the state in twenty years. It was designed to serve the poor and medically underserved in Cheatham and surrounding counties. But at the "certificate of need" meeting, a large corporation opposed the plan. I was dumbfounded. Why would anyone oppose caring for the poor? The opponents had their reasons, of course, but the prayers of the people prevailed. Twenty-five years later, that hospital is still going strong, and Karen and I have made the area our home.

TODAY'S RX

Serve someone who is in poor health or who is poor financially or spiritually. You will create joy in two lives—theirs and yours.

Jesus, help me to model your ministry of serving those in need. Show me how I can be of better use to help those who are poor, lonely, or sick. Thank you for modeling this for me through your great love.

HE DIDN'T LEAVE YOU

Do not be afraid or discouraged, for the LORD *will personally go ahead of you. He will be with you; he will neither fail you nor abandon you.* DEUTERONOMY 31:8

Frank and Ginny were truly soul mates. People often remarked that they seemed like a match made in heaven—even after fifty years of marriage. Everything was going well—until Frank passed away.

"He left me. He left me. I can't believe he left me," Ginny said, sobbing. She was brokenhearted beyond consolation. Her better half was gone, and she felt as if she couldn't go on without him.

"Mom just walks around the house looking for Dad," her two daughters told me. "We know that we'll all see him again one day. But the way Mom is acting, we're afraid she's going to see him soon, and we don't want her to go before her time."

Ginny was in great health for her age, but the past month had taken its toll. She had lost weight and wasn't eating enough to sustain herself.

"Ginny, you're dehydrated and malnourished," I said. "Your family tells me you aren't eating or sleeping."

"He left me. He left me. I don't want to continue."

"Look, Ginny, I understand the pain you're feeling. But Frank is with Jesus. He hasn't left you. He's helping to prepare a place for you."

Ginny obviously needed some rest. I admitted her into a local rehab unit, and we surrounded her with encouragement, love, and comfort. The staff prayed for her and made sure that she ate and slept. Her children visited every day, and I stopped by to pray with her and make sure she was thriving.

Three weeks later—to the day—she got up, packed her bags, and went home. She had stopped crying and started living. We could all see that her attitude and emotions had been renewed.

"You know, Dr. Anderson, each day I have here on earth is a blessing," she said. "I also think that each day is granted to us for a reason. I know now that each day brings me closer to Frank and to Jesus."

For Ginny, the turning point seemed to come from realizing that Frank hadn't left her; he'd only gone on before her. That realization restored her will to live.

TODAY'S RX

Whatever your current trials, know that God is close to the brokenhearted. Take one step at a time with him.

God, thank you for wrapping your arms around me when I'm lonely and grieving. Help me to sense your presence each day on earth, and continue to plant the hope of heaven deeper in my heart.

SEEKING WITH FOCUS

Seek the Kingdom of God above all else, and live righteously, and he will give you everything you need. MATTHEW 6:33

Today's Scripture verse contains a promise: If we seek God first and above all else and live accordingly, our needs will be satisfied.

To *seek* is to journey and to quest. Seeking is something that must be done daily and without distraction. When my kids were little, they played hide-and-seek. The child who won was always the one who was the least distracted and most single-minded while searching for the others. We need that same kind of focus when we seek God's Kingdom.

To live righteously is to live like a bird dog who faithfully points toward the object of its master's desire. The dog never thinks about shortcuts or beating around the bush. Instead, the dog locks steadfastly onto the target and goes straight toward the desired destination. Likewise, we should be straightforward in our words and actions. This includes treating others as we would like to be treated.

As for our needs, God says that he will give us what we need. When we think about how God cares for our needs, it's easy to think of him as a genie in a bottle who grants us wishes when we hand him our list. But who knows what we actually need better than God?

Our children may continually ask for sweets, but as loving and wise parents, we provide for their greater need—a balanced and nutritious diet. Parents know what their children need better than their children know themselves. Even when our children unceasingly insist that they need something different, we, as their parents, focus on what is best for them.

Seek.

Live righteously.

Receive what God gives you to meet your needs.

TODAY'S RX

Follow your bird dog instincts, and keep your focus on God.

Clear my mind of distraction, Lord. Help me to seek you each day by lifting my requests to you and focusing on your Word.

THE TALK

The L*ORD your God will change your heart and the hearts of all your descendants, so that you will love him with all your heart and soul and so you may live!* DEUTERONOMY 30:6

Dwayne wasn't a zombie, but he was certainly a dead man walking. His cholesterol was over 300 with an LDL (the bad kind of cholesterol) reading of nearly 200. He refused to take his blood pressure medicine because he said it made him feel tired and weak, so his blood pressure was often dangerously high. And if that weren't enough, Dwayne also smoked. In fact, he had smoked two packs a day for more than thirty years.

"Dwayne, we need to talk about your health," I said.

"Yes, sir," he said, lowering his head. Dwayne had heard it all before, and he didn't need evidence that what he was doing was unhealthy. His father and uncles had died in their fifties from massive heart attacks.

"You've already outlived every male relative by three years or more. You're in your midfifties now, but you've dodged some bullets to get here." He shifted in his seat, and I could see he was sweating. "It's only the good Lord who has kept you alive and brought you to this point. But if you want to walk your daughter down the aisle when she gets married, you need to make some changes."

"You're right. I know my heart is going to give out if I don't change my ways."

As Dwayne and I talked, he agreed to quit smoking, lose weight, eat better, and start taking his blood pressure medicine. Though he was anxious and sweating at the beginning of our conversation, he seemed agreeable to the plan at the end.

"Thanks, Doc, for the heart-to-heart talk. I love my family, and I want to be around for them."

Two years later, when Dwayne came for his annual checkup, he showed me a photo of himself with a beautiful young woman. He had stopped smoking, his blood pressure was normal, and he was fifty pounds lighter.

"You look great, Dwayne!" I said. "Where was the photo taken?"

"At my daughter's wedding," he said with a grin. "Thank the Lord!"

Dwayne had known he was living on borrowed time, and he had decided to get right with himself—and with the Lord who had protected him.

TODAY'S RX

You only have one heart. Care for it spiritually, emotionally, and physically.

Father, you've blessed me with life and given me this body to care for. Help me to treat it right and not take it for granted. Thank you for caring for me always.

WE WORK BECAUSE OUR HOPE IS IN THE GREAT HEALER

We work hard and continue to struggle, for our hope is in the living God, who is the Savior of all people and particularly of all believers. 1 Timothy 4:9-10

"Code 10, Room 7. Code 10, Room 7."

In the blink of an eye, a sleepy Sunday morning in the emergency room went from calm to controlled chaos as staff members grabbed instruments and equipment and organized under my direction. Though it may have looked like bedlam, it was well orchestrated, with each professional doing his or her part. My role was to be the maestro with the baton, calling in the other players at the exact moment when their skill and expertise were required. Leading the charge to save the man's life, I gave my orders:

"Chest compressions at 100 per minute."

"Breathing pattern ratio of thirty compressions to two ventilations."

"Charge the paddles to 360 joules. Clear . . ."

"Continue compressions."

"Epinephrine IV. Charge the paddles to defibrillate a second time."

When the man's heart was finally shocked back into a normal sinus rhythm, the staff and I breathed a collective sigh of relief and offered silent prayers of thanks. The patient could finally be moved to the ICU.

Before everyone returned to normal duty, I thanked each member of the code team. Without their professionalism, dedication, and experience, the outcome would not have been the same. Furthermore, I knew that each person believed he or she was there to serve a much larger purpose.

I am proud to be a part of a group of Christian health professionals who understand that God is the one who ultimately heals. We're blessed to be his hands and feet—occasionally used to carry out his healing work—and we're blessed that he utilizes our gifts for his glory. Though I may have directed the players, God orchestrated their lifesaving talents and their instruments into a symphony of healing. In playing our respective parts, we all had a role in something bigger than ourselves.

Where in your own sphere of influence is God able to use the gifts he has given you for his purpose and his glory?

TODAY'S RX

If God ever calls you to use CPR, just remember that 100 chest compressions per minute is the same rate and rhythm as the Bee Gees' song "Stayin' Alive."

God, help me to be your hands and feet so that I may reflect your goodness and love to those around me. May I use my gifts well and bring you glory.

STILL TICKING

Those who control their tongue will have a long life; opening your mouth can ruin everything. PROVERBS 13:3

Gene was ninety-four when he entered the nursing home. He was a quiet and calm man who was more likely to observe others than to interact with them. On his first day there, I sat down to talk with him.

"How do you feel?" I asked.

"I feel pretty good for ninety-four," he said.

"So what's the secret to living this long and still feeling good?"

"I guess the good Lord wanted me to live this long; otherwise, I don't know why. I'm ready anytime he calls me home."

Our conversation moved to questions about a living will and whether he wanted the staff to perform CPR if his heart stopped.

"I don't see the need," he said. "If the good Lord wants it to keep ticking, it will keep ticking."

Years later, it was still ticking. I stopped by the nursing home one day for a special celebration.

The nurses referred to Gene as Rip Van Winkle because he slept a lot. But he didn't mind the nickname; when they said it, he just grinned. I watched the nurses fuss over him, getting him a fork and a napkin while he sat back and took it all in. He had a gentle spirit and never complained about anything. Medically, he was as healthy as they come; the only thing I'd ever prescribed for him was a daily multivitamin.

The nurses began to sing and held out a cake for Gene to blow out the candles—he was celebrating his one hundred and fourth birthday. He'd been in the nursing home for ten years and now was officially the oldest patient I'd ever cared for.

The party that day was just like Gene's life, all calm and quiet, nothing loud or flashy. The nurses handed Gene a plate with birthday cake and ice cream. He took a bite of the cake and smiled at us with a toothless grin.

When I think of today's verse, I think of Gene. Perhaps we're all born with a limited number of words, and when we use them up, we're done. But if we spend them as wisely as Gene did, we'll live a long and happy life as well.

TODAY'S RX

Speak carefully. What you say matters.

Give me the wisdom to know when to remain quiet and when to speak, Lord. Guard my tongue, and help me to speak words of life and encouragement to those I interact with today.

JEALOUSY AT WORK

A peaceful heart leads to a healthy body; jealousy is like cancer in the bones.
PROVERBS 14:30

There's a link between peace and health. And there's a link between jealousy and disease. These links aren't uncommon. As a doctor, I see them at work all the time. Maybe you have too.

I've had countless patients who were physically healthy but felt sick. They complain of fatigue, an inability to sleep, or depression. Sometimes their blood sugar or blood pressure readings are higher than normal. But I often find that the cause of their symptoms has less to do with a physical problem than with an emotional one. They're not sick; they're carrying around hurt and anger that they can't seem to get over.

We think of jealousy as an emotion between lovers, but in my medical practice, I've found that jealousy is much more common in the workplace than in the bedroom. The green-eyed monster can come out when a coworker gets a raise or promotion. This kind of jealousy churns the entire time the person is at work.

When our hearts are full of negative emotions, the stress-related hormones start flowing. If untreated, everything from weight gain and inflammation to anxiety and depression can result. Jealousy may start slowly, but if we don't keep our thoughts in check, those feelings can turn into a dark force that eats away at us until our negativity adversely affects our health. That's when we go to the doctor.

To be healthy and happy, we need to have balance in our lives and in our work. We also need to focus on the peace and joy that God has promised us. If we want to be truly healthy, we must let the anger, fear, and jealousy that we feel melt away. My patients who live peaceful lives generally have better health than those who don't. They remain calm during times of stress, they think positive thoughts even when things aren't going well, and they take life as it comes.

Setting aside our negativity can make us better team players at work. Then we can truly applaud those on our team who succeed. That kind of positive attitude might be exactly what the boss is looking for.

TODAY'S RX

To be healthy, work to live, and live peacefully, rather than jealously living to work.

Lord, help me to let go of the anger and jealousy that consumes me at times. Replace these feelings with feelings of peace and contentment, allowing me to be a light to my family, friends, and coworkers.

GOD WILL MAKE A WAY

Jesus looked at them intently and said, "Humanly speaking, it is impossible. But with God everything is possible." MATTHEW 19:26

Today's verse reminds me of a time in my life when I truly wanted to serve the poor, but the odds were against me. I had been accepted into medical school, but coming from a poor family, I didn't have any money to pay for my tuition or living expenses. The two most obvious options were to take out a very large loan or join the military. A third option was to join a relatively new program called the National Health Service Corps (NHSC). The program would pay for my tuition and books and give me $500 per month for living expenses. In exchange, I would be required to practice primary care medicine in a poor, rural county for a specified time. It took me less than a Mississippi minute to sign on the dotted line.

When I finished my residency, a clinic in Ashland City, Tennessee, invited me to work there. It was a perfect fit. But when the official NHSC notice arrived in the mail, Ashland City wasn't on the list. It didn't make any sense. Why wouldn't the federal government want a doctor in a community that had only two doctors serving twenty-five thousand people?

Karen and I felt that God was calling us to Ashland City, but if it wasn't a certified NHSC site, I could incur fines of more than $300,000. There was no way we could afford that. So we began to pray.

The local community leaders sent me to Washington, DC, to beg the NHSC to reinstate Ashland City. But the official word was still *no*. Karen and I had a difficult decision to make, but God's guidance and the needs of the community made us choose Ashland City, come what may. Essentially, I defaulted on my loan. I was told to expect a certified letter in the mail in the next few weeks detailing my fines.

Two weeks later, the expected letter arrived. I began to sweat as I opened it. To my surprise, the letter said, "Congratulations! You have been assigned to Ashland City, Tennessee. Please report for duty on July 1, 1983."

TODAY'S RX

Be ready to follow where God leads. Some things only he can make possible.

Father, thank you for unexpected blessings and for making the impossible possible. You are a miracle worker, and I'm grateful for how you've worked miracles in my life.

HOW LONG?

I am on the verge of collapse, facing constant pain. . . . Do not abandon me, O LORD. Do not stand at a distance, my God. Come quickly to help me, O Lord my savior.
PSALM 38:17, 21-22

"How long will it take until I feel better?" It's something we all want to know when we're not feeling well. Have you ever asked that question and received a less-than-satisfactory answer? Maybe your doctor wasn't forthcoming with a prognosis, or maybe the specialist, after looking at your test results, was afraid to tell you that your condition might not improve.

Chances are, if you're in pain, you've already considered what life might be like if you never felt any better. What hope is there in a situation that doesn't promise an end to the pain?

As a doctor, I've treated patients with chronic, debilitating, and progressive illnesses. For some of them, there is no cure or answer this side of the veil. In those cases, I do my best to prescribe medication to take the edge off the pain and to allow the patient to live life as fully as possible. Even in the direst of circumstances, I don't want anyone to give up hope for healing.

I've often found that even when people's bodies are wracked with pain and their hope in the health-care system is declining, their faith in God may be vibrant and growing. Frequently, at these times, patients find new hope and a renewed appreciation and love for family and friends. They develop a deeper longing for, and trust in, our heavenly Father. The trust they once reserved for their doctors and medical science is now fully placed in God.

If you're suffering right now, I pray that God will lift up your weary soul and give you strength for the day. I pray you will take each day and each breath with the knowledge that he loves you and that he is in control, even when you're struggling. Though healing may not be available for you here and now, hope is still accessible. If you trust in Jesus, one day, in the blink of an eye, you will have a new pain-free body, and the suffering and anguish of this world will be gone.

TODAY'S RX

When your pain has no end, take one breath at a time, and know that your suffering can draw you closer to Jesus.

Jesus, I don't always understand your ways, especially when I'm hurting and my world seems upside down. Reassure my heart of your love in these moments, and fill me with your presence.

FAITH TO HEAL WITH SPIT, MUD, OR JUST PLAIN WORDS

He spit on the ground, made mud with the saliva, and spread the mud over the blind man's eyes. He told him, "Go wash yourself in the pool of Siloam" (Siloam means "sent"). So the man went and washed and came back seeing! JOHN 9:6-7

If a man complained to you that he had something in his eye and couldn't see, what would you do to help him? You might take a look to see if you could remove whatever was obstructing his vision. Or maybe you'd help him flush his eye with water.

Chances are good that you wouldn't say, "Hold still while I spit on the ground, make some mud with my saliva, and apply it to your eyes. That'll fix you right up!" Yet that's exactly what Jesus did.

This seems like such a crazy thing for him to do. In so many other cases when he healed people, either he reached out and touched them, or he simply healed them with a word. But in this case, Jesus used two very unlikely, and very unlovely, things to help the man see.

When analyzed chemically, both mud and spit have some medicinal properties. Saliva comes from one of the more bacteria-infested areas of the body. Its purpose is to sterilize the dirty food (and sometimes even dirt itself) that finds its way into our mouths. The enzymes in our saliva begin to break down the food, disrupting the cells of the bacteria.

If the man's blindness were due to something on the surface of his corneas, it might make sense to utilize the abrasive properties of mud by rubbing it on his eyes. As doctors, we often must debride diseased tissue from an area before we will see new and healthy growth. That's essentially what laser procedures do, and we use them all the time for treatment of various eye conditions.

Jesus knew exactly what this man needed and treated him with the most appropriate—though unlikely—elements. But the healing was no less miraculous. We could not simply repeat his actions and expect the same outcome, but we can be certain that Jesus could have healed the man's eyes with a word—and that the same healing is available to us.

TODAY'S RX

Consider that Jesus may use unusual methods, tools, or people to heal you.

Father, your power is made perfect in our weakness, and you continue to show that power in numerous ways. Thank you for healing our sicknesses and disabilities through whatever means necessary.

DESTRUCTION PREVENTS HEALING

There is no healing for your wound; your injury is fatal. All who hear of your destruction will clap their hands for joy. Where can anyone be found who has not suffered from your continual cruelty? NAHUM 3:19

For those who turn away from God, there is no healing for their wounds. Unfortunately, that was the case with a man named Ryder. Historically, there hasn't been a lot of violent crime in our neck of the woods, but with the growth of Nashville, urban sprawl nudged more criminals our way who were looking for small-town hideouts. For years, stories had circulated in our rural community about the terrible things Ryder had done in the past. But one sleepy night, the rumors proved to be true, and our town was the setting for a drug deal gone bad.

The details were never entirely clear. Either Ryder or his buyer got angry. Shots were fired. The buyer ended up on the floor, and Ryder fled the scene.

The local police caught up to him a few minutes later, and a high-speed chase ensued. During the pursuit, Ryder failed to negotiate a curve on a two-lane country road. His car rolled down an embankment and hit a tree.

The shell of a man who was delivered to our emergency room that night was the product of years of poor choices, drug use, violence, and now murder. Though we did everything we could for him medically, in the end there was nothing we could do to save him. His sins had caught up with him once and for all.

When news of his sudden death became known, our town was overwhelmed—not with grief, but with relief. One benefit of living in the country is that we largely avoid the trouble that comes to other parts. Ryder's remains were quietly transported back to where he'd come from, and no one seemed to notice he was gone. Today, when I think of wounds that will never be healed, I think of Ryder.

TODAY'S RX

Live your life so that your wounds will be healed and your neighbors will grieve when it's your time to go.

Jesus, thank you for the promise of new life in you. May I always be grateful for your sacrifice on the cross. I know that it's only through you that I am washed clean of my sin.

COMPLIANCE IS EASIER IN RELATIONSHIP

Restore to me the joy of your salvation, and make me willing to obey you. PSALM 51:12

In the medical field, the term *compliance* is used to describe a patient's willingness to obey and adhere to the instructions given by a physician. Research and experience indicate that the simpler the instructions, the more likely a patient is to conform. For example, we know that one pill per day is about 90 percent more likely to be taken than, say, a pill four times per day.

Often, when patients realize that noncompliance is hurting their health, they will come back to their doctor and ask if there is something that is easier to take or simpler to remember. Having a good relationship with your doctor makes compliance easier.

The human will is the key to both obedience and disobedience. The author of today's psalm realized that his will alone was not enough to make him obey, so he asked for God's help. But he also recognized that obedience is more likely when we are in a relationship with the one requesting our compliance.

When I was young and my father asked me to do something, I was as likely to whine or back talk as any other child. But my attitude changed on days when my dad would take me along to check on the progress of his agricultural students' projects. I loved doing those checks, and my dad and I got along great. I knew that he appreciated our time together too. If he asked me to do a chore after we got home from one of those trips, the obligation was easier to fulfill, and I rarely complained.

In the same way, when we are connected and in relationship with our heavenly Father, it is easier to obey him and to follow his decrees. Perhaps that's why he has made compliance so simple and clear for us. All he asks us to do is love him and then love our neighbor as much as we love ourselves. When we comply, there is great joy for both of us.

TODAY'S RX

God wants to restore the joy of your salvation and build your relationship with him. All he asks from you is your love—which includes obedience and trust. Healing comes with our compliance to the healer's instructions.

Father, give me a spirit that longs to draw near to you and obey you. Take away any tendency I have to grumble and complain, and replace it with a desire to know you more completely.

ON EAGLE'S WINGS

Those who trust in the LORD will find new strength. They will soar high on wings like eagles. They will run and not grow weary. They will walk and not faint. ISAIAH 40:31

It was past sundown when the pathologist called me at home to tell me the bad news about my patient Patrick. She had reviewed his blood test, and the results weren't good.

"Your patient has acute leukemia and a very aggressive type of it," she said.

Earlier that day, I had diagnosed Patrick with anemia and admitted him to the hospital. But I couldn't escape the feeling that something else was going on with what should have been a straightforward diagnosis. I thanked her for calling, but inside I felt sick. The results were much worse than I had expected.

I didn't sleep well that night as I thought about giving Patrick the news in the morning. I wrestled with what to say—especially because I didn't know the state of his spiritual journey.

The next morning, on the twenty-mile drive to the hospital, my heart was still heavy. Just then, as the sun peeked over the horizon, I saw a bald eagle perched on top of a large hickory tree. It was almost directly above a cross that marked the spot where another patient of mine had met the Lord a few years earlier. In my thirty years of traveling that route, I had never seen an eagle in that part of the county. Their habitat was farther north, near the river.

As I got closer, I marveled at the eagle's grandeur. And as I passed by, I remembered today's verse, and it gave me the encouragement I needed to tell Patrick that the Lord would lift him up and give him strength during his upcoming journey.

The conversation I had been dreading went much easier than I had anticipated. Patrick told me he had been walking with the Lord for more than thirty-five years—ever since a nearly fatal tractor accident when he was sixteen.

I told him about seeing the eagle, and we talked about all the ways that God had already lifted him up. Then we prayed together. I knew that, regardless of how Patrick's journey turned out, he would find his strength in the Lord.

TODAY'S RX

If you need new strength to run and not grow weary or to walk and not faint, put your trust in the Lord.

God, thank you for displaying your magnificence and power through your beautiful creation. Let it be a reminder to me always of your great love for me.

THE BLESSING OF PEACE

My child, listen to me and do as I say, and you will have a long, good life. PROVERBS 4:10

God has a funny way of answering our prayers. My wife, Karen, used to pray for our children that God would use them for his Kingdom in the uttermost parts of the world. Now that they're all grown, I remind her of that prayer every time I have to buy a plane ticket to visit them.

Our eldest, Kristen, fell in love with a young man from Northern Ireland—which, as you probably know, has been a place of unrest for hundreds of years. Though the conflict is often depicted as a war between Catholics and Protestants, it seems they are really fighting for power, not religion. Both sides want to control the land and the government. Unfortunately, at times those power struggles have led to armed conflict.

As we landed in Ireland for Kristin's wedding, I thought about the history of violence in her new home country. As part of the wedding ceremony, we set aside time to pray—not only for the region, but also for the safety of our daughter, our new son-in-law, and his family. But most of all, we prayed for peace. At the time, I had no idea how quickly God would answer that prayer or how he would eventually answer it twice.

The next day, as we said our good-byes to Kristen and David and boarded the plane back to America, the BBC announced the withdrawal of British troops from Northern Ireland. Peace soon followed. It was an answer to the prayers we had prayed just the day before.

Seven years later, on my birthday, God answered our prayers for peace again when Kristen gave me a very special gift—my first grandchild. They named him Callum, which means *peace.*

Today's proverb comes with a promise. If we will listen to God and do as he says, we will have a long and good life. This verse has been repeated down through the generations of my family.

TODAY'S RX

Today, I leave you with a traditional Irish blessing:

> *May the road rise up to meet you.*
> *May the wind be at your back.*
> *May the sun shine warm upon your face;*
> *the rains fall soft upon your fields*
> *and until we meet again,*
> *may God hold you in the palm of his hand.*

Lord, please restore peace where there is unrest in this world,
and protect all who have put their trust in you.

THE BEST ADVICE COMES FROM A GREAT TEACHER

Teach me how to live, O LORD. Lead me along the right path, for my enemies are waiting for me. PSALM 27:11

My daughter Kristen and her husband, David, were both brilliant students. Before their first child was born, they read as much as they could about how to take care of a baby. But they were also wise and willing to take counsel from those who had been down the parenting path before them. As a mother of four, my wife, Karen, knew a few tricks she could pass on to Kristen. And Kristen knew that her mother was a trustworthy teacher.

When it comes to caring for our health, it's easy to be deceived by the promises of a new diet or a medication that guarantees extraordinary results. A wise doctor can help us check out the claims and discern whether the treatment is safe or whether it may have unintended or harmful side effects.

Things that are bad for us don't always start out looking bad. They can sometimes be manipulated and falsely advertised as something that is good for us. Over the years, we've learned that soft drinks, tobacco, human growth hormone, and weight loss pills, for example, fall into this category. A good doctor should always take time to answer questions so that patients can be assured that the prescribed treatments will help them—not only to get better temporarily, but also to live better over the long term.

We are all students who need help to live our lives to the fullest. We need someone who has gone before us and has the knowledge to show us the right path to take. Who better to guide us through life than our Creator?

There are many diversions that can lead us away from God and a healthy way of living. Satan is a deceiver, and he tries to attack us from all angles. But God knows the right path for us to take, and he loves us enough to guide us. When we trust him to lead us, he will not lead us astray, and he will protect us from our enemies.

TODAY'S RX

Read and apply God's Word, and listen to wise counsel to avoid the pitfalls of life.

Thank you, Father, that the wisdom and instruction you give through your Word never changes—that it's the same today as it has been for centuries. Help me to study the Bible and learn from it so that I may know you better.

BLESSED ASSURANCE

Jesus traveled throughout the region of Galilee, teaching in the synagogues and announcing the Good News about the Kingdom. And he healed every kind of disease and illness. MATTHEW 4:23

Being a country doctor means I need to travel a bit to see all of my patients. While I no longer make house calls, I still visit three nursing homes, two hospitals, and two clinics.

In the course of my visits, I see a number of familiar diseases—somewhere between thirty and forty—on a regular basis. But occasionally I am caught off guard with a rare disease or a symptom pattern that doesn't seem to fit. In those cases, I enlist the help of specialists to assist me in diagnosis and treatment.

We often need to coordinate care between a series of specialists who have different interests in the outcome of the patient's health. Or we may have to coordinate treatment between two separate health-care facilities. For example, someone in a nursing home may need to go to the hospital for surgery. Or someone from a clinic may need to spend time at a rehabilitation hospital until he or she has recovered and can return home. Fortunately, in many parts of the United States, we are blessed with some of the finest specialists and subspecialists in the world.

More than at any time in history, we can predict good outcomes for patients who follow their treatment plans. We have the resources in people, technology, and medication to give a lot of positive prognoses. But even with that, we can't 100 percent guarantee a specific outcome.

If we want complete assurance about our physical, emotional, or spiritual health . . . well, only Jesus can offer that. He is the only one who has ever been able to heal us completely.

TODAY'S RX

Draw close to the Lord. Not only is he able to heal you, but "the peace of God, which transcends all understanding, will guard your hearts and your minds in Christ Jesus" (Philippians 4:7, NIV).

Jesus, I offer up to you all that has me feeling unwell today. Please bring strength to my bones and energy to my mind. Thank you for your healing touch.

A MESSAGE FROM A DEAD WOMAN

The promise is received by faith. It is given as a free gift. And we are all certain to receive it . . . if we have faith like Abraham's. For Abraham is the father of all who believe . . . because Abraham believed in the God who brings the dead back to life and who creates new things out of nothing. ROMANS 4:16-17

"Eunice, it appears you're having a heart attack," I said to my patient, a woman in her late sixties. "We need to send you to the hospital in Nashville so we can get a cardiologist to look at you."

Later that day, I received a call from the cardiologist, Dr. Wong, telling me that Eunice had died in the operating room.

"I had a resident with me," he said, "and we worked on her for at least an hour. I was about to let her go, but my resident wanted to practice running a code, so I let him while I supervised."

It was hard to hear the details of Eunice's death, and I started to think about what I needed to tell her family.

"But an hour into running the code," Dr. Wong continued, "and two hours from the time she flatlined, her heart kicked in and started beating by itself."

"Are you saying she's alive?"

"I'm saying she was dead for two hours, and now she's alive. I have her on a vent in the ICU, and she's in a coma. I'm not sure how much functioning will come back."

Three days later, Eunice woke up, and they took her off life support. Then she asked to see me.

When I walked into her room, I was surprised at how good she looked.

"Dr. Anderson!" she said, "I have a story to tell you." She told me about seeing Jesus and her family in the most beautiful place one could imagine.

"Jesus said he wanted me to come back here for two reasons. The first was to encourage you and to tell you to stay the course. I don't know what that means, but that's what he told me to tell you."

I teared up because I knew what it meant. My family had been thinking about moving, but God wanted us to stay right where we were.[4]

TODAY'S RX

Trust God that he can restore life and make all things new.

Just as spring follows winter, God, I pray that you breathe new life into me this season. Thank you for how you make all things new.

HE HEALED EVERY ONE

After leaving the synagogue that day, Jesus went to Simon's home, where he found Simon's mother-in-law very sick with a high fever. "Please heal her," everyone begged. Standing at her bedside, he rebuked the fever, and it left her. And she got up at once and prepared a meal for them. As the sun went down that evening, people throughout the village brought sick family members to Jesus. No matter what their diseases were, the touch of his hand healed every one. LUKE 4:38-40

No matter what disease a person had, Jesus healed everyone! Even today, with our modern medical system, designer drugs, and technological tools, we cannot boast this kind of cure rate.

Many diseases still are considered incurable, and others have only a fifty-fifty chance of being cured. Even with the most established treatments, we don't always know who will respond and who won't. Sometimes, we have to try a second treatment option, or a third, because the first one failed to work.

For example, most infections are treated successfully today. But in Bible times, the simplest of infections could have had life-threatening consequences because antibiotics weren't yet available. While not always the case, some infections that cause a fever can resolve when the body's immune system kicks in. However, serious systemic infections can overcome the immune system, causing a toxic condition called *sepsis* and possibly resulting in death. But under the healing hands of Jesus, the viruses or bacteria were rebuked and ran for the hills, just like the demons did when Jesus commanded them to leave.

Today, we are learning that many of our "gold standard" treatments are failing because the disease microbes are developing a resistance to many antibiotics. With Jesus, there was no resistance, only complete healing of every disease he encountered.

As a physician, I am increasingly in awe of our Lord's power, not only over the spiritual world but also over our physical world. I pray that his healing hands will touch you today and give you the strength and courage for your own healing journey.

TODAY'S RX

Even if you have been told you have a difficult case, remember, nothing is too difficult for Jesus. He alone can heal you completely.

God, I trust in you for complete healing for anything that comes my way. Help me to always be prayerful, thanking you for my health when I am well and seeking your strength when I am ill.

A WITHERING WEED BLOSSOMS

Ask me and I will tell you remarkable secrets you do not know about things to come.
JEREMIAH 33:3

A well-dressed young woman, full of life and energy, sat on the exam table. When I entered the room, she stuck out her hand and firmly shook mine.

"Remember me? I used to see you years ago, right after my car wreck. I was a handful back then. Do you remember me?"

There are lots of reasons why patients are memorable to their doctors. It might be their personality, the particulars of their disease, or even their faith in the face of adversity. Mindy was one I remembered because she had been such a mess! Even before the auto accident—caused by a drunk driver—her life had been like a train wreck. And she'd lost more than just her leg in the accident; she'd also lost her self-respect.

I was genuinely happy to see her again. "Mindy! Where have you been? It's been . . . what . . . five years since I last saw you?"

As her doctor, I had worked to help her heal from her physical wounds, but she had much deeper wounds in her soul. You see, Mindy was the drunk driver who had caused the accident. Fortunately, she hadn't injured anyone else.

Back then, her physical and emotional pain had required a number of specialty consultations with orthopedists, psychiatrists, and pain management physicians. I was her primary care physician for backup and crisis management—which meant I saw her a lot.

"Did you move?" I asked.

"No. I was on the streets, looking for my next fix to escape the pain. But even on the streets, I kept thinking about how you would encourage me to look to God when everything seemed lost. I finally took you up on it and went into rehab. And I got saved. I've been clean for a year. Now I'm studying to be a drug and rehab counselor, finishing up this semester."

"It's so great to see you doing so well!" I said.

"So many people were praying for me and encouraging me. Those were all seeds that took root, and now the Holy Spirit has helped them sprout and grow.

TODAY'S RX

Pray for and encourage those in need, even in the worst circumstances. You never know when those seeds, planted deep in the human soul, will sprout and grow.

Holy Spirit, work in the lives of my family and friends who are struggling right now. Make your presence known to them and help them to see their need for you. Thank you for faithfully following after them.

THE STRENGTH OF OLD AGE

Lord, remind me how brief my time on earth will be. Remind me that my days are numbered—how fleeting my life is. You have made my life no longer than the width of my hand. My entire lifetime is just a moment to you; at best, each of us is but a breath. Psalm 39:4-5

Marty showed up for his checkup with a paradoxical set of complaints: "It seems like the harder I work at trying to stay healthy, the more I fall apart."

I had heard similar stories from patients before, and I asked him to explain what he meant.

"At sixty, there seems to be a diminishing return to my efforts," he said. "I go for a run, and my feet ache for two weeks. I lift weights, and my shoulders lock up. I think I'm doing all the right things, but I just end up injuring myself."

Marty had always been healthy. He ate well and exercised regularly, but over the past few years, his activity and his age seemed to be catching up with him.

"It does seem as if all your healthy living is working *against* you, not *for* you," I said. "But not all of us are made for the Olympics. Even world-class athletes age out of their ability to perform the amazing physical feats they once did."

When my patients face their own mortality or their growing inability to do what once came easily, I remind them that God has a plan for each of us to live a predetermined number of days and not a day beyond. When we were younger, our bodies healed faster, recovered from exercise better, and burned more calories. As we age and adopt a slower pace, we don't see the same gains and achievements we once did. With each decade, we have to adjust our diet and exercise to fit our aging bodies. As I remind my patients, it was the slow and steady tortoise who ultimately finished the race.

TODAY'S RX

Boast not in your own physical strength; boast in God, who is the strength of your life.

Though I'm not capable of doing what I once was, God, help me to be grateful for each day you've given me. Show me where my new strengths lie as I get older, and allow me to use my gifts for your glory.

WAR AND PEACE

You will keep in perfect peace all who trust in you, all whose thoughts are fixed on you!
ISAIAH 26:3

When we think of peace, we often think of a world without war or violence. But for some people, the war that rages isn't in a foreign country somewhere; it's in their heads. When Kari came to see me, her thoughts were warring against her body.

"I don't know what's going on," she said. "I can't sleep. My mind keeps running over things that I should have done, should be doing, or have done wrong. I keep obsessing about this or that. I've tried counting sheep, but then I obsess about how the sheep look. I have so many crazy thoughts running through my mind."

As Kari spoke, her words seemed to race in motion with her thoughts.

"Let me ask you a few questions," I said. "First, are there ever times when you feel overly energetic, even though you may not have slept in the preceding three or four days?"

"Yes!"

"Do you have habits of checking, double-checking, and maybe even triple-checking the same thing?"

"How did you know?"

"Have you also had days or seasons with no energy and feelings of doom or dread?"

"Yeah, but I just figured I'm tired from all that I've got going on."

"Kari, I think you may be struggling with bipolar disorder."

A fairly common disease, bipolar disorder affects 2.6 percent of the population. Many people struggle for years with undiagnosed or misdiagnosed bipolar disorder. And often the typical symptoms of depression are what cause a patient to finally seek a doctor's help.

In Kari's case, we started her on one of the newer atypical antipsychotic medications, which helped her thoughts become more streamlined and less chaotic. As a result, her mind quieted and peace was restored—something she hadn't experienced for years.

The last time Kari was in my office, she said, "I thank God for this new life he's given me. My thinking is no longer scattered like the wind, and at night, I can finally rest. My life now has a sense of peace and tranquility that I didn't even know existed."

TODAY'S RX

If your life is like a seesaw, always up or down, and you can't seem to balance out, it may be time to see your doctor.

Father, be with those who are fighting an illness right now. Take away their distress, and give them peace of mind. Thank you for seeing the bigger picture and knowing their route to recovery before anyone else.

BRINGING HEAVEN DOWN TO EARTH

Your unfailing love is as high as the heavens. Your faithfulness reaches to the clouds.
PSALM 57:10

When I was a boy, I would often lie on my back and stare up at the sky, counting the clouds as they floated by. Occasionally, I'd be startled out of my daydream by a fighter jet doing a flyover.

Craig Air Force Base was just a few miles from where I grew up. The base was used to train fighter pilots for the war in Vietnam. On any given day, a jet screaming by at lightning speed could disrupt a quiet, pastel sky. Sometimes the planes seemed no more than a few hundred feet above the ground. I could actually read the insignias as the jets flew overhead.

If I kept watching, they would sometimes do the most astounding thing: They would suddenly change trajectory and shoot straight up through the cumulus clouds until they disappeared near the darkness of the upper atmosphere. To me, it was nothing short of a miracle—though it may have been a technical miracle. The more I watched the pilots do their work, the more I began dreaming of becoming one myself.

For years, I'd heard preachers talk about how mighty the heavens are. They preached sermons on how God's faithfulness could reach the clouds. I wanted to leave the bounds of earth and reach out and touch the face of God. A fighter jet seemed like the most logical step to get there. How else could a farm boy reach the heavens?

Years later, I pursued my dream, but I never managed to take off. When my eyesight proved faulty, I flunked out of flight school because I couldn't see the clouds.

God was faithful, though, and he started a new work in my soul. On my journey to becoming a doctor, God revealed to me that heaven is not some faraway place beyond the clouds. Rather, it is a very real place that stretches back to us here on earth. We don't have to run toward heaven and eternity because heaven is much closer than we realize. The veil between this world and the next is thin. We don't have to run toward heaven because heaven walks alongside us here and now.

TODAY'S RX

We are much closer to heaven than most people think. Our last breath here will be our first breath there.

Lord, help me to remember that you aren't a distant, faraway God, but that you're present with me each day of my life, walking beside me until the day comes when I will see you face-to-face.

PRAYERS AND PRAISE

Pray in the Spirit at all times and on every occasion. Stay alert and be persistent in your prayers for all believers everywhere. Ephesians 6:18

Art fidgeted on the exam table, and I could see he was uncomfortable. "Did you get the results of your scans back yet?" I asked. He'd recently undergone surgery for renal cell carcinoma and had been awaiting test results to see whether it had spread.

"No, and I'm scared. They said they saw a spot on my liver and on my other kidney, and they seemed concerned about it."

"They should have the results back in a few—"

Art interrupted me before I could finish. "I haven't prayed in a long time," he said. "Now, I'm praying every day because I need something. I'm not sure that's okay. Do you think God hears my prayers? And does it matter that I'm just asking him for stuff? Ever since I found out about the cancer, I just feel like praying more. Does he listen, even though I didn't pray before?"

Art's sudden burst of questions reminded me of my own spiritual journey. I told him how, for years, I had walked around in a spiritual desert, and I hadn't prayed or talked to God at all during that time.

"But here's the thing, Art. God loves his children. He wants us to come to him with our needs. And just like the good Father he is, he sometimes grants our requests. Other times, he has something better planned for us, but he is always pleased when we come to him. I know you're worried, and God knows it too. He knows everything in your heart. Whatever the outcome of your scans, he will be right there beside you."

"I know you're right, but I feel as if the only time I pray is when I am scared or worried."

"Art, just keep talking to your heavenly Father; that's what he wants more than anything."

A week or so later, I received a call from Art filled with thanks and praise to the Lord for an encouraging test result. And he had made some decisions about his future prayers.

"Regardless of whether my cancer is gone for now or gone for good, my praise and my prayers won't ever stop."

TODAY'S RX

Take a moment to talk to God today; he wants to hear what is on your heart.

God, I confess that oftentimes my prayers are a list of needs and little else. Help me to remember you in times of joy as well, praising you for all the good you've done in my life.

A HEALTHY AND GLAD HEART

No wonder my heart is glad, and my tongue shouts his praises! My body rests in hope. For you will not leave my soul among the dead or allow your Holy One to rot in the grave. Acts 2:26-27

"It's kind of late for a farmer to be sleeping in, isn't it?"

Brett opened his eyes, yawned, and smiled. He was usually up and out before the rooster crowed, but he'd had heart surgery the day before and was still recuperating.

Brett had grown up on a meat and potatoes diet—usually with dessert to polish it off. And like many of my patients whose diets had placed them at an increased risk for premature heart disease, his unhealthy eating habits had caught up with him. At forty-two, he was much too young to have undergone heart surgery.

"Brett, your heart surgeon gave me a call yesterday. That surgery saved your life. He said you needed a four-vessel bypass and that you had a 99 percent blockage in the left coronary artery—that's what we call a *widowmaker*. You're a lucky man to have this much heart disease and not much muscle damage."

"I am thankful," Brett said. "That widowmaker almost caused me to meet my maker! But I know that God has a different plan for my life."

"You're right. He does, but you're going to have to make some different choices about your health—specifically, your diet."

"I know. You've been preaching to me about diet, exercise, and especially watching my portions. Being in the ICU gives a man a lot of time to think. I realize that instead of my friends and family gathering at my bedside right now, they could be gathering at my graveside. Not only am I going to make changes, but I am going to make sure everyone I know realizes they need to make changes too."

Brett was faithful to his word. He made a major overhaul to his life and became an evangelist to his friends and family, not only for God's goodness, but also for good health. Each day, when he gets up before the rooster crows, he thanks God for his second chance.

TODAY'S RX

When faced with a major blockage in your heart or in your soul, look to God for a way to bypass the damage and start a new life.

Lord, you are a God of second chances, allowing people to be reborn into new life with you. Thank you for not giving up on me, and instead showing me the way.

A METAMORPHOSIS TO A LONG LIFE

I will reward them with a long life and give them my salvation. PSALM 91:16

While reading Psalm 91, I couldn't help but think about the world we live in today and all the arrows that seem to be fired at us. We each face the enemy in different ways. For some, it's through illness. For others, it's grieving the loss of a loved one. For those who watch the evening news, it may seem as if the entire world is at war.

Yet, throughout Psalm 91, God reveals himself as our protector and defender from the evil one. He promises us long life and salvation if we follow him and his words.

During my years as a country doctor, I've come to believe that having a long life means something different than what we might first imagine. I've had the privilege of standing in the foyer of heaven and watching as many have left this world and been gathered under the wings of salvation, delivered into eternity and their forever home.

It reminds me of a caterpillar that is born into this world as an egg but becomes a larva and learns to find nourishment and sustenance on the plant leaves near where it was born. Then one day, the larva begins its metamorphosis. We can't see what happens in this chrysalis transition stage, but big changes are happening, until finally the majestic butterfly bursts forth.

This butterfly no longer has the limitations of the caterpillar. It can fly far from where its life began. But for the butterfly to have wings, the caterpillar must give up life as he knows it so that the completed being can be free to fly.

Our lives here on earth are a foreshadowing of what is yet to come, and what is yet to come is beyond our imagination. Why would we not want to become like butterflies? Why would we postpone our forever life as a completed work to glorify God? Do we stubbornly sit out in the cold simply because we don't want to accept the open door into the warm, protected home of our Savior?

TODAY'S RX

As we give ourselves to God, he will transform us into glorious beings who will live with him for eternity.

Father, refine me as I live out my days on earth. Help me to shed my sinful behavior and put on your truth. I long for the day when I am a fully new creation in you.

CRAVINGS THAT KILL

Such a prayer offered in faith will heal the sick, and the Lord will make you well. And if you have committed any sins, you will be forgiven. JAMES 5:15

Ramon stood five feet six inches tall but weighed more than 300 pounds.

"I can't lose weight," he told me at his annual checkup, "because of my job. I'm a night watchman, and it's so boring. All I do is sit and watch the monitors all night. There's a doughnut shop on one side and a pizza place on the other, and they both deliver."

A year later, when Ramon returned, he was proud to tell me about the "extreme" changes he'd made to his diet. "I started ordering the whole-wheat crust, and now I order a dozen doughnut holes instead of the regular glazed doughnuts. That's healthier, isn't it?"

"That's fine, if your goal is to go from 6,000 calories a day to 5,000 calories a day," I said. "But that's not going to get you healthy. If you want to get healthy, you have to change your habits and not justify your addiction by saying that you're overeating less."

The Bible warns that gluttony is a sin, and in Ramon's case, his physical illness was a direct result of giving in to temptation. "I'm going to suggest that you completely eliminate doughnuts, pizza, and any other white foods, such as bread, rice, potatoes, pasta, sugar, and any form of flour."

"But, Dr. Anderson, if I do that, what will I eat?"

I recommended that he replace those foods with fruits, vegetables, and lean meats like fish and poultry. But he wasn't having any of it. So I wasn't surprised when he showed up in my office a year later having once again gained weight.

"Ramon, you're over 350 pounds. That's just too much for someone your size."

A few months later, Ramon had a heart attack, resulting in a four-vessel bypass. By the grace of God, he survived and began a major overhaul of his life.

The next time I saw him, he had lost fifty pounds and was continuing to lose a pound a week.

"So I assume you've cut back on pizza and doughnuts?"

His response was telling: "Now, if I take even a bite of them, it's like poison, and I spit it out."

TODAY'S RX

Don't try to justify an addiction. Surrender your will to God, and get help to get well.

God, help me to make good choices when it comes to diet and exercise.
Give me the strength to avoid unhealthy foods and to treat my body well,
supplying it with the nutrients it needs to function as you've designed.

GOD IS GOOD ALL THE TIME

May all who search for you be filled with joy and gladness in you. May those who love your salvation repeatedly shout, "God is great!" PSALM 70:4

When I read today's verse, I smiled as I thought about the psalmist and his friends jumping up and down, shouting, "God is great!"

God is great. But there are times in our lives when the last thing we feel like doing is shouting for joy. When Ray entered my office, I could see he was having one of those days.

"Tell me what's going on," I said.

"After losing my son, I feel as if I've lost my joy. There's nothing in the world that makes me happy anymore. It's like I'm seeing the world in black and white. People irritate me, and the family members that I can stand to be around tell me I should seek help. That's why I'm here."

"I know it hurts to lose a son."

Ray began to cry. "Nothing hurts worse."

As we talked, I explained to Ray what was happening to him. "When we're under a lot of stress like you've been, it's as if the chemicals in our brains get used up by the stress. Without those chemicals, we perceive the world differently. These are the same substances that help us with our sleep, appetite, and memory."

"I haven't slept well since he died," Ray said. "My diet has gone down the tubes, and I can't even remember what I had for breakfast."

We talked about some solutions and eventually agreed that he should start on a Selective Serotonin Reuptake Inhibitor to help restore the chemicals in his brain.

"But there's something else that can help you even more than the medicine," I said.

"What's that?"

"From experience, I know we have two choices during times of great grief. We can run from God, as I did when I was a young man, or we can run *to* him. He's waiting for us with open and loving arms. Because I waited so long to run back to God, I can say without a doubt that running to him is a whole lot better than running away."

TODAY'S RX

If your perspective is out of balance because of grief or suffering, search the Psalms to shine the light of truth into your heart.

Lord, thank you for this reminder that you are good all the time. I may not feel joy in all seasons, but I know you're beside me even in my despair. Thank you for speaking words of affirmation and love to me through your Word.

GOD'S ODDS

This hope will not lead to disappointment. For we know how dearly God loves us, because he has given us the Holy Spirit to fill our hearts with his love. ROMANS 5:5

At forty-three, Mark had every reason to live and yet one reason that might prevent him from doing so.

Mark's daughter was getting married in six months. She had planned her wedding for the following year but moved up the date when Mark was diagnosed with pancreatic cancer.

Fortunately, the cancer had not spread, and the oncology surgeon felt that Mark might have a chance of surviving with something called the Whipple procedure—a major surgical operation involving several organs. If Mark hoped to be at his daughter's wedding, this was his only option. Without it, the odds of surviving this type of cancer for more than a few months were close to zero.

As we talked about possible complications and outcomes, Mark asked me, "Will I be going through the motions just to get to the end of it all and still have cancer? Could I end up dying anyway before the wedding?"

With God, I believe there is always hope for healing, but I never want to give my patients false hope in medicine. So I gave Mark my honest assessment.

"Dr. Paulo is one of the best, and I trust his judgment in this area. I don't think you'll be disappointed with your decision. But this journey isn't going to be easy."

At Mark's six-week postsurgical checkup, he was twenty pounds lighter and beginning to eat without pain. "I wouldn't suggest this as a diet plan," he said, "but if it gets me to the church for my daughter's wedding, I'm glad I went through with it."

A few weeks ago, Mark was back in my office for his annual checkup, and he was unusually talkative. "When I went through my surgery, my family loved me even when I was at my worst. I'm beginning to understand God's love for us because I saw it reflected in my family's love for me during those dark days."

"How long ago was the surgery?" I asked as I flipped through his chart.

"It's been three years, and not only was I able to walk my daughter down the aisle, but last month I received another gift."

Mark handed me a photo.

"My grandson!" he said, grinning.

TODAY'S RX

With God on your side, the outlook is always favorable.

Holy Spirit, fill me with your presence today. Help me to have a positive outlook on all I'm facing, and give me hope for my future.

APRIL CHECKUP

I often think about Jesus' life here on earth as a series of seasons. His birth was like a spring awakening that opened our minds and hearts to see what new life with the Father looked like. He lived among us for a growing season. As he walked and talked among us, training his disciples to continue God's work here on earth, they grew in knowledge, wisdom, and understanding. As a result of their witness, we continue to grow in these areas as well. The harvest is described in the book of Acts when so many people came to acknowledge Jesus as their Lord and Savior.

But there was another season—a time when the authorities of the day decided that Jesus' presence was a threat. Though he wasn't guilty of anything, they convicted and condemned him. They flogged him and mocked him, spat on him, and ultimately hung him on a cross to die. This was the winter season of his time on earth. A time when it seemed as if everything was dead and would never blossom or bloom again. But three days later, Jesus rose from the dead, and forty days after that, he ascended into heaven. His resurrection was proof that, despite the seasonal cycles of life, he had the power to overcome it—all of it, including death. When we put our faith in Jesus, there is no winter. After we die, we instantly move into an eternal spring of joy. Because Jesus conquered death, we are new creations who will blossom with him in heaven.

April is a month that contains promises. Though summer is still a ways off, we see the beginning signs of it everywhere. April showers promise future blooms. The early blossoms give rise to hope for a fruitful growing season. Even Jesus' death on the cross was the beginning of his promise that we would one day be with the Father. As you read this, the Easter season is either beginning or drawing to a close for you. In either case, it is still appropriate to think about what the holiday means. Too often we spend the time leading up to this holiday worried about ordering a ham for dinner, buying new clothes, or hiding candy-filled eggs. Our society has commercialized Holy Week much like it has Christmas, and as a result, we've missed the meaning of Jesus' coming to earth to give his life for us.

This year, take time to read your favorite Gospel account of Jesus's life, or read all four and compare them. Get the kids involved by reading before dinner. Or read aloud to a senior whose ability to read has diminished. When you remind others of the reason we celebrate Easter, you will remind yourself of a promise made long ago.

My prayer for you during this month is that you will slow down and remember the most important event in history, or as I like to think of it, "his story," the story of Jesus.

April Booster Shot: April's unpredictable weather sometimes catches us out in a storm. Drive carefully; take your time, and realize that it is often the storms of life that cause us to seek the firm foundation of Jesus, who is our shelter in time of need.

A TALE OF TWO BROTHERS

The human spirit can endure a sick body, but who can bear a crushed spirit?
PROVERBS 18:14

Ron and Billy Kern were brothers who were separated by more than their two-year age difference. Ron, who was the elder, had cerebral palsy, whereas Billy had been blessed with good health.

When their parents died, Billy took over as Ron's caregiver, and about that time, they also became my patients. Dutifully, the two men showed up together for regular appointments. Both had inherited hypertension and hyperlipidemia from their parents, but both conditions were under control with medication.

Each time they came in, I was struck by how Billy, the "healthy" brother, seemed more distant and less engaged. I would have expected this from Ron, who was confined to a wheelchair; but Ron was always engaging. He had a hearty laugh and a contagious smile.

One day while I was working in the ER, the EMS radio alerted us to the impending arrival of a forty-five-year-old white male who appeared to have had a heart attack. The EMTs were performing CPR en route.

When the ambulance arrived, I learned that the patient was Billy. He'd had a massive heart attack, and there was nothing we could do to save him. A neighbor brought Ron to the hospital, and I met him in a private room to give him the bad news.

"I'll help you figure something out," I said. "In the meantime, I'm going to admit you into the hospital so we can help you until we sort out the details of what's next."

Over the next few days, we did some research and found a Christian care center that had a room available for Ron. He'd already had such a tough life that I was worried about how he'd take the news that he would now essentially be institutionalized. But I needn't have worried. Though he grieved the loss of his brother, Ron was his usual, happy self.

The day we moved him from the hospital to the care center, he was grinning from ear to ear.

"This will be a new adventure," he said.

Five years later, Ron is as funny and engaging as ever. He's a perfect example of today's verse: Though his body is sick, his spirit is lively.

TODAY'S RX

Laugh a little today. Laughter gives life to all who enjoy it.

Lord, I take great comfort in knowing that though I won't always feel happy, I will always have joy, thanks to your Son, Jesus Christ, and the hope that he is to the world. Thank you for sending him to earth and for his sacrifice on the cross.

THE MOURNING DANCE OF JOY

The young women will dance for joy, and the men—old and young—will join in the celebration. I will turn their mourning into joy. I will comfort them and exchange their sorrow for rejoicing. JEREMIAH 31:13

After a family tragedy, months passed as our family struggled to find the joy we had known before the accident. It seemed as if we were stuck in the sorrow of our past, and our shared grief somehow blocked our ability to think about the future.

One of the counselors we saw at the time suggested that we take up a new hobby—something mindless and repetitive that would engage both the right and left sides of our brains. At the top of her list of suggestions was ballroom dancing. We had all taken a few dance classes, and Karen was already a great dancer, so we agreed that dancing would be our new family hobby.

We started out slowly, and some of us (meaning me) were slower than others—mixing up left and right feet or stepping on our partner's toes. But after a month of lessons, we could all do the rumba. After six months, we could all do the cha-cha. But it took us only a few minutes into our first lesson for us to laugh at ourselves.

I'm not sure if it was the dancing that saved us or the laughter, as we tried to learn each new dance. But each new step helped us put our past behind us as we began to anticipate our future. Our dancing may not always have been graceful, but the hobby was our saving grace. It helped us to live in the moment and restore a proper balance to our lives.

After a year of lessons, we decided we'd had enough with trying to learn new steps. But even though the hobby ceased, the laughter continued. Today's verse reminds me of how important it is to find pleasure in the moment. At the time, dancing helped exchange our sorrow for joy. Even today, the shared laughter over those dancing lessons remains.

TODAY'S RX

So you think you can't dance? Put one foot in front of the other and soon you'll be dancing, or at least laughing at your own attempts. Either way, joy will restore your soul.

God, just as Scripture says, there is a time and season for everything—both joy and sorrow. Thank you for walking with me in all seasons and for giving me much to be joyful about.

GOD MAKES THE WEAK STRONG

Hammer your plowshares into swords and your pruning hooks into spears. Train even your weaklings to be warriors. Joel 3:10

I had been asked to stop by the nursing home to see an elderly patient who had become despondent. Catherine had recently had a stroke, but I knew she could recover from it. The problem was that she didn't seem to want to.

When I entered the sparsely furnished room, Catherine looked ashen and pale—a rag doll wrapped in twisted sheets. She pulled the covers over her head when she saw me. I glanced at the nurses, and they nodded. Everything about her demeanor suggested she'd given up.

"Why are you hiding from us?" I asked. "We're just trying to help you."

Catherine mumbled something that I couldn't hear. Her voice was barely audible—more like a whisper.

The reason she didn't feel well had nothing to do with her stroke. She and Thomas, her husband of fifty years, had lost all their valuables in a flood a few years earlier. And recently, Thomas had gotten ill and died.

"I know you want to join Thomas," I said, tenderly taking her hand. "But your time hasn't come yet."

The stroke hadn't taken her life, but it had certainly disrupted it. Her speech was distorted, and the right side of her body was now weakened and crumbling before our eyes.

"God has further plans for your future with us. He wants you to pick up your plowshare and hammer it into a sword and fight for this new journey—this plan for your life." I wasn't sure why I said those words, or what they meant to her. But I hoped they would encourage her.

As we continued to talk, she took her fist and pounded the bed. After a few minutes, she pushed herself up and got out of bed. When I left, she was sitting in a chair by the window, where the sunshine could pour into her soul and dry her tears.

Catherine wasn't transformed overnight, but God definitely performed a miracle in her life. I saw it, and so did the nursing staff. Catherine hammered away at her recovery until she was well enough to return home, strengthened and ready for battle.

TODAY'S RX

Never give up, and never give in to the whisper of despair. When you're weak, allow God to make you strong for the fight.

Father, help me to keep my eyes on you when I'm weighed down with grief. I know it is when I am weak that you are strong. Thank you for revealing yourself in new ways to me during this time.

HIS SPIRIT WALKS WITH US

You have not received a spirit that makes you fearful slaves. Instead, you received God's Spirit when he adopted you as his own children. Now we call him, "Abba, Father."
ROMANS 8:15

"Doc, I'm afraid to go to the big city hospital. Can't you do the surgery here? I've never really traveled outside of Cheatham County, and it worries me."

Many of my patients are salt-of-the-earth country folks who don't get out much. The anxiety of an unfamiliar place, along with the fear of a life-threatening illness, can easily overwhelm them. Sometimes their fear paralyzes them, and they don't take the actions they need to get better. Occasionally, they outright refuse lifesaving treatment because of their fear.

As a way to help them, I started accompanying my most fearful and fragile patients to the hospital. When accompanied by a familiar face, their fear abated, and they went willingly.

Often using today's verse, I would pray with them that God would be with us in this strange and unfamiliar world we were entering. That way they could know for certain, even when I left, that God was right there beside them.

Are there fears that paralyze you from doing God's will in your life?

Do you prefer to sit in the comfort of the familiar?

If the God of the universe personally held your hand and guided you, would you be willing to step out of your comfort zone and take up a new task for him?

My patients bravely crossed over barriers they would not have surmounted if they'd had to go it alone. Because they knew that Jesus was walking side-by-side with them, they were able to overcome their very real fears. As their doctor, I've had the privilege of a fifty-yard-line seat, watching and cheering them on as they did.

TODAY'S RX

Step out in faith, one step at a time, and God will light your path.

Lord, when I face obstacles that scare me, help me to remember that you are mighty and all-powerful, taking down giants and parting seas for the benefit of your people. Thank you for always being at my rescue.

THE FORGIVENESS DIET

He forgives all my sins and heals all my diseases. PSALM 103:3

"I eat like a bird, but I look like a hippo!" Patsy said. "Dieting just doesn't seem to work. I think I need bariatric surgery."

At only five foot three and weighing more than four hundred pounds, Patsy was right in some respects. She had tried multiple diets, plenty of plans, and pounds of pills to suppress her appetite. And they all failed. Due to a fatty liver, her liver enzymes were elevated. Her diabetes was poorly controlled, and her high cholesterol foreshadowed a heart attack. She was on a fast train headed over the cliff to a health disaster from which she might not recover. The one bright spot in Patsy's health was that her thyroid was working properly—those tests were normal.

The dietitian confirmed that if Patty was eating like a bird, it was more like a flock of birds. She had to be consuming well over 4,000 calories in her "diet food." I suspected that the problem ran deeper than her fat cells.

"Patsy, tell me about your childhood and growing up with your parents and grandparents."

She happily told me stories of what sounded like a perfect family life until "Uncle Bob" moved in. Then her eyes darkened as she described how much she and her sister hated Bob.

"Why?" I asked, though I already suspected the answer.

"He hurt us, and I couldn't tell anyone, or he would hurt my sister. Even though he's been dead for five years, I still see him in my nightmares. I can't forgive him for what he did, and I blame myself for all of it."

Her answer didn't surprise me; it also gave me the key to her binge eating disorder. "Before we discuss surgery, I'd like for you to see a psychologist and start the healing process of forgiving your uncle and yourself."

Patsy agreed. Though the physical weight didn't come off quickly or easily, relieving the emotional weight helped her to get off the train that was bound for the cliff and board a new one that was slowly climbing toward a healthy life.

TODAY'S RX

Sometimes, we need to restore our emotional health before we can fix our physical health. If you need to forgive someone, or forgive yourself, ask God to help you forgive just as he has forgiven you.

Jesus, may I always remember your sacrifice on the cross when I'm tempted to remain angry with someone who has done me wrong. Your death was the ultimate display of forgiveness freely given to those who didn't deserve it. Thank you for your great love for me.

GIVE US EARS TO HEAR

One of them struck at the high priest's slave, slashing off his right ear. But Jesus said, "No more of this." And he touched the man's ear and healed him. LUKE 22:50-51

One reason I love the Bible so much is because the stories in it are so rich and layered.

Take, for example, the scene described in today's verses. Jesus is about to be taken away by the Roman army and sentenced to die on the cross. Peter tries to stop this from happening by cutting off the ear of the high priest's servant. When I read that the man's ear was slashed off, I can only think of how close the sword was to the man's vital organs. His brain, eyes, and carotid artery were just a slip of the sword away from where Peter slashed him.

Had Peter's sword killed the slave, I'm sure Jesus would have raised the man from the dead and healed his mortal wounds. Perhaps some people would have believed in him as a result.

To me, though, it seems fitting that the blood spilled that night was from a lopped-off ear. It is symbolic of a world that had stopped listening. Jesus was the Word, and the people were no longer hearing him. The world was as deaf to Jesus as the man whose ear filled with blood. They could no longer hear what the Savior had to say.

It was also symbolic that Jesus' last act of healing was to heal the wounds of an enemy who had come to capture and kill him. After Jesus' touch, the blood stopped running, the ear was restored, and the man could once again hear clearly. To me, this act represents the redemption that was coming to the world after Jesus' blood flowed from his crucified body. When he died, he healed us all.

TODAY'S RX

Don't let the words of our Lord fall on deaf ears. Declare them to restore a lost world.

Lord, open my ears to hear your voice today. Help me to be still and listen for all you have to say.

THE GIVER OF LIFE IS ALSO THE GREAT HEALER

If you will listen carefully to the voice of the LORD your God and do what is right in his sight, obeying his commands and keeping all his decrees, then I will not make you suffer any of the diseases I sent on the Egyptians; for I am the LORD who heals you.
EXODUS 15:26

At the end of a long day, I entered John's room and sat down beside his bed. He was asleep as I silently prayed, *Please, God, don't let him die yet.*

John's wife and kids were all Christ followers, but he had never seen a need for God. Now the acute heart attack he'd had earlier that day was likely going to be terminal.

Please, Lord, just a little more time, I prayed.

I thought about all the times when John had visited my office. Though I'd known him for years, I didn't know if he'd ever listened to my pleas to turn his life around. It wouldn't have surprised me if he hadn't. After all, he had never listened when I asked him to quit smoking and drinking. I had also warned him that the stress from his executive position was taking a toll on his health. And now it appeared to have worn out his heart.

As I finished my prayer and left the room, I knew it might be the last time I'd see John. Only the healing hand of God and the care of an excellent cardiac surgeon could save him now.

A few weeks later, I got a call from the cardiac rehab director. "I need to make a follow-up appointment for John."

Stunned, but elated that he'd made it through the surgery, I set up an appointment for the following week.

When John arrived at my office, I was prepared to have another hard conversation about his lifestyle with him. I also wanted to delve into the spiritual realm with him again. But he surprised me by introducing both topics first.

"The Lord spoke to me last night. And I'm ready to hear whatever wisdom you have for me."

John accomplished some amazing medical, physical, and lifestyle changes over the next few years. But the most astonishing change was how God had transformed him into a new creation.

TODAY'S RX

Show your appreciation for the gift of life by dedicating your days to the Giver of life.

Nothing is too challenging for you, Father. You soften the most stubborn hearts and bring people back to you. Thank you for softening my heart and allowing me to be your child.

THE STORM OF FEAR

God has not given us a spirit of fear and timidity, but of power, love, and self-discipline.
2 TIMOTHY 1:7

"The feelings of fear used to attack me in the middle of the night," Cindy said, biting her lower lip. "But now, it's worse."

"Can you tell me about the first time this happened?" I asked.

"It started when I was a teenager. One night we had a bad storm that spawned a tornado. It destroyed homes in the town next to ours. Ever since, whenever a storm comes, I feel as if someone is attacking me—like they're holding me down, and I can't catch my breath."

At first, Cindy thought that her feelings were a normal response to that frightening first storm. But when the feelings started happening randomly—and more often—she grew concerned.

"Now, I can be driving down the road, and I'll have to pull over and get out of the car because I feel like I'm going to suffocate. This fear has paralyzed my life. I've lost two jobs and several friends because I'm afraid to leave my house."

When God created us, he gave us a fight-or-flight response to help us avoid danger. When we're under stress, physiological systems kick in to help save us from the threat. Whether it was a caveman confronted by a saber-toothed tiger or a modern man or woman confronting a burglar, our bodies were designed to either react or run.

In stressful situations, chemicals are released that increase our heart rate and blood pressure. Our breathing quickens, and our pupils dilate to take in as much light as possible. Blood that used to go to our digestive tract is rerouted to our muscles. As a result, we're ready to fight or take flight.

In some cases, the system doesn't work properly, and our bodies react even though the perceived threat is an internal one. In Cindy's case, her system had malfunctioned, causing her to suffer from a panic disorder and agoraphobia, a fear of open spaces.

Fortunately, with proper medication and concurrent behavioral therapy, this disorder can be controlled, and a patient can return to a relatively normal life.

God did not give us a spirit of fear. If you are struggling with excessive fear, seek help. It is available.

TODAY'S RX

Fear not. The God who calms the storms and raging seas is with you and will help you live in peace.

Lord, your Word tells me not to be afraid but to trust in you with all my heart. Help me to remain faithful, knowing that you're directing my path and showing me the way. I desire to live a life that is obedient to you.

DAMASCUS ROAD

Repent of your sins and turn to God, so that your sins may be wiped away. ACTS 3:19

I'll never forget one Fourth of July camping trip I took in the Tennessee mountains. As darkness fell, I read the Bible by flashlight, seeking answers to questions I had buried for years. As soon as I finished my reading, my eyes closed, and I fell into a deep sleep. This slumber was different from any I had ever experienced. It was as if my mind were tumbling and free-falling, like a waterfall I'd seen earlier that day. An overwhelming peace filled my entire being, and everything seemed right with the world.

When my mind came to rest, I opened my eyes to the most fantastic countryside imaginable: Everything was vivid and brilliant. I inhaled the most fragrant scent—light and pleasing, like a mixture of citrus and lilac. I heard a trickling noise behind me and turned to see a running stream. As I moved toward the stream, I felt an icy but refreshing spray.

I heard an unmistakable voice calling me from a distance—though it didn't make an audible sound; instead, it resonated inside of me and echoed outside, as if I'd heard it with my heart and soul. It was easily the most compelling yet comforting voice I had ever heard.

Though the circumstances were different, a man named Saul in the Bible had a similar experience. As a zealous persecutor of Christians, Saul was on his was to Damascus to arrest any believers he could find there. However, along the road, a light from heaven shone down on him, a voice called to him, and he found he'd been struck blind. But as he followed the irresistible call of the Lord, he regained his sight and became an ardent follower of Jesus. We know him today as the apostle Paul.

Paul and I are very different people, living in very different circumstances. Yet the Lord reached both of us in a similar way. Without warning, he appeared to us and spoke to us in an unmistakable voice. He healed our blindness so we could see the truth in full, vibrant color. We were both transformed and dedicated the rest of our lives to his Son, Jesus Christ.

TODAY'S RX

How did Jesus call you to himself? How did you respond? Pray that he would reveal himself to you today in an unmistakable way.

Thank you for meeting me where I'm at today, Father. It's a comfort knowing you never lose sight of me as I journey through life. Continue to reveal yourself to me so that I may know you and love you more fully.

A PILL AND A PRAYER ARE BOTH GOOD MEDICINE

A cheerful heart is good medicine, but a broken spirit saps a person's strength.
PROVERBS 17:22

"No matter what I do, I'm tired all the time," Beth said. "Even when I try, I can't seem to get up before noon. What do you think is causing all of this? Last night, I was looking at my symptoms on the Internet, and it kept saying that tiredness could be caused by a problem with my thyroid or that I could be anemic. Do you think that's the case?"

Beth looked worried. She also looked tired. "We'll do some blood work to assess those possibilities," I promised. "But first, start by telling me about your sleep habits."

"Usually, I go to sleep around midnight or one, but most nights I can't fall asleep, so I get back up and try to do something until I get tired."

"What else is going on in your life?"

"I don't know. I feel as if all I do is worry about what's going to happen next. They're laying people off at my husband's workplace, and I'm afraid he could be next. When he's under stress, he doesn't take good care of himself, so I worry about his health. The kids haven't been doing very well in school, and my mom hasn't been feeling well. Also, next month I'll be working a lot of overtime—and I'm not looking forward to that."

I was starting to get the picture. Though Beth was certainly busy, there was a lot more going on with her emotionally—and her anxiety was keeping her awake at night. Her fatigue was probably not due to a physical cause but rather a worried heart and broken spirit.

As promised, I ordered some tests and lab work, and it all came back perfect, as I had anticipated. After I explained to Beth that there didn't seem to be a physical cause for her exhaustion, we discussed some options for dealing with her anxiety. She decided to try medication and prayer.

Within two months, I could see the positive results of both. I knew she was on the mend when she bounded into my office and started talking about all of the great things the Lord was doing in her life.

TODAY'S RX

When worry and the cares of the world break your spirit, turn to the Lord to find joy, hope, and peace.

From day to day, God, there are always new concerns and worries. Be with me when my heart panics and my thoughts become a jumble. Calm me with the truth of your Word, and help me to remember how you've always been faithful in the past.

THE BLESSINGS OF BEING PRESENT

The Lamb on the throne will be their Shepherd. He will lead them to springs of life-giving water. And God will wipe every tear from their eyes. REVELATION 7:17

Last year, our rehab unit placed first in the company for patient satisfaction. After the news was released, I wanted to find out more, so I started asking the employees, "Why are patients so happy with their care here?"

Their answers were very similar.

"We're a family. We take care of our patients just like they're a part of our own family."

"We're a close-knit group here."

"Everyone works together—the nurses, therapists, aides, housekeepers, dieticians, and pharmacists."

I beamed with pride as each person I asked told me a story about how someone else had lived up to this very high standard. I was surrounded by a group of humble do-gooders. Not one person thought our unit received the award because of something he or she had personally done. These people were living examples of Jesus' command to do unto others as you would have them do unto you.

To me, it was an up-close look at how being like Jesus starts with the smallest kindnesses done for the least among us. I was inspired by stories of a housekeeper who brought water to a thirsty patient even though it wasn't his job and of a nurse who stayed a few minutes past the end of her shift to listen while an elderly stroke victim, who had trouble getting his words out as he talked, described his last fishing trip.

Life-giving water not only quenches our thirst in the moment, but it gives life to everything it touches. In this busy world, we can often miss the blessing of giving and receiving God's life-giving water. Slowing down can be a refreshing oasis from our overscheduled world, but it can also be used to refresh someone else. The blessings found in taking time to wipe the tears from our neighbor's eyes and having a cup of coffee together are the very things that God can use to refresh our weary souls.

TODAY'S RX

Make it a point today to slow down and connect with other people. The person you help might be you.

Jesus, I take such comfort in knowing that someday you will wipe every tear from my eyes. Help me to display this same affection for others and comfort them in their times of need.

TWO-FOR-ONE PRAYER

I tell you the truth, anyone who believes in me will do the same works I have done, and even greater works, because I am going to be with the Father. JOHN 14:12

Harold had smoked most of his adult life. He had what we call, in medical terms, a fifty pack-year history of smoking—two packs of unfiltered cigarettes per day for twenty-five years.

He'd been coughing up mucus for years, but when he noticed it had become tinged with blood, he hurried in to see me at the office. "My dad had lung cancer, and I think I might have it too," he said.

I sent him for chest X-rays and prayed for a miracle, but I wasn't surprised when the test revealed an ominous looking spot.

"The X-ray results are worrisome," I said to Harold. "But in order for us to be certain, we'll have to do some further testing. A CT scan and a biopsy will tell us what's really going on."

I scheduled Harold for the first available test slot and arranged for a follow-up appointment with a pulmonologist three days afterward to discuss the results. In the meantime, I continued praying for Harold's health.

A few days later, I got a call from the radiologist who had performed the tests. I was stunned when he told me that the CT scan couldn't locate the spot—the same spot we had both clearly seen on the X-ray the week before. When Harold went to his follow-up appointment three days later, the pulmonologist reviewed Harold's chart and recent test results and agreed that the mass on the X-ray was no longer there. When I received the news, I thanked God for healing Harold.

A few days later, Harold had a bronchoscopy to diagnose the reason for the blood in his sputum, but the results also came back negative.

At Harold's next appointment, we discussed what had happened.

"Dr. Anderson, I went to church and asked them to lay hands on me and pray for my healing," Harold said. "And you know what? I don't have the mass, and I no longer crave cigarettes. I guess I got two healings that day!"

TODAY'S RX

If you need a miracle, pray. God still performs miracles—and sometimes they're even doubly healing.

Lord, I confess that oftentimes my sin keeps me from pursuing you. Help me to change my unhealthy ways and look to you for strength in the midst of temptation.

THE BEST PARTY

Trust in the LORD *and do good. Then you will live safely in the land and prosper. Take delight in the* LORD, *and he will give you your heart's desires. Commit everything you do to the* LORD. *Trust him, and he will help you.* PSALM 37:3-5

Things weren't going well in Tommy's life, so I asked him about his faith.

"That stuff never interested me, Doc. I grew up on the wrong side of the tracks, and the church was never my friend. I don't relate to all that goody-two-shoes stuff."

I chuckled. "That's not what it's about. In fact, most Christians aren't Goody Two-shoes. We all fall short of God's perfect will for our lives. Me, I spent years walking on the wrong side of the tracks. I didn't even believe in God. But now I know that even when I didn't believe in him, he was watching out for me and keeping me safe."

"That's fine for you, but I've been bad for too long. I don't see myself ever getting into religion. I like to party too much, and God doesn't seem to want us to have any fun."

"I hear you. I used to think that way, too, especially on those late nights when I closed down the bar. But now my fun is found elsewhere, though I still enjoy an occasional glass of wine."

"You do?"

"You may have heard that Jesus turned water into wine at a wedding party. He loved a great party! In fact, I can't wait to join him at the party in heaven. I'm sure it will put to shame any celebration here on earth."

"People party in heaven?"

"Yes, but probably not the way you're thinking. One thing we have to understand is that God wants what's best for us—not to take away our fun. As your doctor, I tell you not to drink so much because I want you to live a long and healthy life filled with real fun."

"Hmm. I never thought about it that way."

"When I was in college, I was headed in the wrong direction, but I had an encounter with Jesus that turned me around and gave me a new life. It's not about religion or going to church. It's about having a personal relationship with Jesus Christ—that's when the real fun starts!"

TODAY'S RX

If you haven't yet accepted your invitation to God's forever party, do so today.

Father, thank you for loving me like a parent and wanting your best for me. Forgive me when I go my own way and do not listen. Help me to be obedient to you.

THE LIFE PRESERVER

The LORD is close to all who call on him, yes, to all who call on him in truth. He grants the desires of those who fear him; he hears their cries for help and rescues them.
PSALM 145:18-19

Belfast, Northern Ireland, was the birthplace of two very remarkable things. The most recent was my grandson, Callum, but it was also the birthplace of the RMS *Titanic.*

In 1912, the *Titanic* was the largest cruise ship ever built, and its construction was considered a wonder of the world. Most experts believed it was unsinkable, and it was expected to break every transatlantic crossing record on its maiden voyage. But late on the evening of April 14, 1912, the ship collided with an iceberg in the North Atlantic. Within three hours, the unsinkable ship had sunk, killing more than 1,500 people.

When the ship departed from Southampton, United Kingdom, it had more than 2,200 people aboard but only enough lifeboats for half.

On a recent trip to Northern Ireland, Karen and I visited the Titanic Museum in Belfast. As we walked through the corridors, a sense of reverence overcame me. The recording of the last message sent was an urgent SOS to whatever ships were in the area. I thought of how there must have been a flood of desperate prayers as those 1,500 men, women, and children called out to God to save them before they took their last breath.

Reflecting on those desperate cries for help, I realized that although those people perished, God heard each voice that cried out. He answered their prayers, not by bringing them safely to New York City as they had planned, but by bringing them directly to his dwelling place for them in heaven.

Today's verse reminds me that even amid great tragedy, God's arms are outstretched to all who want to be saved.

TODAY'S RX

In times of trouble, trial, and tragedy, we have two choices: We can either run away from God or we can run to him and receive his protection and healing—even when the outcome is not what we expected.

God, there is so much pain and tragedy in this world. Sometimes it feels as if there is little hope. Rescue this broken world. Help us to see your light and remember that you are near.

FAMILIAL BLESSINGS

I will pour out my Spirit on your descendants, and my blessing on your children. They will thrive like watered grass, like willows on a riverbank. ISAIAH 44:3-4

In today's verses, the Lord makes a promise to Jacob and his descendants. He assures them that he will do more than protect them. He will also bless them so they will thrive and grow.

As parents, there are things we can do to bless our children and grandchildren and help them thrive. I've been in the same practice, treating many of the same families, for almost thirty years, and it's given me a great perspective on what familial blessings can look like.

For example, one of the first families I met had kids who grew up and brought me their own children to treat. Now, the second generation is bringing the third, so I've had the opportunity to watch three generations of the same family thrive and grow.

Because of our history together, whenever a member of this family comes into my office, it's always a special treat. I don't see them as much as I would like, but from a health perspective that is a good thing. The last time one of the daughters was in my office, I had the chance to ask her, "Why is it that your family has always been so healthy?"

"None of us smoke or drink. We eat fruits and vegetables that we grow ourselves. We all eat dinner together, and we pray before we eat. And Momma and Daddy told us never to miss a Sunday at church."

For generations, this family has been healthy and hardy. They come in for routine physical exams and those required for school or sports, but that's about it. Even their blood work has remained remarkably consistent throughout the generations.

Recently, the family matriarch died. She was in her midnineties. If all my patients lived such long and healthy lives, I would go broke. But knowing this family as well as I do has only enriched my life by their kindness to all and their love and devotion to one another.

A family with good health habits flourishes and stays healthy for generations. What we proactively decide to do today can help our descendants to thrive.

TODAY'S RX

Follow God's instructions for living, and teach your children—and your children's children—to do the same.

Help me to remember, Lord, that my actions not only affect me, but my family as well. May I be an example of your kindness and peace and love.

A GENERATIONAL CHAIN OF BELIEVERS

Understand, therefore, that the LORD your God is indeed God. He is the faithful God who keeps his covenant for a thousand generations and lavishes his unfailing love on those who love him and obey his commands. DEUTERONOMY 7:9

For my birthday one year, Karen gave me the gift of genetic testing and a membership to www.ancestry.com, a website that allows people to trace their family tree. The results were fascinating and helped me learn more about the last fifty or sixty generations of my family. The furthest ancestor that I could identify was a Viking who lived in Norway around AD 400.

It's humbling to think about all the generations that came before me. What would have happened if they'd made different choices along the way? What if one of them had married someone else? Would I still be here?

Reflecting on the lives of so many people from so many generations and the number of choices involved was illuminating. For the first time, I realized that, somewhere back in England, one or more of my ancestors had made a commitment to Jesus Christ and started a generational chain of faith.

From the moment of that decision, the Lord lavished his love on every generation that would follow. God has never wavered from the promises he made to that first person in my family who committed to him—even when some of us down through the ages strayed from him. During my own wandering in the desert, he was always there, sustaining me even when I didn't acknowledge him as my provider.

Karen and I have four children, some of whom now have children of their own. God's covenant with my ancestors continues through them. And I have many families in my practice with similar stories of multigenerational faith in which God has been constant and trustworthy. Many of these families are pillars in our community.

One of my daughters lives in Great Britain, where our family's chain of believers began. Recently, while visiting her and my grandson, I once again marveled at how the Lord has shown us his steadfast love for more than a thousand years—and yet, his promise is for a thousand generations, so there is so much more to come.

TODAY'S RX

Your legacy matters. The faith you choose and the example you set for how to follow the Lord may affect a thousand generations.

God, you are faithful. Your love endures forever. You shine your love on all who follow you, and I'm grateful to be your child. Help me to leave a lasting legacy for the generations in my family that are yet to come.

PRUNING FOR A FRUITFUL LIFE

If you remain in me and my words remain in you, you may ask for anything you want, and it will be granted! John 15:7

As a small boy, I used to watch my father prune the peach trees in our orchard. Even when I was very young, he taught me how to tell the difference between the branches that produced fruit and those that were diseased, dying, or already dead. The unhealthy branches could safely be pruned because they would never produce fruit. By the time I was a teenager, I could finger a branch in the dead of winter and know whether it had life teeming inside it or if it would only divert resources from the rest of the tree.

The branches that remained after pruning were our hope for a bumper crop, and we did whatever it took to protect them. If a late freeze was expected, we built a fire in the orchard to ward off the cold. During the growing season, my father kept an eye on each tree for signs of what it needed. More water? More fertilizer? A little more pruning? He spent countless hours nurturing the trees and protecting their yet-to-be-borne fruit.

Jesus is the watchful gardener who tends to our spiritual health. He sees what we need even before we recognize it. And he is quick to offer us protection. But unlike a tree, we can decide whether or not we will live and abide in him. Do we allow him to take care of us, or do we think we know what's best and resist his care? Do we have branches that need pruning—areas of our lives that need to be cut away and discarded?

When we allow the master gardener to tend to us, he never reduces our fruitfulness; he only increases our yield. But when we resist his pruning, we end up hanging on to dead, diseased, or sinful areas of our lives that prevent us from being fruitful.

Jesus invites you to remain in him and allow his truth and wisdom to prune your life and make it more fragrant and fruitful than you can imagine.

TODAY'S RX

In medicine, surgery is much like pruning—we cut away the dead and diseased parts. We need to allow the Great Physician to do the same thing to us spiritually if we want to thrive and bear good fruit.

Jesus, thank you for tending to me so carefully, preserving me through harsh seasons and growing me in others. May my life be fruitful and pleasing to you.

THE PAIN OF GROWING AND HEALING

I pray that your love will overflow more and more, and that you will keep on growing in knowledge and understanding. PHILIPPIANS 1:9

"I don't know what's wrong with me," Gary said. He'd come to my office complaining of weight loss, night sweats, general malaise, and fatigue.

We did the usual in-office exam, and I didn't find anything remarkable. "Looking at your records, I see you were here about six months ago. Everything looked good then, and you were fit and healthy with no complaints. The only thing that's changed is you've lost fifteen pounds."

"Yeah, I'm kind of puzzled about that. I haven't been dieting."

Gary wasn't a smoker or a drinker, and he didn't have a family history that would indicate any problems. Without more clues to go on, the cause of his symptoms could be almost anything.

I ordered lab work and gave him the results a few days later. "It all came back negative, except for your white blood cell count. Yours was twenty-seven, which is about twice as high as normal. Your hematocrit was thirty, which is slightly low. I think I'll have you meet with a hematologist. He'll be able to run some specialized tests to see what's going on."

The next week, Gary was diagnosed with non-Hodgkin's lymphoma, an aggressive type of cancer that needed treatment. The specialist tried different chemotherapy treatments, but they all failed. Eventually, Gary's only option was to have a bone marrow transplant.

For the transplant to work, the treatment had to completely destroy Gary's existing bone marrow so his body wouldn't reject the donor marrow. It's a dangerous treatment primarily used in life-threatening situations. Fortunately, in Gary's case it worked.

Sometimes growth and healing involve rooting out or destroying something that isn't functioning properly for us. This is also true spiritually. If we want new life to grow, we must destroy old habits and destructive patterns of thinking.

The Bible refers to this as pruning the vine so that new life can develop and the vine can produce fruit. Is there something in your life that isn't functioning as it should? Whether it's an old habit or an old way of thinking, consider pruning the dead branches from your life as a way to help you grow stronger.

TODAY'S RX

Though pruning can be painful, the new growth will produce fruit that will make your pain a distant memory.

Lord, examine my heart. Please uproot and destroy the sinful behaviors that have taken hold and are spreading in my life. Replace them with your life-giving truth.

WHISKEY-SOAKED PROMISES

Some were fools; they rebelled and suffered for their sins . . . "LORD, help!" they cried in their trouble, and he saved them from their distress. PSALM 107:17, 19

Friday nights in the ER are usually hopping. One particular Friday had been very quiet, but then it started to rain, and soon the ER was back in business.

The roads in Cheatham County are slick and curvy—a bad combination, especially when mixed with motorcycles and alcohol. Unfortunately, there is a popular bar located near one of those curves. The local watering hole has a regular crowd, but occasionally someone passing through will stop in for a drink. When the whiskey soaks in, people can become a little too brazen, and one of the locals might decide to correct the situation—with his fists.

That's what happened on that rainy Friday evening. A fight broke out inside the bar and spilled out into the parking lot. During the fray, the stranger got punched in the eye. Wanting to avoid a bigger beatdown, he hopped onto his motorcycle and took off. As you might imagine, driving drunk, on a motorcycle, on an unfamiliar road, on a dark and rainy night, with only one good eye, wasn't going to end well. It didn't.

The young man ended up in the ER, where I spent a lot of time cleaning road debris out of his wounds. I couldn't do much for his broken ankle, though, other than to splint it and recommend a good orthopedist for him to see the next morning. I ended up putting more than sixty stitches in his body.

As I finished up, the man said, "You know, I almost got killed out there."

"Yes, indeed. The good Lord had to be looking out for you."

"While you were sewing me up, I decided I need to turn over a new leaf and start going to church like my momma keeps telling me."

"That's a great idea," I said. "I know that Jesus would welcome you with open arms."

I don't know if he kept his drunken promise, but I pray that he did.

TODAY'S RX

If you want to live a happy and healthy life, avoid excessive alcohol, brazen words, motorcycles and curvy roads in the rain, and sucker punches to the eye. For good measure, turn over a new leaf with God.

Father, I confess that my sin and rebellion have taken me down roads that have only led to harm. Forgive me for not looking to you in these moments. Straighten my path so that I may honor you with my life.

THE LORD HEALS YOUR WOUNDS

"I will give you back your health and heal your wounds," says the L*ORD.*
JEREMIAH 30:17

One of my diabetic patients, Jose, was faithful to come to my office every month for a checkup, but he wasn't consistently taking good care of himself. Diabetes is a disease that requires constant monitoring and vigilance. Otherwise, complications can affect the eyes and kidneys. It can also leave many patients with numbness in their extremities. Though Jose's vision and renal function had thus far been spared, he was suffering from neuropathy and small vessel disease. He was completely numb to any sensation in his feet.

He came into the office one day after stepping on a nail. The foot wound had started out as a small puncture, but it had gotten so bad that I was afraid we might eventually need to amputate his right leg. Jose and I prayed together, and he agreed to get back on a proper diet. Together we outlined a plan for aggressive wound care.

Weeks rolled into months, and Jose faithfully kept his regular appointments. Even so, it took almost two years before his foot was completely healed. From start to finish, this was a miracle from God because by all accounts, this was a wound that should not have healed. Jose did his part by remaining steadfast and vigilant with his diabetic care. As a result, he was able to continue walking upright on two feet.

Sadly, not every case has such a positive outcome. Over and over I see the same patients with the same problems flaring up, causing them pain and suffering. Even when they're trying to faithfully follow their treatment plans, the slumbering giant of this disease continues to awaken and raise its ugly head.

If you suffer from a chronic illness, I know that the battle can be wearying. It can take its toll on even the most diligent patient. Often, all it takes is a temporary victory to help heal and reenergize your soul.

TODAY'S RX

Even if the row is long and hard to hoe, God can accomplish anything. Stay close to him and follow his guidance.

God, the journey to healing isn't easy, and I need you for support and strength. Help me to be patient and persevere as I face setbacks that leave me feeling discouraged. Thank you for knowing my needs and holding me in your arms.

GOD STRONG

In your strength I can crush an army; with my God I can scale any wall. Psalm 18:29

My office in Ashland City is perhaps the closest private practice to Fort Campbell, so many of the military families choose us for their health care.

Bo was stationed there when he came to see me. He'd grown up on a farm in Middle-of-Nowhere, Alabama, and in many ways, he reminded me of myself at his age.

On the day he turned eighteen, Bo had joined the US Army, which gave him a measure of independence and freedom from the boyhood chains that tied him to the farm.

"I had to get out," he said. "I wanted to see something other than the hood of that Ford tractor. I didn't want to spend the rest of my life with the smell of diesel choking me to death."

"But you're smoking unfiltered cigarettes?" I asked. "Those will do the same thing."

"My uncle used to smoke unfiltered, and I stole cigarettes from him when I was a kid. I guess I got hooked."

"Bo, you've done what—two or three tours of duty in Iran and Afghanistan?"

"Actually, it's been four. Two in each country."

"So, tell me what's going on."

"Well, I know the big picture of why we're there and what we're doing. But the daily grind is getting to me. I can't seem to sleep, and I keep dreaming that I am deployed instead of here with my family."

As we continued our conversation, it was obvious that Bo was struggling with post-traumatic stress disorder (PTSD) but coping as well as he could. We set him up with a team of counselors on the base to help him understand what the rest of his life's journey could look like and what God originally intended it to be.

Bo had already defeated a foreign army, and now with God's help, he was going to scale the wall back to good health. My prayer for him was that God would give him the will, strength, and fortitude to make it to the other side. Even those who are Army strong need to depend on our stronger God.

TODAY'S RX

If you struggle with the aftereffects of trauma, enlist the help of those who can help you return to full health.

Lord, I know I will not be defeated when I put all my trust in you. Help me to seek you with all my heart and depend on you for strength when difficult situations arise.

MAKING PEACE WITH THE BLACK SHEEP

Make every effort to keep yourselves united in the Spirit, binding yourselves together with peace. Ephesians 4:3

Everyone loves to talk about the black sheep of the family. They're typically the first to be thrown under the bus when anything goes wrong, and we're quick to judge their decisions. Though we say we care about them, our words often betray more gossip than concern.

When the family gets together, the black sheep can often become the elephant in the room. Everyone tries to tiptoe around the awkwardness, not saying what he or she really thinks and certainly not addressing the issue directly. But is this what Jesus would have us do?

In the New Testament, Jesus is portrayed as the Good Shepherd who drops everything to rescue a single wandering sheep. He searches until he finds it, and carries the sheep on his shoulders back to the rest of the flock. By the time the sheep rejoins the others, it is no longer a "black sheep." Jesus has washed it white as snow.

We need to follow the example of Jesus and become good shepherds who welcome the black sheep back into the family fold. We need to love them the way Jesus loves them—and us—offering forgiveness and restoration.

Perhaps the black sheep in your family has an addiction or a psychological illness that disrupts the civility within your home. Call for help if you need it. Professional physicians, counselors, and addiction specialists stand ready to help carry the burden of a loved one's illness. If your family member balks at the suggestion that he or she needs treatment, you may have to curb your tongue. Better yet, express your love and your desire for him or her to get well.

Call a truce, if necessary, to bring peace to your home and family, even if it means signing a treaty after a long-fought war. Opting for peace instead of chaos doesn't mean you approve of everything the black sheep has done (or is doing), but it will help protect the relationship. Remember, Satan is the enemy, not your loved one. The goal should be for words of grace and peace to restore your loved one's heart and soul.

TODAY'S RX

If your family is at war, seek help before it causes further pain and illness.

Jesus, thank you for never abandoning your sheep. Help me to have a heart of forgiveness and grace, so that I may reflect your love to others and have peaceful relationships.

HEALING ON THE SABBATH

If the correct time for circumcising your son falls on the Sabbath, you go ahead and do it so as not to break the law of Moses. So why should you be angry with me for healing a man on the Sabbath? JOHN 7:23

Early in my medical career, I alternated emergency room duties with another doctor. On our designated weekend, we arrived at the hospital on Friday afternoon and stayed until after Monday morning rounds. After the usual chaos of a Saturday night "gun and knife show," Sunday mornings were typically pretty quiet, a time when I could get a little shut-eye to recover from my lack of sleep.

One Sunday morning had started out like most of the rest, until the radio squawked with a call for both emergency medical services and the police. A person of interest from a local bar fight had been located and was now racing through the woods. When the police finally apprehended him, they found he was injured.

Before the suspect could be taken to jail, the EMTs determined that he would need a few stitches, so they brought him to the ER. When they rolled him into the exam room, he reeked of alcohol. I might have failed a breathalyzer test just by being in the same room with him!

The man, who was in his midthirties, had been out drinking all night. After he had consumed too much alcohol, jealousy had overtaken him. A fight over a woman broke out in the bar, rolled out into the parking lot, and ended up in the woods.

Once he was in the ER, I discovered that it would take more than a few stitches to do the job. My ending total was a new record for me—176 stitches! Fortunately, he hadn't lost enough blood to require a transfusion. The police were able to safely transfer him to a holding cell at the jail a few blocks away.

That day, my Sabbath didn't include rest or a traditional form of worship. But I believe that God was honored as I did everything I could to heal that man.

TODAY'S RX

If the ox is in the ditch, you have to pull it out—even if it is on the Sabbath.

Lord, use me as you would see fit to help those in need.
I desire to live a life that is pleasing to you.

DON'T WORRY ABOUT TOMORROW

Worry weighs a person down; an encouraging word cheers a person up. PROVERBS 12:25

Rob was one of those guys who seem to have it all together. He was successful and well liked. But the worry lines on his forehead were like furrows in a freshly plowed field. When he came to my office, he seemed tense, even jumpy.

"I've got fifty things that are bothering me," he said.

"Okay, let's start with number one," I said.

He pulled out a list. "Number one: My thirteen-year-old wants to join the military and fight in a war when he turns eighteen. Two: The stock market is so unpredictable that I may not be able to retire in twenty years like I planned. Three: Insurance premiums keep going up. Four: Same with my taxes. Five: My blood pressure is probably too high. Am I at risk for a heart attack or stroke?"

As Rob continued to read his list, his shoulders slumped as if he had the proverbial albatross around his neck. When he got to number twelve, I stopped him. Most of the things hadn't even happened and maybe never would.

"Rob, let's put your list away."

"But, why? I'm worried that—"

"I can make you a list of my own," I said. One: Your son doesn't even know yet who he wants to take to the middle school dance. Two: The stock market always goes up and down, but over the long term, it always goes up. Three: Taxes and insurance will always go up. Should I continue?"

"No," he said, shaking his head.

"Let's focus instead on things that you can directly affect. For example, despite your list, your blood pressure is still normal at 130/80, so great job on that!"

"Thanks. You have any more great news?"

"I can help you lose fifty pounds, and you won't even feel it."

"Fifty pounds? How would I do that?"

"Hand me your list."

When he handed me the paper, I tore it into pieces and threw it away. "See, don't you feel lighter already? If you take care of what you can take care of, God will take care of the rest." When Rob left, I knew I'd done my job. A few of the worry lines had been replaced with smile lines.

TODAY'S RX

Trust God and live today by faith, moment by moment. Let God worry about tomorrow.

God, when I'm anxious and worried, help me to remember the promise you give in Jeremiah 29:11—that you have plans to prosper me, not to harm me; plans for hope and a bright future. Thank you, Lord, for faithfully providing for me.

VITAL SIGNS OF FAITH

Some people brought to him a paralyzed man on a mat. Seeing their faith, Jesus said to the paralyzed man, "Be encouraged, my child! Your sins are forgiven." But some of the teachers of religious law said to themselves, "That's blasphemy! Does he think he's God?" Jesus knew what they were thinking, so he asked them, "Why do you have such evil thoughts in your hearts? Is it easier to say 'Your sins are forgiven,' or 'Stand up and walk'? So I will prove to you that the Son of Man has the authority on earth to forgive sins." Then Jesus turned to the paralyzed man and said, "Stand up, pick up your mat, and go home!" And the man jumped up and went home! MATTHEW 9:2-7

Today's verses are a great reminder for all health-care workers, myself included.

Before Jesus healed the paralyzed man's physical body, he first took care of the man's spiritual health by forgiving his sins. Only then did he fix the man's seemingly useless legs.

In modern medicine, we often do the opposite. We take great care and skill in fixing people's bodies, but we often don't bother to take their spiritual vital signs. Do they believe in God? Do they have any experiences of his healing work in their lives? Are they afraid of death? Do they have a community of believers in their life praying for them?

We review their physical systems, and we ask how they're doing mentally and emotionally. But we rarely delve any deeper than the obligatory religion check box on the registration form.

Certain religions have specific beliefs and restrictions about which health-care services they want or don't want. If it weren't for those deeply held beliefs, I'm not sure we'd even ask about religion. But what an oversight! A number of studies have shown that if patients are connected spiritually, their physical outcomes improve significantly; that is, it takes less time for them to heal and recover.

I think there's a lesson for all of us in the story of Jesus' healing of the paralyzed man. If we first care for the health of a person's soul, the health of the body will follow.

TODAY'S RX

Check your spiritual vital signs today. Is your heart beating for God? Is the fire of faith burning in your belly? Has the blood of Jesus washed away the burden of your sins?

Father, there are seasons when my spiritual well-being goes unchecked, and I don't take the steps needed to get well. Place it on my heart to pray and be in your Word during these times, so that my faith may continue to grow.

ROLLING THROUGH LIFE

I still dare to hope when I remember this: The faithful love of the LORD never ends!
LAMENTATIONS 3:21-22

"I hear you need some insurance paperwork filled out. How can I help?"

"Ol' Bessie needs a new battery and wheels," Neil said, patting the side of his electric wheelchair. "I've about worn these out."

I looked at the bent rims and worn treads. "Looks like you've been traveling."

"I get around," he said, smiling.

Neil had been a patient of mine since he was in elementary school. He was a good kid but never one to sit still for long. After he graduated from high school, he'd been a promising college student at a nearby university. But that was before the accident.

It all started with a dare. Neil and his frat brothers were out partying one night, and on the way home, somebody bet him that he couldn't get his old Ford pickup up to 100 miles an hour. He had proved them wrong, but he was going too fast as he approached Creekside Curve. Unable to stop in time, he had slid off the road and hit a tree. Now instead of a pickup truck, he drove Ol' Bessie, with a top speed of about four miles per hour.

Bessie might have been slow, but that didn't stop Neil from going wherever he wanted. In the four years since the accident, he'd gone as many places and met as many people as any other twenty-four-year-old I'd known.

"Describe how the accident has affected your daily life," I said, reading from the form.

"Since the accident, I need help with everything. I can push the joystick, and I can talk, but everything else is in God's hands—or in the hands of the angels he's sent to help me," he said, nodding to the young woman assisting him that morning.

"I could have lost my life on that curve, and when I woke up in the ICU, I knew immediately that it was Jesus who'd saved me."

I had heard his story many times, and this was my favorite part.

"I may have lost my previous life, but I gained eternal life. Now I look to Jesus because through him I can do anything. Well, almost anything. I'm still going to need those new wheels and a battery, Doc."

TODAY'S RX

You'll go further in life in the strength of the Lord.

Though my plans are not always the same as yours, Lord, I take comfort in knowing that your plans are best for me. Thank you for intervening in my life and keeping me close to you.

A JOYOUS STAMPEDE OF HEALING

For you who fear my name, the Sun of Righteousness will rise with healing in his wings. And you will go free, leaping with joy like calves let out to pasture. MALACHI 4:2

Back on the farm, springtime is when we'd release the newborn calves from the confines of their calving pens. They'd burst forth from the barn and race toward green pasture, seemingly defying gravity in their pursuit of freedom.

For patients in a doctor's office, the exam room can feel as confining as a calving pen; and for those who are sick, the last thing they feel like doing is frolicking. So I was pleasantly surprised when I entered the exam room one day to see Harvey, a regular patient of mine, who had a rare tumor on his pituitary gland. He seemed surprisingly jubilant considering his health situation.

"Hi, Doc!" he said with enthusiasm. "I just got back from the Mayo Clinic. I think you're going to have to update my chart."

"Okay, why's that?" I said.

"I went there hoping for a cure, but instead the doctors were baffled."

"Why? What happened?"

"Well, before I went, we all prayed for God's guidance for the doctors as they treated my tumor. But my aunt wasn't satisfied with that. She said, 'I'm praying for your complete healing.'"

Harvey's eyes twinkled as he continued. "I'm here to tell you that the miracle my aunt prayed for happened! The tumor is gone! The doctors at Mayo couldn't believe it, but God has cured me!"

Pure joy radiated from his face.

"Sure, I know the tumor could come back someday, but right now I'm convinced that God has cured me. Put that in my chart," he said as he nearly skipped out the door, like a calf bursting forth from the barn.

God wants us to experience the kinds of healings we see in the New Testament. He wants all of us to have freedom from the chains of sin and disease. And when we're healed, he wants us to shout it from the mountaintops and leap for joy.

Though I made the proper notes in Harvey's chart, I didn't have to. The joy of God's faithfulness was something I would never forget!

TODAY'S RX

Today, pray with the confidence that God can open the barn door of your life and release a stampede of joy.

Jesus, I do not thank you enough for the freedom I have in you. You have paid for my sin in full by going to the cross. You have healed me with your love. Because of this, I will praise you all of my days.

HEALING CAN BE A PROCESS

Jesus took the blind man by the hand and led him out of the village. Then, spitting on the man's eyes, he laid his hands on him and asked, "Can you see anything now?" The man looked around. "Yes," he said, "I see people, but I can't see them very clearly. They look like trees walking around." Then Jesus placed his hands on the man's eyes again, and his eyes were opened. His sight was completely restored, and he could see everything clearly. MARK 8:23-25

Jesus could have healed the blind man completely on the first try. So why didn't he? The Gospel of John records a time when Jesus used saliva and mud to cure a blind man. Did he forget the secret mud ingredient this time? Did Jesus mess up?

We can become frustrated when things don't happen the way we want them to—or when we want them to. But I think Jesus did exactly what he intended to do. It's not that Jesus wasn't capable of healing the man instantly. Neither was it because the blind man had done anything wrong. Jesus healed the man the way he did because he wanted us to know something about his healing power.

Sometimes healing doesn't happen instantly. Sometimes healing is a process. I believe that Jesus didn't heal this man on the first try because he wanted to encourage us that even if all we get is a glimpse of the Lord's power, we shouldn't give up.

If your healing hasn't happened in the time, place, or way that you desired or hoped for, keep holding on to the hand of the Savior. Trust him to finish the good work he has started. Not every encounter with God allows us to see him clearly. Sometimes, all we see are blurry visions of "trees walking around." During those moments, it's important to remember that we shouldn't let go; we should continue to let God work.

Whether it is physical healing we're after or just trying to get a better glimpse of what God is doing in our lives, it may take more than one or two encounters before our sight is fully restored. Don't give up on the miracle that God wants to give you.

TODAY'S RX

If at first your prayers do not succeed, pray, pray again!

Lord, it's always in hindsight that I'm able to understand how you've worked in my life. Fill me with your Spirit today that I may trust your ways in the here and now, knowing you are with me wherever I go.

WE'RE AS SICK AS THE SECRETS WE KEEP

Oh, what joy for those whose disobedience is forgiven, whose sin is put out of sight! Yes, what joy for those whose record the LORD has cleared of guilt, whose lives are lived in complete honesty! PSALM 32:1-2

The first thing Jon said to me was, "Dr. Anderson, please don't tell Tammy that I came to see you today."

Jon was a longtime patient, and I knew him well. His wife adored him and trusted him, and together they had two small children. I'd heard that he had recently been promoted at work, and from everything I could see, his life seemed to be going well. But Jon was hiding more than a doctor's appointment from his wife.

"I've gotten myself into a bit of trouble. When I travel to Vegas on business, my buddies and I like to play the tables. Tammy knows that we sometimes stop at the casinos, but I haven't told her how often or how long. Lately, I've been playing higher stakes, and I'm on the verge of losing everything. But there's nowhere to turn. I've thought about suicide, but my insurance policy isn't even enough to bail out my family. I don't know what to do. Can you help me?"

I had no idea the full magnitude of Jon's financial troubles, but I could tell he was in serious emotional distress. If you're in a similar place emotionally, I advise you to seek available help. You're not alone.

"I can help, but it won't be easy," I said. "The first thing you need to do is tell Tammy everything—down to the last penny."

"I know," Jon said as his head and shoulders slumped.

"You also need to find a Gamblers Anonymous meeting and start attending regularly. They can provide the emotional support you need to deal with your addiction."

"Okay," he said.

"Finally, and most importantly, you need to pray. God is the Great Physician; he's always on call, and he can heal you completely if you go to him and admit your weakness.

The next time I saw Jon, he seemed less depressed, and though he wasn't yet out of the woods, he was well on his way to recovery. He had taken my advice, and he was no longer keeping secrets. But I suspect what had helped most was that his wife had forgiven him.

TODAY'S RX

If you've been keeping secrets, repent and ask for forgiveness.

Forgive me, God, for how I have been disobedient to you. Change my heart, and give me control over my words and actions. Thank you for your amazing grace.

TUG-OF-WAR BETWEEN JOY AND GRIEF

I entrust my spirit into your hand. Rescue me, LORD, for you are a faithful God.
PSALM 31:5

I can't tell you how many times I've sat or stood at the bedsides of my patients as they've taken their final breath here on earth. Each time it happens, I'm aware that I'm standing on holy ground.

In those final moments, life and death is a bit like a game of tug-of-war. On one side is a tangible but ailing body with a family who doesn't want to let go. On the other side is heaven with a spiritual body that is free from sickness and disease, and a Savior with outstretched arms, waiting to welcome the patient to his or her forever home.

Knowing what I know of eternity makes it easy to reassure my patients that it is okay to let go of the rope that ties them here so they can run freely into the arms of Jesus.

At the same time, I know that God breathed into us and gave us life here on earth. We should desire to enjoy every breath we have left.

When it comes to the tug-of-war between earthly life and eternal life, I've noticed that the patient often has an easier time letting go of the rope and slipping to the other side than the family who is left behind does. Even after the patient puts down the rope, the family wants to keep tugging, hoping their loved one will return.

The birthing of a new soul into heaven is a special time of joy, but it is also a time of grief. When the tug-of-war between earthly life and eternal life ends, the emotional tugs between joy and grief begin. The grief is just as important as the joy. It is a real emotion for real times that we all experience in this broken world.

TODAY'S RX

Jesus wept at the grave of Lazarus. When the time comes to lose a loved one, so will we. But we also know that there is joy for our loved one on the other side of the veil.

Father, thank you for the gift of life. Help me to make the most of mine and be a shining light to the world.

MAY CHECKUP

With all the activities that transpire before the end of the school year, May can feel like the exhausting final sprint in a yearlong marathon. For those who have children in school, this month can be just as busy as December or perhaps even busier. May is filled with class parties, concerts, athletic team playoffs, and end-of-year banquets. There are graduations from kindergarten, elementary, middle school, high school, and college, as well as all the celebrations, presentations, and parties that go along with them. If you have children who are making a big transition, you want to celebrate their successes and their growth. But you may also feel a little sadness as you realize that your children are moving on to a new stage, and they're becoming more independent. Depending on their age, they might even be moving out of the house.

Throughout the Gospels, we see that when the crowds and activities were most crushing for Jesus, he took a break. He didn't run away or head out on a vacation; he simply withdrew from the commotion temporarily so he could talk to his Father. If the activities and transitions of this month feel overwhelming, see if you can cut back on attending a few events to make time for yourself. Get up a half hour earlier so you can have some extra time to think and pray—or have a much-needed extra cup of coffee. If you're feeling sad or anxious, spend your prayer time pouring out your heart to God, and then stop and listen for his words of wisdom. May is a great time to read the Psalms because David and the other psalmist are so forthcoming about pouring out their emotions to God. It's a great reminder for us to do the same.

In Jesus' day, people walked everywhere they went. Try walking to nearby events. It will give you a few minutes alone, or with your children, to think and reflect. And if you attend all of May's events, be on the lookout for someone else who needs a hug. Lend an ear to those who are having a difficult time with a child's transition—it could be a good opportunity to invite someone for coffee or to your church.

Though May can be a busy month, it is also a time to reflect on how much everyone has grown. Acknowledge and cherish the past, but look forward to the future. As you reflect on whatever changes you face, my prayer for you is that God's blessings will outweigh any past burdens.

May Booster Shot: Don't wait until August for all those back-to-school appointments. Take a moment now to arrange for annual physicals and checkups with your children's doctor, dentist, and optometrist. By getting those appointments on the calendar now, you'll avoid the back-to-school rush and avoid disrupting your summer vacation.

SOUL SURVIVOR

Now may our Lord Jesus Christ himself and God our Father, who loved us and by his grace gave us eternal comfort and a wonderful hope, comfort you and strengthen you in every good thing you do and say. 2 THESSALONIANS 2:16-17

Trey's journey had been most unusual. As I sat down next to him, he began to tell me about it.

"When I was fifteen," he said, "I got drunk and high one night. I was supposed to meet a girl at the crossroads of the main highway and the railroad tracks that ran through town. But she wasn't there, so I just sat down to wait for her. I didn't realize I was sitting in the middle of the train tracks. That's obviously not a smart thing to do, but at the time, I was drunk and high and not thinking clearly."

Trey paused and looked off into the distance, as if remembering something.

"The next thing I remember is a train screeching to a stop. It was as if time stood still in that moment. A light that was so bright surrounded me, and I couldn't see anything else. Then this lone figure approached. It was a man, and he reached out for me. It was my grandfather, and he was asking me if I was ready to go with him."

But Trey's grandfather had died ten years earlier.

"I didn't feel anything when the train hit me. It wasn't until six months later, when I woke up in the ICU with the right side of my skull crushed, that I felt anything at all. I almost died twice."

"What do you mean you almost died twice?" I asked.

The day I woke up was the same day my parents had agreed to remove me from life support. But somehow, Jesus protected me and helped me."

"Wow, that's quite a journey, Trey. How did it change your life?"

"Without a doubt, I knew that it was Jesus who gave me the strength to overcome my injuries. He's been my comfort every day for thirty-five years since it happened. Each day, I wake up looking for him, and he's always right there by me—just like he was when I spent those six months in a coma."

TODAY'S RX

No matter how bad the train wreck, God can put your life back on track.

Father, you are my wonderful hope. Thank you for rescuing me in times of trouble.

CLEAN AND FREE

In one of the villages, Jesus met a man with an advanced case of leprosy. When the man saw Jesus, he bowed with his face to the ground, begging to be healed. "Lord," he said, "if you are willing, you can heal me and make me clean." Jesus reached out and touched him. "I am willing," he said. "Be healed!" And instantly the leprosy disappeared. Then Jesus instructed him not to tell anyone what had happened. He said, "Go to the priest and let him examine you. Take along the offering required in the law of Moses for those who have been healed of leprosy. This will be a public testimony that you have been cleansed." LUKE 5:12-14

Leprosy, also known as Hansen's disease, is a chronic condition that affects the eyes, skin, peripheral nerves, and respiratory tract. Infections and injuries resulting from a lack of sensation can cause everything from wounds to the loss of fingers or toes. Even today, leprosy is difficult to treat, and the scars are permanent.

There are only a few cases of Hansen's disease in the United States today, but from 1894 to 1999, most patients were sent to the national leprosarium in Carville, Louisiana, to be physically isolated from the rest of the population. Currently, treatment is centered on prevention and rendering patients noncontagious by using medications. As a result, patients no longer have to be kept in isolation.

During Jesus' time, leprosy was so highly contagious that people were forbidden to even touch a leper. In many places, lepers had to ring bells and shout, "Unclean!" to warn people. Yet Jesus had no hesitation about touching the lepers he encountered. He reached out and healed them with the touch of his hand.

Though we can now cure Hansen's disease with medications, we cannot reverse the damage already done. Scars don't magically disappear, and missing digits cannot be restored. Yet, when Jesus healed the leper, the man appeared as if he'd never had the disease. This medical miracle points to God's complete control over illness and disease.

Jesus not only wants to heal us physically, but he also wants to heal our social prejudices. By caring for the sick, the outcast, and the downtrodden, Jesus takes those who are unclean and cleanses them physically, spiritually, and culturally.

TODAY'S RX

When Jesus heals us, he cures not only the sickness, but also the social ills that go along with it.

Jesus, I take comfort in knowing that when you died on the cross, you didn't cleanse me of just some of my sin, but all of it. I am a new creation in you, and I thank you for fully restoring my life.

HEALING FAITH

A woman in the crowd had suffered for twelve years with constant bleeding. She had suffered a great deal from many doctors, and over the years she had spent everything she had to pay them, but she had gotten no better. In fact, she had gotten worse. She had heard about Jesus, so she came up behind him through the crowd and touched his robe. For she thought to herself, "If I can just touch his robe, I will be healed." MARK 5:25-28

Lisa came to my office frustrated and exhausted. She was out of money and out of hope.

"I've seen a dozen doctors, and no one has been able to help me. They think I have some kind of neurological problem, but all the tests come back negative. I've used up all my insurance, and I'm nearly broke. Can you help me?"

"I'm not sure I can do more than the other doctors," I said. "But I can pray that God will reveal the problem to us and lead us to a solution."

Looking at her chart, I understood why the other doctors thought she was suffering from a seizure disorder. Still, none of the treatments had worked. Several tests had been repeated multiple times, with inconclusive results. No wonder she was going broke! I scratched my head and prayed. "Lord, help me know where to search for an answer."

As only God would have it, I'd been talking with a cardiologist recently about a new technology at the time—a thirty-day event monitor. I hoped that maybe this new technique would give us the information we needed to diagnose Lisa's mysterious ailment.

For two weeks, nothing happened, but on day fifteen, we captured the data we needed to diagnose a heart condition. Lisa had a pacemaker put in, and she's been doing fine ever since.

In today's verses, a woman who had tried every option and spent every resource in search of healing had only gotten worse. Still, when she heard about Jesus, she believed he could heal her if she could get close enough to touch his robe.

Is that the kind of faith we have? Too often, we take things into our own hands and turn to God only when nothing else works. What would happen if we turned to him *first*?

TODAY'S RX

To be healed, we must have the faith to reach out to Jesus.

Lord, help me to have faith in you. Whether I'm suffering physically, emotionally, or spiritually, show me that all I need is you. Thank you for your great healing power.

NO OBSTACLES TO HEALING

Jesus went over to their synagogue, where he noticed a man with a deformed hand. The Pharisees asked Jesus, "Does the law permit a person to work by healing on the Sabbath?" MATTHEW 12:9-10

A patient came to a Saturday night clinic with symptoms that suggested the possibility of a brain tumor. I wanted an MRI to confirm the diagnosis, but first I thought about the questions the insurance company would ask:

"Is there a less expensive test you can use?"

"Have you talked to the insurance medical director to get permission?"

In this case, it didn't matter, because not only was the patient's insurance company closed for the weekend, but we also didn't have access to any past MRIs or a neurologist to interpret the results. So it's likely that permission would have been denied anyway. Instead, we followed the established protocols and didn't get the MRI until Monday—at which time the diagnosis was confirmed, and the patient began treatment.

Medicine has morphed into something very different from what it was in the days when a doctor and patient worked together to solve a mystery. A third-party payer (the insurance company) has entered the equation, and in many ways it feels like an intrusion into the care and intimacy of the doctor-patient relationship. I understand why it's part of the equation, but the system can be frustrating to sick patients who just want to get well.

Sometimes I envy Jesus' ability to heal all who came to him. My instinct is to help everyone who asks, but often there are artificial barriers to providing treatment. When Jesus healed someone on the Sabbath, he didn't have to get permission from a third-party corporation. And though the Pharisees questioned him, they couldn't stop him from healing. Nor could they stop the flood of people who sought healing from him. Many who sought his healing touch were Gentiles—they didn't even believe in God, yet Jesus healed all who came.

There are no roadblocks to healing when it comes to Jesus. We know that we can confidently call on Jesus to meet our needs—even on the Sabbath. He's never closed for business. His healing isn't limited to a specific group of people. He doesn't need permission. And his resources are unlimited.

TODAY'S RX

Jesus' healing hands are outstretched to all who need his touch.

Help me to have patience, Lord, as I navigate the road to healing. The hurdles I face can be frustrating and exhausting, and I need your strength to persevere. Thank you for going before me and showing me the way.

SET FREE FROM THE LIES

If the Son sets you free, you are truly free. John 8:36

Nothing is more exciting than seeing someone who has been held captive by the enemy's lies set free to live a transformed life.

Peter's story wasn't much different from that of thousands of others who have sought fame and fortune in the entertainment industry.

"I've been a rock musician for years," he said when he came in for treatment. "Made some bad choices over that time."

Recently, his dream had become a nightmare.

"I don't know where else to turn. My voice is shot, and the tremors from the alcohol prevent me from playing my guitar very well. I need help."

In every corner of Nashville, you can find a similar story. Music City is full of the emptiness of broken dreams and unfulfilled aspirations. Hurting hearts are assuaged with alcohol, and emotional pain is numbed with drugs.

As a musician, Peter knew this world better than I did. The years of smoke-filled bars, whiskey shots, and empty beer cans had finally caught up with him.

Miraculously, a thirty-day spot in the rehab unit had opened up that very day, and Peter checked in. I knew many of the staff who worked there, and I was confident that, along with tips on how to stay sober, they would introduce Peter to Jesus when he was ready.

The next time I saw Peter, months later, his smile was something to behold. He seemed happy and peaceful—as if the old demons were gone.

"What are you doing now that you're out?" I asked.

"I've decided to go back to school to become a counselor," he said. "Jesus found me when I was in a very dark hole. He pulled me out, dusted me off, cleansed my heart and soul, and called me his, even though I'd run from him for years. I want to help others find the truth and stop listening to the lies of the enemy."

"Peter, I'm happy to see the transformation that God has done in your life. My prayer is that you'll use your experiences to bring the same life-changing truth to others in Nashville who need to hear it."

TODAY'S RX

Your tomorrow doesn't have to be the same as your yesterday. God's transforming grace is new every morning.

Thank you, Father, for setting me free from a life of hopelessness and struggle. Through your Son, I'm capable of all things, and I praise you for the strength you've given me.

GET TO KNOW HIM

The LORD is good to everyone. He showers compassion on all his creation. PSALM 145:9

"I've always lived my life on the edge," said Ray. "That's why I don't expect I'll live to see sixty."

Ray was fifty-five years old, and he admitted to smoking two packs of unfiltered cigarettes a day and drinking a six-pack of beer every night. He'd also had at least a couple of DUIs and spent time in jail for use and possession of drugs. When he guessed that he wouldn't live to see the age of sixty, it was probably a good guess.

"Here's the deal," I replied. "Only God knows the number of breaths and heartbeats we have left, but you're facing some pretty serious health concerns. Your lungs have been damaged with COPD—chronic obstructive pulmonary disease—and your chest X-ray shows a spot that may be cancerous. I've set up an appointment for you to meet with a pulmonary and thoracic surgeon next Monday."

By the following Thursday, Ray was in surgery, and he returned to my rehab unit the week after that. He seemed liked a different man. He was quieter and showed less bravado.

"You know, Dr. Anderson, I've lived a terrible life, and God is certainly going to punish me for that," he said.

"Let me tell you something, Ray. You don't know God that well. He's not standing by with a sledgehammer, waiting to bash us. No, he showers us with grace. When we're lost and not even looking for him, he pursues us. He shines his blessings on all his creatures—good and bad. When we recognize his goodness and how he has extended his loving-kindness to us, it's natural to want to have a relationship with him. In fact, that's what happened to me many years ago. Had God not found me, I might be standing in your shoes. I just want you to know, it's not too late if you'd like to get to know him better."

"You're right. This cancer diagnosis scared me. When I get out of here, I'm going to church because I want to know him."

That was fifteen years ago, and Ray meant what he said. He just celebrated his seventieth birthday, and his life has become a blessing.

TODAY'S RX

You can't earn God's love, but you can yearn for God's love.

God, I need your grace each day. Thank you for continually pouring it out on me and for pursuing me with your everlasting love.

IN GOD'S TIME, IT'S NEVER TOO LATE

Even when there was no reason for hope, Abraham kept hoping—believing that he would become the father of many nations. For God had said to him, "That's how many descendants you will have!" And Abraham's faith did not weaken, even though, at about 100 years of age, he figured his body was as good as dead—and so was Sarah's womb. ROMANS 4:18-19

The woman in my office reminded me of Abraham's wife, Sarah. She had three beautiful children, and she and her husband had decided to try for a fourth, but after three first-trimester miscarriages, they had just about given up hope. Her obstetrician had told her that her body wouldn't be able to carry another baby.

As she sat in my office, she listed off some vague symptoms of tiredness and nausea and then said, "I know it's unlikely that I'd be pregnant at forty-three, but would you do a pregnancy test just to make sure?"

"Of course," I said.

A woman can still be fertile at forty-three, but this "Sarah" believed it was impossible for her.

We drew her blood, and a few hours later I called her with the result. "The test came back positive. Congratulations!"

As I hung up the phone, I knew she still had many difficult hurdles to face, not the least of which was the first trimester. Would this pregnancy have the same outcome as the last three?

But just as with the biblical Sarah, God showered his grace on this family. Not only did she carry this surprise baby to full term, but she and her husband found new life and joy as the parents of four.

TODAY'S RX

Put your trust in God's wisdom, mercy, and grace. His plans are fulfilled against all medical odds.

Father, I praise you for knowing the desires of my heart and for listening to my requests. You've given me much to be thankful for in this life.

GOD'S GRACE IS FOR ALL

God knows people's hearts, and he confirmed that he accepts Gentiles by giving them the Holy Spirit, just as he did to us. He made no distinction between us and them, for he cleansed their hearts through faith. . . . We believe that we are all saved the same way, by the undeserved grace of the Lord Jesus. ACTS 15:8-9, 11

At times, there are calls from the EMS radio that send shivers down your spine. We got one of those on an otherwise quiet weekend night.

"EMS en route to your facility. MVA. DUI suspected."

As we set up the trauma room for unknown injuries from the motor vehicle accident, we found out there were three victims. One had already been airlifted to Nashville. The other two were being transported by ambulance to our hospital.

The first patient to arrive was the wife of the driver who had been airlifted. When they brought her in, she was crying—not due to her injuries, but for her husband. "Please, doctor, can you find out what happened to my husband? They took him away in a helicopter, and I don't even know if he's dead or alive!"

I nodded at the EMT, and he left to find out the husband's status, while I cleaned up the wife's wounds. She mostly had minor cuts and bruises. While I worked, we prayed for her husband and for God to intervene.

When the EMT returned, he said, "The report is better than we expected. The husband has a ruptured spleen, but they're able to treat it, and everything looks good."

As I walked down the hall to check on the third victim, the drunk driver who had caused the accident, I thanked God for protecting the two innocent victims from greater harm. In the exam room, I found a middle-aged man who was still very inebriated. I checked him out to confirm what the nurse had already determined—there wasn't a scratch on him.

The police requested blood tests, and we decided to hold him overnight to make sure his alcohol levels were safely down before he was taken to jail.

Too often, trauma codes end with the veil of heaven being pulled back to welcome a new soul. But this time, God had been gracious to everyone involved, giving them all more days here on earth.

TODAY'S RX

God shines the light of his mercy on both the evil and the good. Be thankful for his gracious wisdom.

Lord, thank you for pouring out your lavish love on all your people. Help me to reflect that love to all I meet, even those who have hurt me.

NOTHING LASTS FOREVER—ESPECIALLY SUFFERING

In his kindness God called you to share in his eternal glory by means of Christ Jesus. So after you have suffered a little while, he will restore, support, and strengthen you, and he will place you on a firm foundation. 1 Peter 5:10

Tanya hadn't been on the schedule the last time I looked, so I was surprised to see her name penciled in as the last patient of the day. I knocked on the door and entered the exam room. When she saw me, she started to cry.

"What's going on?" I asked, sitting in the chair beside her. She looked tired and thin. "Why are you so sad?"

"I'm not sure I can take another day of this chemo/radiation treatment. I'm only on week three, and it already feels like forever. The oncologist says I need eight weeks, but I don't think I can make it that long. I'm sick and tired of feeling sick and tired."

"Can you tell me more about what's going on?"

"First thing every morning, I throw up everything I ate for dinner the night before. I feel horrible, but I can't go back to bed. I have to get in the car and drive forty-five minutes for another treatment. I've not only lost my hair, but I've lost my appetite. I feel like I've also lost my life!"

"What you're describing isn't unusual. Many people suffer similar side effects. I know it seems unbearable when you're in the middle of it. I've had other patients with the same kind of cancer and the same treatment, and they felt just like you do right now. But they kept fighting, and they made it through, and now they have their lives back."

"I guess I just needed to hear that there's hope, and that this will all be worth it."

"I know you can't see the end yet, but this treatment shows promise. Let's pray for strength and restoration for your body and your spirit."

Tanya and I prayed together, and she seemed reassured and committed to seeing the treatment through.

Suffering in any form is hard to take, but it helps to know that it won't last forever. Even in this broken world, our suffering is only for a little while.

TODAY'S RX

When life is hard, take one step at a time and watch for God's faithfulness in the journey.

Give me strength and energy today, God, to do all that is required of me. Help me to manage my stress and have a positive outlook on my work and responsibilities.

A RENEWED HEART

The LORD will work out his plans for my life—for your faithful love, O LORD, endures forever. Don't abandon me, for you made me. PSALM 138:8

"Dr. Anderson, my ticker is doing that thing again," Derrick said. "I feel it racing, like it wants to jump out of my chest, and then I get short of breath. You don't suppose God brought me all this way just to take me now, do you?"

"Tell me more about what's going on."

"I can't even walk up a flight of stairs without running out of breath. Ever since the heart attack, things have been a little haywire, but I believe this is something worse."

"Okay, let's get you to the hospital, just to make sure it's not."

"That sounds good," Derrick said.

His response nearly floored me. Derrick was the kind of guy who resisted any kind of medical intervention. With his first myocardial infarction, he argued with me the entire time, but now he seemed to have had the wind blown out of his sails—and that concerned me.

At the hospital, we consulted with Derrick's regular cardiologist, who had placed three stents into Derrick's cardiac arteries just six months earlier. After the examination, I told Derrick the news.

"Dr. Johnson says your plumbing is okay. All the stents are still wide open. But the myocardial infarction knocked out some of your electrical pathways. That's why you feel your heart jumping around so much. You're going to need a pacemaker and a defibrillator. Dr. Steinfeld will be here in a few minutes to explain how it will work. Until he gets that done, we have to keep you in the ICU to make sure you stay safe."

Derrick looked defeated. "I'm kinda worried that I won't make it through this one."

I shared today's verse from the book of Psalms with him. "Just like your doctors have a plan for your physical heart, God has a plan for your spiritual heart, too. More than anything, he wants you to trust him."

Derrick was quiet for a moment. "Thanks, Dr. Anderson."

Derrick's surgery went smoothly, and a few months later, he stopped by for a blood pressure check. All he could talk about was the miracle that God had done in his heart—literally and figuratively. God had not abandoned Derrick, and Derrick was grateful.

TODAY'S RX

A healthy heart is a thankful heart. Thank God for his faithfulness today.

Father, thank you for faithfully caring for me every day. Provide me with energy and rest and healing today, and show me how best to take care of myself.

SEEING HIS ANSWER

Abraham never wavered in believing God's promise. In fact, his faith grew stronger, and in this he brought glory to God. He was fully convinced that God is able to do whatever he promises. And because of Abraham's faith, God counted him as righteous. And when God counted him as righteous, it wasn't just for Abraham's benefit. It was recorded for our benefit, too, assuring us that God will also count us as righteous if we believe in him, the one who raised Jesus our Lord from the dead. ROMANS 4:20-24

You've hoped and you've prayed. You've given and forgiven. You feel as if you've done everything God has asked of you, yet the disease still ravages your body unabated. In that dark moment, ask yourself a different question: What if God's answer to my prayer is not the same as what I'm asking for?

If God answers your prayers differently from how you want him to, does that mean prayer doesn't work? Do you give up on him?

God is the potter, and we are the clay. God molded us into being and breathed life into us. Without him, we would not be here to ask these questions.

Does the clay tell the potter that he isn't doing it right?

At first, Abraham doubted God's promise that he would become the father of nations. In fact, he doubted he would become the father of even one. God eventually answered Abraham's prayer, but it wasn't how or when Abraham expected.

How would history be different if Abraham had stayed true to God's promises and hadn't had a son with Hagar? The conflict between the descendants of Abraham's two sons continues to this day.

Do we also risk future problems when we twist God's promises to fit our own desires? I know at times I've prayed for healing for my patients because that's what *I* wanted. Later, I discovered that their cancer had spread. Did God not answer my prayers?

Sometimes God's miraculous healing is to bring the patient's soul back to life, even as the body withers away. Is that not an answer to prayer?

Pray for God's will and not your own. Whatever answer comes, believe that it is God's complete and perfect will.[5]

TODAY'S RX

God is faithful to answer our prayers, and his plan is perfect. Sometimes we have to adjust our expectations.

Help me to remain faithful to you, Lord, when my prayers seem unanswered. Do not let me fall away. I know all the days of my life are in your hand, and I take comfort in that.

A NEW HOME AWAITS

You have decided the length of our lives. You know how many months we will live, and we are not given a minute longer. Job 14:5

The news wasn't good. The test results revealed that Gregory wouldn't be around much longer. He'd fought long and hard against the cancer, but the cancer had spread and was starting to shut down his organs. I needed to be the one to deliver the news to him—one of the least favorite parts of my job.

I entered his room just as the late evening shadows began to stretch from his window toward the white sheets of his hospital bed. I pulled up a chair next to him and gave him the news he was expecting.

"We know our time on this earth is short, and I'm afraid, Gregory, that yours is coming to an end. We've fought hard together to battle this cancer, but it has finally won."

"There is nothing else to do?" he asked.

"We've turned over every stone. The best doctors at the Mayo Clinic and the MD Anderson Cancer Center have seen you. They've both told you the same thing. There isn't anything more we can do."

"I guess that means that death has won."

"Over the past five years of this journey, we've talked about how death is the key to life. Jesus died so that you may live for eternity. Though your life ends here on earth, there is a forever home waiting for you in heaven with our Lord and Savior."

"So my days on earth are numbered, but my days in heaven will be innumerable."

"That is true for all of us who have accepted Jesus as Lord. We have prayed for your body, mind, and soul to be healed for the past five years. Now you will see that healing completed."

"I want to live each day here that I can, but I also look forward to seeing Jesus."

"As you live out your remaining hours, I think you will begin to see the new life that awaits you with Jesus, and you will look forward to your new home. Just know that your last breath here will be followed by a breath of the sweet air of heaven."

TODAY'S RX

Our days on earth are numbered, and we all face death. But with Jesus, we will embrace a new life.

Lord, when my time comes to leave this world and see you face-to-face, give me peace. Help me to let go of earthly cares and to be ready for the joys of heaven.

SPILL YOUR JOY

I have told you these things so that you will be filled with my joy. Yes, your joy will overflow! John 15:11

Jesus died on the cross to restore our broken relationship with our heavenly Father. We no longer have to worry about whether we measure up to God's perfect laws because Jesus has supplied our righteousness. We also no longer have to be concerned about the future because Jesus has already taken care of it. He is the eternal well of joy, and he wants us to celebrate with him, be filled with his glory, and have our joy increase.

We know that Jesus enjoyed parties because his first miracle took place at a wedding when the hosts ran out of wine. If Jesus were as solemn and serious as we sometimes make him out to be, he probably would have avoided the fun and allowed the party to end so that he could get back to doing the *important* things he came to do.

But Jesus didn't want the party to end. Instead, he helped it continue by turning water into the most delicious wine the guests had ever tasted. Talk about bringing joy! Imagine how the servants must have felt as they watched the host and his guests celebrate.

Jesus is the source of our joy. We don't have to ask whether our cup is half full or half empty, because Jesus has filled us until our joy runs over the brim. As we allow him to pour into us, our cups will continually overflow. The joy that spills out of us will flow to our neighbors and throughout our communities. Eventually, our joy will flow to the next town, the next state, and the next country, until the entire world is soaked in the joy of Jesus.

TODAY'S RX

When your glass seems empty, look to the Lord, and he will fill it to the brim with joy.

My heart is full when I worship you, God. Your spirit fills me with joy and delight. Allow me to be a source of encouragement and light to those I see and meet with today.

WHOLLY FORGIVEN

Since God chose you to be the holy people he loves, you must clothe yourselves with tenderhearted mercy, kindness, humility, gentleness, and patience. Make allowance for each other's faults, and forgive anyone who offends you. Remember, the Lord forgave you, so you must forgive others. COLOSSIANS 3:12-13

The Alday family had helped build the church they attended, and they were cornerstones of the community. Jimmy and Jerry were hardworking, God-fearing young men and two of the best Christian examples I've ever known. They never tolerated cursing or any kind of disrespect—especially toward women. God was very much a part of their lives in both the big and little things. They were always quick to credit God if something good happened.

The Aldays were distant cousins, and we spent summers together selling watermelons at the Farmer's Market in Atlanta. They tutored me in how to trust God and be thankful for everything. They wanted me to grow up to be more than a good man; they wanted me to be a godly man.

When I was sixteen, my dad showed up at the door of my history class one day with horrific news. Jimmy and Jerry had been murdered, along with their brother Chester; their father, Ned; and Ned's brother, Aubrey. Worse yet, Jerry's wife, Mary, was missing.

The next day, I learned that Mary had been found dead in the woods. Two prison escapees were later found and convicted of the crime, but my world had already flipped upside down. For years, I carried a grudge in my heart as I ran from God. Over the next seven years, I became an atheist and didn't pray once. My spiritual life was a dark abyss. The light had gone out in my heart, and all my relationships were self-centered.

But one day, Jesus revealed himself and his plans for me in a dream. All at once, I understood his forgiveness and was able to pray, "Lord, please forgive me for the hatred I have for the men who murdered my family and friends." Instantly, the fire of heaven reignited my spirit, and I began to live fully again in body, mind, and spirit.

If unforgiveness has been a barrier in your life, pray that the Lord of forgiveness will once again shine his light in your heart.[6]

TODAY'S RX

Broken people break. Forgiven people forgive. Forgive and be whole.

Jesus, help me to lay my burdens at your feet. I've shouldered them for too long, and they've kept me from having a heart that beats for you. Reignite my spirit today.

TELLING GOD'S STORIES

I lift my eyes to you, O God, enthroned in heaven. We keep looking to the LORD our God for his mercy, just as servants keep their eyes on their master, as a slave girl watches her mistress for the slightest signal. PSALM 123:1-2

One afternoon, after finishing my rounds at the hospital, I called my wife to tell her I'd be home as soon as I stopped by the nursing home. After seeing the patients I'd gone to see there, I was on my way out the door when one of the nurses stopped me.

"Dr. Anderson? I'm sorry to bother you, but can you check on Coach before you leave?"

Her request was so nonchalant that I assumed Coach probably needed company more than he needed a doctor. But I was happy to do it. He had been one of my first patients, and we'd been friends for more than twenty-five years.

How are you feeling?" I asked Coach as I entered his room.

"I'm really good, but I'm getting tired of this world. I'm ready to go."

"I understand," I said. "But we can take assurance in knowing that, even before we were born, God recorded the number of our days on earth in the book of life."

My words were meant to encourage him, but he didn't seem to be paying attention. Instead, he was looking past me, up and to the right, in what I've come to call "the gaze of glory." I've often seen it with patients who are about to leave this world.

I pulled up a chair and sat down. Coach was smiling from ear to ear, as if he had heard something wonderful.

"If you're gazing at glory, that's good," I reassured him. "We'll all be okay if you go on ahead. We'll be joining you soon enough."

As soon as I spoke those words, Coach's breathing changed. It wasn't much longer before I sensed the parting of the veil between earth and heaven, like someone opening a door on a spring day, and Coach stepped ever so gently into eternity.

Had I left the nursing home when I planned to, I would have missed saying *bon voyage* to Coach. In that moment, I was reminded of the importance of keeping our eyes on God and being responsive to the nudge of the Holy Spirit.

TODAY'S RX

You are part of God's unfolding story. Take a moment today to tell someone what he is doing in your life.

Father, what a comfort it is to know that every day of my life is recorded in your book. Help me to use my days wisely and to continue telling your story to the world.

HOLDING TIGHT TO HOPE

Let us hold tightly without wavering to the hope we affirm, for God can be trusted to keep his promise. HEBREWS 10:23

I've had the privilege of escorting many of my patients to heaven's front door. When I am with them during their last moments on earth, the environment in the room changes. A peace that surpasses all understanding enters the room, and a calm takes over. In these moments, I know God is preparing to welcome them to their forever home.

I witnessed this happen again recently.

I was at the hospital making my regular rounds, and my next patient was in an adjacent building. While walking down the enclosed corridor between the buildings, I heard a code alert on the PA and realized it was for my patient. I quickened my pace.

Marco was so ill that he appeared much older than his forty-five years. His lungs were in such bad condition from smoking that he had been on oxygen for nearly a year. Yet, when the ambulance crew had picked him up to bring him to the hospital, they reported that he was smoking with his oxygen on.

We had tried everything we could to untangle him from his addiction to tobacco but without success. When I heard the code alert, I knew that his lungs were likely failing for the last time.

I thought about the conversations we'd had over the past few years. He'd never been open to talking about his spiritual health—until last year. That's when he had accepted Jesus and started getting involved in his local church—as much as his health limitations would allow.

When I entered Marco's room, it was controlled chaos as the code team did its work. When they realized I was there, all eyes were on me for guidance.

I knew that Marco wanted us to try CPR, but he didn't want to be placed on life support. He was content with God's timing. After a short trial of CPR, we called time of death. As everyone else left the room, I lingered to feel God's presence. He had kept his promise to Marco to heal him for all eternity. Someday, he'll keep the same promise for us, as well.

TODAY'S RX

Make time today to record your end-of-life instructions. Decisions made in advance allow everyone there to be fully present in the moment.

I can only imagine how it must feel to be fully restored in body, mind, and spirit, Lord. Thank you for the promise of eternal life with you. Help me to sense your presence while I live out my time on earth and to draw near to you for your comforting embrace.

THE ENEMY IS CANCER

The eternal God is your refuge, and his everlasting arms are under you. He drives out the enemy before you; he cries out, "Destroy them!" DEUTERONOMY 33:27

When we read today's verse, we know from its context that the armies fighting against the Israelites are the enemies that God drives out. Though this was written in Old Testament times, this verse is still applicable today. In my medical practice I hear God cry out, "Destroy them!" in a very different way.

Here's one example:

Bryant came in to get the results of a bone marrow test.

"The report confirmed our worst fear," I said. "I'm sorry to say . . . it's leukemia."

"But I was in six months ago, and all my blood work was normal."

"You're right. There was no hint of it at that time."

"So, how long have I had it?"

"It's hard to say. This is a fairly aggressive form of leukemia, but the good news is that we've caught it early on. I'll get an appointment for you to see the oncologist in the morning, and we will do what we can to defeat this enemy." Before he left, I promised to pray for him.

A week later, a letter from the oncologist confirmed what I had told Bryant. It was definitely leukemia, but being in an early phase made it treatable. The day after the oncologist examined him, Bryant started his treatment, and we all prayed for the best.

Six months later, Bryant stopped by my office.

"Great news, Dr. Anderson! The leukemia is in remission. And the oncologist is very hopeful."

We chatted about the good news, and before Bryant left, he said, "The Lord has given me new strength and new hope. Thank you for praying for me."

God hears our prayers, and he desires to drive out our enemies, even if they are unseen rogue cancer cells.

TODAY'S RX

Prayer can be the weapon that fights even the worst diagnosis. Remember, with God all things are possible—even driving out cancer.

Lord, you are the ultimate source of power and strength. Thank you for giving me courage to battle my illness. I look forward to when I stand victorious in your sight.

NO ONE CAN STAND IN THE WAY OF GOD'S HEALING

One day while Jesus was teaching, some Pharisees and teachers of religious law were sitting nearby. . . . And the Lord's healing power was strongly with Jesus. LUKE 5:17

Consider the scene described in today's verse. Jesus was teaching, and the Pharisees were sitting nearby. They weren't there to learn from the great teacher; they were there to catch him doing something against the law of Moses. Instead of absorbing his teaching, they took note of every infraction against the prevailing religious system of the day.

The verse tells us that God gave Jesus the power to heal. In fact, in the verses that follow, Jesus heals a paralyzed man. But consider for a moment how the Pharisees' presence must have affected both Jesus and the crowd. Perhaps there were some who needed healing, but they were afraid to come forward because they knew the Pharisees were watching. And as Jesus taught and healed, he must have been aware of what the Pharisees were saying about him. The religious leaders should have done everything they could to help their fellow citizens receive healing. Instead, they actively worked against Jesus.

Are there people who have tried to block your healing? Has someone who should be on your side prevented you from getting the treatment you need?

These days, it seems that all the Pharisees work for insurance companies. The healing practice of medicine has never before seen such scrutiny.

Daily, if not hourly, I am drawn away from seeing patients in order to answer questions, fill out another prior authorization form, or defend why I have chosen a specific course of treatment. With the implementation of the Affordable Care Act, the expense and delay from these third-party adjudicators has escalated exponentially.

Have you and your doctor had to go to battle against these modern-day Pharisees? It can be very disheartening. The paperwork and phone calls can feel overwhelming to sick patients and their families. But keep faith in your health-care provider. He or she truly wants to see you get healthy. Don't give up. Though it is often frustrating, I've found that persistence and reason can prevail.

Finally, remember that Jesus didn't allow the Pharisees to prevent him from doing God's healing work. If it is his will, he will heal you without their help.

TODAY'S RX

If you're facing an insurance battle, pray for perseverance and keep on trusting.

Father, I take comfort in knowing that my healing process is in your hands. You alone know what stands before me, so I ask for patience and peace as I journey through.

KING DAVID'S SICK DAY

The LORD nurses them when they are sick and restores them to health. PSALM 41:3

Have you ever been so sick that you thought you were going to die? Over the years, I've had many patients who were so ill that they weren't able to see me until after they started feeling better. A few have even remarked that they would have to get better to go to their own funeral!

Though we don't often think of biblical characters as having to take a sick day, in Psalm 41 we see King David doing just that. He was lying in his bed because he didn't feel well. I don't know how dire his condition was, but those closest to him were saying they didn't think he would make it. So what did David do? He cried out to the Lord in prayer.

The Lord listens to our prayers and lamentations when we are ill and in need of being nursed back to health. I know he does because I've experienced the healing power of prayer many times.

Recently, while making my rounds at the hospital, I stopped by the bedside of a patient who was very ill. We had tried several different kinds of medication, but nothing seemed to be working, and he continued to deteriorate. That day, he asked me to consult not as a doctor but as a friend.

"Would you pray with me for God to relieve me from my pain and sickness?" he asked.

I had been praying for him silently since I had admitted him, but that day we spoke prayers of healing out loud together. Gradually, from that moment on, he began to feel better.

Some might say that the medication had finally kicked in, but I would beg to differ. "The earnest prayer of a righteous person has great power and produces wonderful results" (James 5:16).

TODAY'S RX

If you are ailing, petition God for healing, early and often.

God, please bring relief to those who are suffering and healing to their bones. Take away their pain and restore them to full health. I, too, need rest and ask for your comforting presence over me this day.

A LACK OF RESOURCES, BUT NO LACK OF FAITH

At that time Jesus prayed this prayer: "O Father, Lord of heaven and earth, thank you for hiding these things from those who think themselves wise and clever, and for revealing them to the childlike." MATTHEW 11:25

In my career as a country doctor, there have been times when I felt as if the big-city doctors, with all of their specialties and resources, unfairly judged those of us who work with the rural poor.

For example, in the earliest days of my practice, whenever I referred patients to the regional hospital, I would receive a standard letter updating me on the patient's status. Often, these letters would list things that should have been done but weren't—maybe a battery of tests or lab work.

When I read those letters, I felt as if the other doctors were judging me—as if they assumed I didn't know that additional testing should be done or that somehow I wasn't competent to make the diagnosis. The truth was that the tests in question weren't available anywhere in the county where I worked. I had to send my patients to a doctor in the city who had access to the regional hospital and additional resources. When I could, I called ahead and personally spoke to the doctor. But I often felt as if these specialists unreasonably expected us to diagnose rare and difficult diseases without the proper means.

Certainly some of the judgment I felt at the time was in my own mind. I was a neophyte doctor who was still learning the ropes. As I became more familiar with the system, I tried harder to communicate that our limitations were due to a lack of resources, not a lack of knowledge. And I no longer read their letters as judgments of me. The hospitals have changed as well. Today they are more likely to express their gratitude for our collaboration and thank us for the preliminary work we've done with the patients.

Whatever I lack in material resources, I make up for in faith. I depend on Jesus to provide healing for my patients in ways that go beyond our limitations. While the proud may trust in their education and medical advancements, the rest of us trust in God.

TODAY'S RX

God's healing power is our number one resource for healing. Have the faith of a child that our heavenly Father can heal us.

God, soften my heart so that I may have childlike wonder again.
Remove whatever it is that prevents me from putting all of my trust
in you. Thank you that there are no limits to your healing power.

HEALING OUTSIDE THE BOX

When Jesus returned to Capernaum, a Roman officer came and pleaded with him, "Lord, my young servant lies in bed, paralyzed and in terrible pain." Jesus said, "I will come and heal him." MATTHEW 8:5-7

Though I've read the story of the Roman officer many times over the years, I am still astonished that he came to Jesus for help.

The Roman soldiers assigned to Palestine despised the locals. Being relegated to such a backwater outpost of the Roman Empire wasn't good for their career prospects. So they took out their frustrations on the Jewish people. Under such circumstances, it was almost unfathomable for one to ask a local healer for help.

In order for this officer to come to Jesus, he must have exhausted all other options and exceeded the expertise of the Roman doctors.

But how had he come to believe that Jesus could heal the servant? Why would he think that asking Jesus would be any more effective than anything he'd already tried?

I believe he must have witnessed Jesus' healing power or at least heard about some of the healing miracles Jesus had performed. Because of this, he had faith that Jesus could heal his servant, even when all other remedies had failed. And it was his faith that compelled him to approach Jesus, despite the social taboos.

It's easy for us to get stuck in a certain mind-set or set of beliefs about how healing happens. For many doctors, the thought of asking a practitioner of alternative medicine for help would be as foreign as a Roman officer asking a Jewish rabbi for help. Early on in my own practice, for me to believe that chiropractors and acupuncturists, for example, had something to offer my patients, I first had to witness their healing prowess. Only then did I feel comfortable inviting them to join me in treating my patients. Since then, I've had many positive and enlightening experiences with alternative healing practitioners, and I have become more open to collaboration.

Are you stuck in a belief system that is preventing you from getting healing or getting healthy? Challenge yourself to faith that someone outside of your usual circle may have something to add to your healing.

TODAY'S RX

God can use many different practitioners for healing. While continuing to trust God, open your mind to new ideas and new techniques.

Father, you are the creator of the universe. Your power is not confined. Help me to remember that when I feel boxed in and let down by the usual routine. Show me the way.

GRANDMA'S HOPE, GOD'S MIRACLE

I pray that God, the source of hope, will fill you completely with joy and peace because you trust in him. Then you will overflow with confident hope through the power of the Holy Spirit. ROMANS 15:13

"I'm having pain in my right side," said Trina. "I have indigestion and a lot of gas that seems to get worse when I eat a fatty meal. What do you think is wrong?"

Trina was a classic gallbladder case. She presented with the four *F*s we use to diagnose it: forty, fertile, fat, and flatulent. Though her presentation was textbook, something about her case seemed different.

I started by testing her gallbladder. The test results showed a tumor in the pancreas, but it was barely visible on the ultrasound. I ordered a CT scan, which revealed that Trina had a large tumor covering her abdomen. I sent her for consultations with gastrointestinal and oncology surgeons, and they both agreed: A Whipple procedure was Trina's only hope; otherwise, she would have less than a year to live. But the Whipple procedure wasn't a guarantee. It is a complex operation that would remove parts of her pancreas and small intestine, along with her gallbladder.

When we met in my office to discuss her options, Trina said, "I've prayed and prayed and decided to go through with this. Not so much for me, but because I'm raising my two grandsons, and they need me to be here for them."

"Trina, I know this decision isn't easy, but I'm confident that God will honor your prayers. He will sustain you and fill you with peace, hope, and joy, even during the difficult days ahead."

Trina had surgery a few days later and came through without any problems—which, considering that her condition was much more complicated than originally diagnosed, was something of a miracle. From the initial diagnosis through a very complex surgery, God had heard and answered our prayers.

Four years later, not only has Grandma Trina been cured, but she is also filled with hope for the future as she watches her grandsons grow into the men God intended them to be.

My faith has been strengthened as well. I know that the Lord must have some mighty plans for those young men because he miraculously preserved Grandma Trina to raise them.

TODAY'S RX

God is able. With him, even the most difficult journey is possible.

Help me not to despair, Lord, when the road ahead is scary. I know you are able, and I trust that you will carry me through the heights and depths of this journey. Thank you for being near.

MIND OF GOD

May you have the power to understand, as all God's people should, how wide, how long, how high, and how deep his love is. Ephesians 3:18

The human mind is truly a miracle. No other creature's brain has the capacity for abstract thought. Look around at the countless examples of what men and women have first imagined and then built. Where did this unique thinking machine come from? What separates us from the rest of creation? Why is it that we've been given the ability to read and write the words on this page?

These brains of ours are such an amazing gift that I feel we have a responsibility to use them in equally amazing ways. Do we use our minds to know more about our Creator? Do we work to expand our understanding in every direction so we can comprehend the love he has for us? Do we use our ability to understand in order to help one another live fuller, more God-directed lives?

In the medical world, most professionals—whether they are believers or not—use their minds to help others. This is true in many other professions as well, such as teaching. Too often, though, people have used their ability to imagine and create to cause disruption and destruction in the world. What a waste of such a miraculous gift!

If I had a prayer for all of humanity, it would be that we recognize how privileged we are to have such power to think and imagine and that we would all use that power to meditate on the idea in today's verse. But even with a lifetime of mental concentration, I am not sure that we could ever fully comprehend the love of God. Remember, it was the loving mind of God that created our beautiful brains in the first place and gave us the ability to think about him.

TODAY'S RX

Expand your mind so you can know how much God loves you.

God, expand my mind through your Word so that I may know you better. Help me to use my words and thoughts for good, not evil, and provide me with opportunities to continue growing in my knowledge of you.

RELIGHTING A CANDLE IN THE DARKNESS

He reached down from heaven and rescued me; he drew me out of deep waters. He rescued me from my powerful enemies, from those who hated me and were too strong for me. They attacked me at a moment when I was in distress, but the LORD supported me. He led me to a place of safety; he rescued me because he delights in me.
2 SAMUEL 22:17-20

Twelve-year-old Cami had been kicked out of the house for being pregnant. The man who had gotten her pregnant paid for an abortion and drove her to the clinic.

She'd lived on the streets ever since. When Cami came to the ER with various illnesses and injuries, I could only imagine the horror of her everyday life. Over the next few years, she had two more abortions, and I saw her in the ER after each one.

It wasn't surprising that Cami soon found herself in the deep waters of addiction. The drugs helped to numb the pain she was living. The next time I saw her, I could see the despair in her eyes.

"Can you help me?" she asked. "I have nowhere to go. My going price on the streets isn't even enough to feed myself."

In my mind, this was as much of an emergency as any heart attack or stroke. "Of course, we'll do what we can," I said, "but it won't be easy."

We admitted her and started her on antidepressants. Then we began to detox her system from the other drugs. "I'm going to call social services to help you find a safe place to land when you leave here," I said.

It wasn't easy watching Cami go through withdrawal, but deliverance from that bondage was necessary to restore light in her dark life.

When she left the hospital, she had a clean mind and body, some resources to start a new life, and a lot of our prayer. But she also left with all the ghosts of the past, and her journey would not be easy. Only with God's help could she make it the rest of the way.

When I saw her six months later, she was a new woman—completely clean and sober, with a job and a place to live. Best of all, she had recovered something she'd lost long ago: her self-respect

TODAY'S RX

When life is at its darkest, trust God to relight the candle.

As Psalm 119:105 says, "Your word is a lamp to guide my feet and a light for my path." Thank you for your wisdom and direction, Lord. Continue lighting my path, so I may know the way to go.

GONE AHEAD TO OUR TRUE HOME

When you go through deep waters, I will be with you. When you go through rivers of difficulty, you will not drown. When you walk through the fire of oppression, you will not be burned up; the flames will not consume you. For I am the LORD, your God, the Holy One of Israel, your Savior. I gave Egypt as a ransom for your freedom; I gave Ethiopia and Seba in your place. ISAIAH 43:2-3

Gerald and Alice had moved more times when it wasn't their choice than anyone should ever have to.

In 2010, they survived the Tennessee flood but lost their house and everything in it. They were thankful that their lives had been spared, but they faced an uncertain future with only the clothes on their backs.

They worked hard and managed to scrape together enough money to buy a doublewide trailer, which they parked on the site of their former house. They were proud of their new place and once again felt at home.

But then tragedy struck again.

One night while Gerald and Alice were sleeping, a fire started in a back room. It swept through the mobile home into their bedroom and ignited an oxygen tank that assisted Gerald's breathing. Miraculously, they escaped unharmed; though, once again they had only the clothes on their backs—the pajamas they were wearing that night.

A few months later, Habitat for Humanity provided them with a new house on a new lot where they could start fresh. But their time together didn't last long. Not long after they moved into their new home, Gerald's health problems, which he had battled for so many years, finally took his life.

When Alice came in to see me, I wasn't surprised that she was burdened with sadness. But then she told me about Gerald's last few days.

"He told me that God was truly God, and he was thankful because God had spared us from so much. I agree. We've been blessed."

Once again, I marveled at her strength and the strength of her faith. "How are you doing now that he's gone?" I asked.

"He's not gone," Alice said. "He's just up ahead, and I know where he is. He's in heaven. And there's no doubt in my mind that he's helping Jesus prepare our forever home."

TODAY'S RX

Beyond every disaster here on earth, God is ready to repair what is broken.

Father, your arms are a safe shelter. May I always run to them in times of need.

LIVING IN THE NOW BUT LOOKING FORWARD TO THE NEW

We are citizens of heaven, where the Lord Jesus Christ lives. And we are eagerly waiting for him to return as our Savior. He will take our weak mortal bodies and change them into glorious bodies like his own, using the same power with which he will bring everything under his control. PHILIPPIANS 3:20-21

Next up on the day's schedule was an appointment for two brothers. Seeing two siblings at once isn't unusual in my family practice, but when I opened their charts, I saw that these brothers were a special pair.

The boys were busy bantering when I walked in, but their mother was on a mission. She got right to the point.

"Robby and Randy need a new primary care physician to help manage their muscular dystrophy. Our old doctor retired, but he said you should be able to take care of them."

"I'd be honored and delighted to do that for you," I said.

"Thank you for working us into your practice," she said. "Ever since their dad died a few years ago, we depend a lot on our family and friends to help us."

The boys were intelligent and kind, and I could see they had not let their disability get the better of them. They used every ounce of battery juice and every inch of tire tread on their wheelchairs to explore the world around them.

"Both boys are trapped in crippled bodies by that terrible disease," their mother said. "But there's also a light that shines from deep within both of them."

"That's because we know that one day we'll have new bodies," Robby said.

"We can't wait for Jesus to give us new legs, so we can run to meet him," Randy added.

"I get it," I said. "And I'm here to help you have the healthiest journey you can until the day you exchange those wheels for strong legs."

Eventually, we all have parts of our mortal bodies that don't work the way we'd like. For most of us, it isn't as drastic as muscular dystrophy. But we can all look forward to the day when our mortal bodies are transformed and renewed. Until then, I want to live every day like these brothers—aware of my limitations, but living life fully in spite of them.

TODAY'S RX

Even as you wait for a new body in eternity, live your life to the fullest.

Jesus, thank you for my body—for its strengths and its weaknesses. Its strengths help me to live more fully for you, and its weaknesses help me to depend on you. May I always treat my body with care.

HEART HEALTH

Christ will make his home in your hearts as you trust in him. Your roots will grow down into God's love and keep you strong. Ephesians 3:17

Over the past thirty years, cardiology has changed more than any specialty I've seen.

During the 1980s, the idea of angioplasty was developed. This procedure calls for passing a narrow tube, called a catheter, up to the heart through an artery in the groin. From the digital pictures it provides, cardiologists can see whether everything is working properly.

If there is a blockage, doctors can use a procedure called balloon angioplasty, in which a small balloon is inserted into the catheter and threaded along until it reaches the clogged vessel. There, it is inflated to flatten the plaque that is causing the blockage and help increase blood flow.

Later, stents were developed and introduced to keep blocked arteries open long term. The stent uses a small, metal mesh tube that acts like a scaffold to provide support for a blocked blood vessel.

These are just a couple of examples of the new technologies and medical devices that are now available to keep the heart alive. When I hear about each new development, I'm reminded of something a very wise heart surgeon once told me: "Protect your heart; you've only got one!"

I think the writers of the Bible could relate to that statement. Perhaps that's why they use this vital organ so often as a metaphor for spiritual things. Our physical strength is derived from our heart. When the heart malfunctions, everything else starts to fail. Spiritually speaking, our heart is also central to our spiritual strength. If Jesus lives in our hearts, it seems that everything else—mind, body, and soul—works together in harmony. This allows our love for God, and for others, to grow rich and strong.

TODAY'S RX

Protect your heart (physically and spiritually). You've only got one!

Make your home in my heart, Lord. I offer it to you.

MIRACLES OF FAITH

Jesus turned around, and when he saw her he said, "Daughter, be encouraged! Your faith has made you well." And the woman was healed at that moment. MATTHEW 9:22

The EMS radio squawked, "Forty-five-year-old . . . white . . . female. Emergency transfer to your facility. ETA of five minutes. Heart rate: 175. Shortness of breath. Chest pain.

When the patient arrived and was hooked up to a heart monitor, the information on the screen led us quickly to a diagnosis of supraventricular tachycardia—an abnormally rapid heart rhythm.

"You're having a cardiac arrhythmia," I said to the anxious patient, "and we're going to give you some medication to temporarily stop your heart."

She looked at me like I was crazy. "You're going to stop my heart? What if it doesn't start back up?"

Her question was valid. It crossed my mind every time I did this procedure. But my training and experience gave me confidence that her heart would restart. It was my job to instill that same confidence in her so I could do what I needed to do to help her.

"God designed your heart with a reset button, kind of like your computer. You may feel a little funny when your heart stops, but if you trust the knowledge he has given us, soon your heart will be back in rhythm."

We gave her the medication, and for the next few seconds—though it always seems like an eternity—we watched the flat line on the monitor. About five seconds later, we got the first beat. Gradually, the patient's heart rate increased to thirty beats per minute—then forty, sixty, and finally seventy as it resumed a normal sinus rhythm.

When I think about that day, I realize that the patient had tremendous faith in me and in the science of medicine—and that allowed us to treat her and heal her. Every day, God asks us to place our trust in him and allow him to do what he knows is best so we can be healed.

But how often do we question his plan? How often do we choose to put our faith and trust in something else? God has given us much medical knowledge that we can use to heal the body. The Bible reminds us to put our faith in Jesus, who is the ultimate healer.

TODAY'S RX

When life seems out of control, allow God to reset your heart.

God, so often I race through the day until I've run myself into the ground. Help me to be still and have a quiet heart so that I may live in the rhythm of your grace.

RENEWED ATTITUDE

Throw off your old sinful nature and your former way of life. . . . Instead, let the Spirit renew your thoughts and attitudes. Ephesians 4:22-23

From the outside, Logan resembled many of my other patients. He was average height and build, had brown hair, and worked with his hands. He seemed to carry a little extra anger along with a little extra weight. Even his diagnosis was pretty common: hypertension and diabetes mellitus.

But if you could have peered into Logan's thoughts, you would have seen that they were anything but ordinary—as I found out one day when he opened up to me. He was in my office for what seemed like an ordinary checkup, until he began to tell me about his inner life. His thoughts were dark and roiling—like a storm forming in the distance.

"Sometimes, I wake up in the middle of the night, and I think my family would be better off without me," he said. "Most nights I fall asleep thinking the same thing."

As we continued our conversation, I asked a few probing questions. He revealed a past emotional injury that, years later, he still couldn't release. As a result, over time, his attitude had begun to crumble, and depression had begun to fill the void in his spirit.

Recognizing that he needed help, he was willing to start right away with a combination of medication, therapy, and counseling. My prayer was that he would let the Holy Spirit renew his mind in ways that he had been unable to do himself.

A few weeks later, Logan's counselor reported that they had been able to excavate the old emotional wound and had begun cleaning it out by discussing it. Logan was back on the road to recovery, and with that came a real change in his attitude.

TODAY'S RX

If your thoughts are stuck in the buried past, allow the Holy Spirit to clean house and renew your attitude.

Holy Spirit, cleanse my thoughts and unclutter my mind of past hurts. I need your help to clear a pathway to forgiveness and acceptance. Thank you for showing me the way.

ASK IN HIS NAME

This same God who takes care of me will supply all your needs from his glorious riches, which have been given to us in Christ Jesus. PHILIPPIANS 4:19

Being in a strange place can be nerve-wracking—especially if you're eighty-eight and accustomed to living on your own in familiar surroundings.

Raye was a proud woman who had always been independent. She lived alone and drove herself to the store. But one night, she tripped over Trixie, her precious poodle, and fell and broke her hip. The experience of falling had frightened her, but staying in the hospital frightened her more.

"Hi, Raye, I'm Dr. Anderson. I'm the medical director here," I said. "The nurses told me about your fall and that you are concerned about staying here."

"Doctor, I'm afraid," she said timidly.

"Afraid of what?" I asked.

"I'm afraid I might need something, and I won't be able to get it."

"Do you need something now?"

"No, but I might tomorrow or in the middle of the night," she said with a worried look on her face.

"I know this is a new place for you. I'm hoping and praying that everything goes well as you rehabilitate your fractured hip," I said, trying to reassure her. "But in case it doesn't, I'll tell you what I tell all my patients. All you have to do is push that call button and ask for what you need. If they don't have it, you tell the nursing staff to call me, and I'll do my best to get you whatever you need."

Raye eased back into her pillow. "Thank you," she said.

For the next few days, she was confused and had trouble remembering where she was when she woke up. Fortunately, her family was nearby and very supportive during her stay in the hospital. She recovered nicely from her fracture and eventually was able to go home.

Jesus makes the same promise to his followers that I make to my patients. If you need something, ask for it in his name, and trust that he will give it to you. Even when we aren't feeling needy, there is great comfort in knowing that we have someone we can ask if we do.

TODAY'S RX

Don't be afraid to ask Jesus for what you need. He promises to "supply all your needs from his glorious riches."

Jesus, thank you for providing for my needs and blessing me with many physical comforts. Help me not to be afraid when I stumble and fall but to call on your name for healing and support.

VACATIONING WITH GOD

This good news—that God has prepared this rest—has been announced to us just as it was to them. But it did them no good because they didn't share the faith of those who listened to God. HEBREWS 4:2

God wants us to rest and not be on the treadmill of life all the time.

The other day, Karen and I took this advice for ourselves. We were going to exercise together with the help of a video. When we turned it on, the first thing the instructor had us do was breathing exercises.

"Take slow, deep breaths. Exhale and relax at the sound of my voice. Set aside the worries of your day."

The tape was a great reminder to slow down and savor life, even when we were about to get our heart rates up. Slowing down is something I often advise my patients. "Take time to breathe," I tell them. "Stop and reflect on what's going on in your life."

Recently, I read a book that referred to "adding space to your life." I like that description because too many of us don't have space in our lives, unless it's a special occasion.

For example, vacations are often planned as times of rest. They are times to sleep, rest, renew, and reflect without the burden of work or worrying about the usual things that trouble us.

Though many of us are not very good at taking these kinds of pauses, we should be. After all, God created us to rest. If you consider that God created human beings on the sixth day and then on the seventh day, rested, you might say that he created us to start resting on the very first day of our lives.

Even more important, he invited us to rest *with him*.

Think about that for a minute. The creator of the universe had a vacation planned, and he created us just in time to share that vacation day with him. What's more, he invites us into that peaceful garden of rest every seven days.

Are you too busy to stop? Is there something more important in your life than vacationing with the creator of the universe? He is inviting you to rest with him. Will you accept his invitation?

TODAY'S RX

Today, take a moment to breathe deeply. With each breath, thank God for wanting to spend his day of rest with you.

God, you tell me in your Word to be still. Help me to pause and reflect on your goodness today, taking slow breaths and meditating on your promises.

JUNE CHECKUP

For many, June is the first month of summer. School is out, and graduations are over. When I was young, I spent my summers on a farm in South Georgia, where June marked the beginning of the harvest season. The first fruits of that harvest were watermelons. They were our cash crop and our first opportunity to dig ourselves out financially from a long and frugal winter.

This first fruit also connected me to the men and women in my life who raised me much like they did a watermelon crop. They tended to my needs and helped mold me into a man until I was ready to be cut from the vine and be off on my own.

For many, this month begins the toil of yard work. The grass is growing and needs to be mowed. Annuals need to be planted or trimmed. You and your kids will likely enjoy a few sunsets at the ballpark, whether they're playing T-ball or watching the major leaguers hit a home run. Young children will want to catch lightning bugs and butterflies and put them in a jar so they can be observed. Older kids may be preparing to attend camp. And the whole family is talking about a vacation that will involve beaches, lakes, or mountains.

With so much focus on the outdoors, now is a great time to take your Bible reading outdoors. Let the kids see you reading and studying in a lawn chair while they play nearby. Better yet, get them a children's Bible, and let them read along with you. Focus your reading this month on all of the ways that Scripture describes nature—from Genesis to Revelation. As you read, look for the metaphors, signs, and symbols of God's handiwork in the outdoors. Use this as a time to teach your children that, like the finger paintings they made at school, God colors the sunset each night with hues of pink and gold, creating a living light show just for us.

Summer also reminds us of how each bug, bird, and butterfly is also part of God's creation and that our responsibility is to care for the earth. Start a recycling program at home or at your church. Volunteer at an animal shelter. As you spend time in caring for God's creation, remember that not a single sparrow falls to the ground without your Father knowing it; and yet, you are more valuable than an entire flock of sparrows. Spend relaxed time with those closest to you this summer. Love well. Make new friends. And most of all, enjoy the creation God has given us.

June Booster Shot: For outside activities, be prepared with sunscreen, insect repellent, Band-Aids, plenty of water to prevent dehydration, and lots of hugs and kisses.

CONFESSION IS GOOD FOR THE SOUL

If I had not confessed the sin in my heart, the Lord would not have listened.
Psalm 66:18

Whether you have an appointment for your annual physical or you're visiting the doctor because you don't feel well, it's important to be honest about what is happening in your life. It's important to tell your doctor everything, even when it is uncomfortable. You may need to confess areas of your life that are holding you back from health. Your doctor has to know the real you to guide you back to a healthy state.

Sometimes my nurses are surprised that patients will tell me things they haven't told anyone else. But in order to have open communication with anyone, there has to be a place for confession. It's a good thing when patients tell me their secrets; it means they trust me.

The same is true with the Great Physician. He wants us to share our deepest and darkest secrets with him, not because he doesn't already know them—he does—but because he wants to forgive us completely. First we must ask for that forgiveness through confession.

God is always there, and he is always willing to listen to the desires of our hearts. However, sometimes things get in the way of our relationship with our heavenly Father. The barriers between ourselves and God can quickly be removed if we start our prayers with confession. Then, if we'll let him, God can do miraculous things in our lives, including healing us to the depths of our being.

Jesus is knocking on the door to your heart. Open the door to him and confess what's been going on in your life. You will not only feel better if you do, but you'll also open the door to healing.

TODAY'S RX

Find a trusted friend, family member, or spiritual leader and confess anything that is holding you back from the life that God desires for you.

Lord, help me to be honest with you about my sins. Help me to be honest with myself, with my loved ones, and with my doctor. In doing this, help me to find a path toward you, toward honesty, and toward better health.

I WAS BLIND, BUT NOW I SEE

They went right into the house where he was staying, and Jesus asked them, "Do you believe I can make you see?" "Yes, Lord," they told him, "we do." Then he touched their eyes and said, "Because of your faith, it will happen." MATTHEW 9:28-29

Have you ever been blind to an opportunity and didn't see what you were missing until it was too late? In today's verses, Jesus asks two blind men whether they believe he is capable of helping them see. Because of their profession of faith, he heals them.

Most people are born with good vision. For those of us who aren't, we have corrective lenses to help us see what we're missing. So it may be hard for us to imagine how these blind men felt when Jesus restored their sight and suddenly they could see for the first time.

When I was eighteen, I wanted to be an Air Force pilot. As a part of the eligibility requirements, I had to pass a physical and have good stamina and perfect eyesight. Having grown up on a farm, working six days a week from daylight until past dark, I knew I had the physical attributes. And because I could shoot a squirrel on the run at 150 feet with a .22 rifle, I was confident about my eyesight. Though the exam proved more challenging than I expected—only half the applicants made it through—I passed with flying colors.

Two years later, when I went back for my final exam before starting flight school, I was stunned when I didn't pass the vision test. My eyes had deteriorated to 20/100, and I was no longer eligible to be a pilot. My career path had flown off course, and my future was dark. And the same could be said for my spiritual life at the time. Blind to my future, and blind to God, I followed the advice I was given and went to medical school.

It wasn't until Jesus opened my eyes on the night I gave my heart back to him that I caught my first glimpse of his future plan for me to help the sick and the poor. Looking back on my life now, I can clearly see that God was with me the whole time.

TODAY'S RX

Ask Jesus to open your eyes and give you a vision for what he has planned for your life.

Open my eyes to my future, Lord. Show me the plans and purpose you have for me. Help me to be obedient to your calling and serve you with all of my heart, soul, and strength.

SECRET PAST

It was our weaknesses he carried; it was our sorrows that weighed him down. And we thought his troubles were a punishment from God, a punishment for his own sins!
Isaiah 53:4

"Darrell, I'm so sorry to hear of your dad's passing," I said. Darrell's father had been one of my patients in the nursing home, and he'd recently died.

"I wish you had known him in his prime," Darrell said. "He was a strong and courageous man."

"I know he struggled those last few years."

"Yeah, I'm sorry he gave everyone at the home such a hard time. The Vietnam War caused a dramatic change in him. He wouldn't tell us much about it, but every now and then, something would slip out."

"What do you mean?"

"He would say things like, 'It was bad,' and, 'Bad things happened, but it was war.'"

"Darrell, we now have a name for that. We call it PTSD or post-traumatic stress disorder. It happens when people have seen something they can't stop remembering. Many of our soldiers have come home with vivid memories of the trauma they endured on the battlefield, and they have to deal with it. It can be hard for them and their families."

"All these years, we always thought Dad went crazy because of something he'd done. Frankly, we thought God was punishing him for some crime he'd committed that no one knew about. It wasn't until after he died that we found out Dad had not done anything bad. In fact, it was quite the opposite. He was a medic, and he was decorated for bravery multiple times for saving others."

Darrell's story of his father's valor gave me a glimpse into the past of a difficult patient. But Darrell's dad wasn't the only one who had a secret past. Many of my patients have lived lives that they've kept from their friends and family. We may not hear their stories until after they're gone. Sometimes the bravest people don't have the courage to tell their stories while they're alive, and we can draw the wrong conclusions if we're not careful.

TODAY'S RX

Don't judge a book by its cover. Treat everyone you meet with compassion.

Protect those who serve our country, God. Give them courage and strength to fight the good fight, and provide healing for them physically, mentally, emotionally, and spiritually.

TRUSTING THROUGH THE STORMS

Give all your worries and cares to God, for he cares about you. 1 PETER 5:7

When our kids were young and I worked a late shift in the ER, Karen always had them tucked into bed before I got home. If the weather was bad, I might come home to find one or more of them curled up in my bed. A storm that had lots of thunder and lightning or a howling wind might mean I would find three or four kids in the bed.

When I would tiptoe in, I'd find them all snuggled up under the covers, looking like puppies, with arms and legs splayed so that they could reach out and touch Karen if they got scared.

Other nights, I would come home and our bed would be empty. I would find Karen cuddling a child in his or her bed. Usually that meant the child was sick or had had a really bad day.

That's part of what makes mothers so special. They care for their children when they're sick and worried. In those moments of fear or illness, it's not enough for a mother to say she'll be down the hall. The sick or worried child wants to be able to reach out and touch Mama for comfort.

Most nights, the kids slept in their own beds after Karen sang a lullaby to them. If I was home, I would hear her soothing voice filling the house with song. One of my favorites, and one that still lingers in my grown children's minds, is based on Psalm 56. The lyrics describe putting our trust in God when we're afraid.

Those simple words gave my children the strength and courage to conquer their fear and sleep in peace. When we're afraid, Jesus wants us to cast our cares on him—especially in the midst of a storm.

TODAY'S RX

The songs in Scripture calm the storms of life. Find a song based on one of the psalms, and sing it or play it the next time you're in a storm.

Jesus, you are truly a Good Shepherd, who makes me lie down in green pastures and walk beside still waters. You calm my fears. Thank you for your comforting embrace.

AN ENCOURAGING WORD CALMS THE SOUL

Don't use foul or abusive language. Let everything you say be good and helpful, so that your words will be an encouragement to those who hear them. Ephesians 4:29

Though I was at the opposite end of the hall, I could hear the cursing as if it were right next door to me. When I walked down to the room, I found a man in an orange jumpsuit handcuffed to the bed and screaming obscenities at the top of his lungs. It was a frightening scene, and I could only imagine what those in the waiting room were thinking. Fortunately, the EMTs and police officers were already in the room, trying to subdue the man and his mouth.

Once I got close to the bed, I could see the man's wild eyes darting about, looking for a way to escape or cause havoc. A closer look revealed that he'd been in a knife fight. He had several cuts and wounds that needed attention, but his volatile behavior and the potential for more violence was scaring away the people who could help.

As one of the officers was warning me, I suddenly realized that I recognized the prisoner. "Greg? It's Dr. Anderson. I'm here to help you."

Greg turned toward me, ready to shout some more expletives in my direction, but when his eyes met mine, he seemed confused.

"I know your mom and your grandma," I said. "Should I call them to come help?"

As soon as he recognized me, Greg became still and silent. When he spoke, it was now in a normal voice and no longer profane or vulgar. "You don't have to do that," he said.

I approached him and started examining his wounds.

"How's your family doing?" I asked.

"They're all right."

"How'd you get yourself in this predicament?"

As he relayed some of the bad decisions that had led to his injuries and arrest, Greg became remorseful, which made him much more approachable, and with help from my staff, I was able to finish patching him up.

When I was done, he waited calmly for the officer to once again handcuff him.

"My life ain't been easy," he said before he left. "I'm appreciative of all you've done and for not judging me."

TODAY'S RX

Everyone deserves a kind word. Today, pass along some encouragement to somebody who needs it most.

Father, help me to remember that those who hurt others with words and actions have often been deeply hurt themselves. Show me how to be a light to these people, offering them kindness, grace, and mercy.

GOD'S DIET

By these instructions you will know what is unclean and clean, and which animals may be eaten and which may not be eaten. Leviticus 11:47

Recently, a flood of diet cookbooks have suggested the health benefits of returning to the Levitical dietary laws. My wife, Karen, is a registered dietician and is familiar with many of these books.

From a religious standpoint, one of the reasons the Israelites were given dietary laws was to set them apart from the surrounding nations. God wanted them to be known as a holy people. What better way to distinguish them than by what they ate or didn't eat?

There may have been good dietary reasons to follow the laws as well. During that time in history, many of the restricted foods had significant health risks associated with them. For example, pork carried trichinosis, a parasitic disease caused by the roundworm *Trichinella spiralis.* If the larvae are eaten in undercooked pork, humans can be infected with roundworms. Usually, the disease is self-limited and has flu-like symptoms. However, it can affect the heart and lungs and be fatal in patients with a compromised immune system.

Likewise, seafood restrictions can be traced to other toxins and infections found in certain kinds of fish.

We no longer worry about these dangers because our cooking practices have changed. We use thermometers to test the temperature of meat to make sure it is thoroughly cooked. In those rare instances where a food makes us sick, we often have medications available for treatment. The Israelites didn't have any of these resources.

Just because some things have changed doesn't mean we should ignore the Bible's dietary advice. Most of us would be better off if we ate the way Adam and Eve ate in the Garden of Eden—where all their food was grown for them.

When I read the Levitical dietary laws, I see them as a promise from God to his people that he will care for his children if they will follow his laws. The Lord ensured the safety of the Israelites even when they did not have the technology or knowledge to know of the dangers that lurked on their plates. To me, this is a promise that God will continue to care for us—even in our ignorance or lack of resources.

TODAY'S RX

God puts a protective barrier around his children. Respect that barrier to live a healthy life.

Lord, thank you for providing for my most basic needs and for protecting my body from toxins and parasites. Your perfect law keeps me from harm. Thank you for your gentle guidance and direction.

AMAZING FAITH

When Jesus heard this, he was amazed. Turning to the crowd that was following him, he said, "I tell you, I haven't seen faith like this in all Israel!" And when the officer's friends returned to his house, they found the slave completely healed. LUKE 7:9-10

Whenever I've seen a mother and child at the same time for treatment—whether it's in the ER after an accident or in my office when they both have strep throat—the mother always wants her child to be taken care of first. If there's only enough money for one prescription, the child always gets the medicine.

This innate desire to sacrifice ourselves for someone we love is exactly why airlines always tell us to do the opposite. You know the drill: *Put on your own oxygen mask first, and then help your child.* They know that, in a midair emergency, our God-given instinct to care for our children first could be harmful to both parent and child.

In today's verse, the Roman officer follows his instincts, despite the fact that asking a Jewish rabbi for help could prove to be dangerous. By asking Jesus to heal the slave, the officer had to go outside of the Roman hierarchy. For a Gentile with a high-level military position, this action could have cost him his job—or worse.

When I read this story in the Bible, I see the same sacrificial instincts as a mother caring for her child. I realize that the officer is not a parent to the slave. However, his loving concern and intuition to do whatever was needed reminds me of a mother's love.

Jesus was amazed at the man's faith. In fact, it's the only story in the Bible in which we're told that Jesus was amazed by someone's faith. And what's so remarkable is that it wasn't the faith of a Pharisee or another Jewish leader; it was the faith of a Roman military officer—an outsider to the Jewish faith.

For whom are you willing to sacrifice? Would Jesus be amazed at your faith in him?

While we were yet sinners, Jesus willingly sacrificed his life for us. The only proper response to his amazing grace is for us is to have an amazing faith in him.

TODAY'S RX

Have faith that Jesus needs only to speak a word in order for you to be healed.

Jesus, I desire to have faith that amazes you. When I come to the end of my life, I long to hear you say, "Well done." Help me to live out your commands and have a sacrificial spirit to those I meet.

LOSING EVERYTHING BUT A PROMISE

As for me, I look to the LORD *for help. I wait confidently for God to save me, and my God will certainly hear me. Do not gloat over me, my enemies! For though I fall, I will rise again. Though I sit in darkness, the* LORD *will be my light.* MICAH 7:7-8

Loretta was raised with money and manners, and it showed in the way she held her head high and walked with confidence. She was always dressed to perfection and very well put together. But when her husband of fifty-five years died, so did her elegance. She seemed to lose her edge, and she cried a lot.

Her loss was monumental, and as time went on, she began to lose weight and energy. We started her on antidepressants, but she remained depressed. The medication only slowed her downward spiral.

One busy day in my office, Loretta missed her appointment. I made a mental note to call and check on her when things slowed down, but before I could phone her, I received a concerned call from emergency medical services. Loretta had been found on the floor at home, where she had lain for more than fourteen hours before someone found her. That alone could have been a terminal event, but even more concerning was the result of the fall—a left intertrochanteric hip fracture. To have the slightest hope of recovery, Loretta would need surgery and extensive rehabilitation. I wasn't sure she had the emotional and mental fortitude it would require.

I prayed with her during this acute phase, and the Lord answered our prayers. Loretta made it through surgery and was transferred to the nursing home for rehabilitation. At first, her sadness continued, but eventually she started to get her old swing back. I knew things were headed in the right direction when she began putting on makeup before my scheduled visits to the home. Soon, the physical therapy department was praising her steps toward recovery. Three months later, she was back on her feet, and her smile was as radiant as ever.

"I'm proud of the progress you've made," I told her.

"Dr. Anderson, I lost everything, except for the promise that God would save me," she said. "And you know what? He did."

TODAY'S RX

When you fall, look up. God is there, and he has the power to heal and restore you.

God, help me to view my condition through your eyes—that it is temporary and that greater things are yet to come. Thank you for restoring my spirit.

RELEASE FROM CAPTIVITY

You are free from your slavery to sin, and you have become slaves to righteous living.
ROMANS 6:18

We are all slaves to something or someone. And every slave has a master. The question is, do we have the right master? In today's verse, Paul alludes to our former enslavement to sin, even as he reminds us that Jesus came to unlock our chains and set us free.

One of my biggest regrets is that I never looked for the key to unlock the chains that kept me enslaved to my career. Because I grew up in a poor family, I felt a lot of pressure to work hard and provide for Karen and our four children so that they wouldn't struggle the same way I had growing up.

But there were times when I took that sense of obligation to the extreme, often working more than eighty hours a week. And even then I felt pressure to work longer. No one was forcing me to do this; it was all self-imposed. I rationalized my overwork by saying I was merely doing what God had created me to do.

The problem was that God had also created me to be a husband and father. But I was trying to serve two wrong masters: my career and my family. Each time I gave in to one, it seemed to take away from the other. If, instead, I had focused on serving God—both at work and at home—I would not have been enslaved to my own, or someone else's, expectations. I would have been free.

Are you caught in the same tug-of-war? Is the rat race enslaving you to the point of physical or emotional exhaustion?

If so, push back. Claim the freedom to serve Christ and Christ alone. Service to Jesus is never about being chained or enslaved. Serving him is an expression of our love and gratitude to him for freeing us from our enslavement to sin.

Only recently have I been able to unchain myself from unhealthy ways of thinking and embrace freedom. As a result, I've set sail on a new course. I urge you to join me. Seek the only master who is worth serving, and he will set you free.

TODAY'S RX

If you must strive for more, strive for more of God—and allow him to truly set you free.

Father, what a relief it is to know that a life pleasing to you is not one of constant strife and struggle. I rejoice in the freedom to walk in your ways, released from the bondage of sin. Thank you for your great love for me.

THE RULE FOR A LONG LIFE

You must serve only the LORD your God. If you do, I will bless you with food and water, and I will protect you from illness . . . and I will give you long, full lives.
EXODUS 23:25-26

Today's verse can be confusing, can't it? It says that the one rule for good health is to serve only the Lord our God. And yet we've all known people who have served him faithfully and died too young.

I've sat at the bedsides of young patients who were terminal and thought, *How is God's promise being fulfilled here?* But what has surprised me the most in these cases is the clarity and fullness of the short lives of these patients. Once they enter their final home, they have a vision of a longer, fuller life. God can and will fulfill his promises in the grandest way possible, even after our mortal bodies are gone.

Today's verse tells us that there were built-in rewards in God's covenant with Israel. If the people of Israel served the Lord, he would bless them with food and water and protect them from illness. Yet, during their exodus in the wilderness, the people were beset by many temptations to sidetrack their faith in the Lord. Even with the promise of prosperity before them, the Israelites fell away from God time and time again.

How often do we do the same thing? Doctors tell us what to do to have a long and healthy life, yet even with the simplest of instructions, we find their advice difficult to follow. How much more difficult would it be to follow a long list of dos and don'ts created by our Creator?

The Great Physician tells us that there is only one rule for good health: *Serve only the Lord your God.* Even today, this promise will result in healthier living and a better life.

TODAY'S RX

Serving the Lord has a gift attached. He will give us a long and full life, even if we only glimpse a portion of that life now.

Father, I confess that my attention is often divided, and I devote my time to worldly pursuits. I pray that you will help me serve you—and you alone. Thank you for the promise of your blessing.

LAST BREATH

I have fought the good fight, I have finished the race, and I have remained faithful. And now the prize awaits me—the crown of righteousness, which the Lord, the righteous Judge, will give me on the day of his return. And the prize is not just for me but for all who eagerly look forward to his appearing. 2 TIMOTHY 4:7-8

Nights on the farm in South Georgia were so quiet that even the roosters slept later than sunrise. But not my Aunt Sophie. She was up before the roosters. We would hear her in the kitchen, cracking eggs into the sizzling black cast-iron frying pan.

Over the years, there was another sound that signaled morning—my uncle's smoker's cough. In the beginning, it wasn't a big deal, but as time went on it became distastefully loud, scaring us all awake.

"Uncle Luther, someday those cigarettes are going to catch up with you," I said to him more than once.

His answer was always the same. "You're probably right. I try to quit about twenty times a day."

A few years later, our fears were realized when an X-ray revealed that Uncle Luther had lung cancer in his right middle lobe. The surgeon felt confident he could get rid of it by a simple lobectomy.

As a doctor, I now know that when someone has moderate COPD from forty years of smoking, there is nothing simple about a lobectomy. Fortunately, Luther survived the surgery, but afterward, he was only about half the man he used to be. As summer passed, he depended more and more on others to help him with the chores.

By the next summer, he was tethered to an oxygen tank in the house. We prayed together more that summer than any other, and I spent a lot of time talking with Uncle Luther about life and death. But as his physical body weakened, Uncle Luther's faith only seemed to grow, and he looked forward to his forever home.

I wasn't at his side when he died, but I'm certain that his last difficult breath on earth was followed by a deep inhalation of joy in heaven.

Uncle Luther lived by today's verse above, fighting the good fight until the end. When he finished the race, he was no longer winded; instead, he was very much fulfilled.

TODAY'S RX

Keep your eye on the prize—your forever home—and finish the race well.

Lord, give me the strength to fight the good fight, finish the race well, and remain faithful to you throughout my healing process. It is only by your grace that I'm capable of persevering.

LAUGHING LAST AND BEST

When Jesus arrived at the official's home, he saw the noisy crowd and heard the funeral music. "Get out!" he told them. "The girl isn't dead; she's only asleep." But the crowd laughed at him. MATTHEW 9:23-24

Some medical discoveries, when first introduced, were thought to be crazy and downright laughable.

When I began my clinicals at the University of Alabama at Birmingham, my first attending physician was Dr. Basil Hirschowitz, a prominent gastroenterologist who, along with two colleagues, invented the first fully flexible fiber-optic endoscope.

Who would have imagined that a flexible tube could be passed into the intestines and be used to diagnose disease? I'm sure that many people laughed at Dr. Hirschowitz as he worked out the details of his invention. Yet even today, all these years later, it is still the gold standard in diagnostic treatment. We would be hard-pressed to make some diagnoses without it.

More recently, two men went to extraordinary lengths to prove their theory that peptic ulcer disease was caused by bacteria—rather than by too much stomach acid, as the medical community had believed for hundreds of years. In the early 1980s, two men working in Australia hypothesized that these ulcers were instead caused by the *helicobacter pylori* bacterium. They did several studies and tried to get their results published, but the medical establishment only laughed at them.

On June 12, 1984, one of the researchers, Barry Marshall, purposely consumed the bacterium and became ill. He then took an antibiotic, and it relieved his symptoms. This discovery saved countless lives that otherwise would have been lost to bleeding ulcers or stomach cancer. But it took Marshall's bold step of testing his theory on himself to stop the laughter.

When Jesus came to the house of a girl who had recently died and told the crowd that the girl wasn't dead, they laughed at him. But Jesus had the last laugh when he took the girl by the hand and she stood up. If people weren't talking about Jesus before this, they certainly were afterward!

If someone tells you that your faith doesn't change things or that praying for healing is a waste of time, don't stop believing or praying. It won't be the first time doubters laughed and were proved wrong.

TODAY'S RX

Put your faith in the God who can raise someone from the dead.

Jesus, your miracles are evident to this day. Nothing surprises you, and nothing is beyond you. Thank you for providing healing through the medical advancements we have today.

GOD OF THE IMPOSSIBLE

Is anything too hard for the Lord? I will return about this time next year, and Sarah will have a son. Genesis 18:14

Some things in life seem too hard even for the Lord to do. In those moments we ask, "Is the God of the impossible still with us? Can we still experience miracles like those found in the Old Testament?"

One day, a patient of mine named Bill asked me to visit him at the hospital, where his wife, Carole, was dying.

"The specialists say there's nothing they can do for her," Bill said with tears in his eyes. "They said it won't be long, and all we can do is wait for her to die."

Across the room, Carole lay in bed, too weak to talk. I watched her fight for every breath. The surgeons had concluded that she was too weak for surgery, and they recommended hospice care.

Hospice is designed to keep terminally ill patients as comfortable as possible in their final days, to make sure their health-care wishes are carried out, and that they don't suffer needlessly. Patients typically leave hospice only when they die.

I discussed Carole's final wishes with her and Bill. She had a living will and a do-not-resuscitate order. I knew that CPR would likely be painful and futile. Before I left that night, the three of us prayed that God would keep Carole alive so she would have more time with her family.

The next morning, I was surprised to hear that she was still alive. The day after that, she seemed a little better. A week later, her breathing was noticeably less labored and color had returned to her cheeks. I called a cardiovascular surgeon who was using some new, less-invasive techniques, and he agreed to see Carole.

Over the next few months, I received occasional updates from Bill as Carole made progress. A year later, at Bill's annual appointment, I was surprised to see a woman I barely recognized sitting with him. Carole's appearance had improved so much that she looked much younger than I remembered.

She glowed as she told me that she'd recently done something we all would have said was impossible a year earlier: "I danced with my son at his wedding!"

TODAY'S RX

Our God is still the God of the impossible. Pray with the knowledge that nothing you face is too big for him.

Father, I praise you that nothing is impossible in your sight. Thank you for working miracles to this day, and for giving me hope to continue persevering.

THE SOURCE OF HEALING

Moses made a snake out of bronze and attached it to a pole. Then anyone who was bitten by a snake could look at the bronze snake and be healed! NUMBERS 21:9

The Caduceus and the rod of Asclepius are both ancient symbols that represent the healing arts. The Caduceus depicts two serpents coiled around a winged staff; the rod of Asclepius has a single snake wrapped around a rustic staff. On their own, these symbols have no healing powers; rather, they were used as beacons to pointing the way to places where health care was available.

In today's verse, the bronze snake that Moses fashioned is a symbol of the ultimate Healer—God. But problems arose when the people began worshipping the symbol rather than the source. When they left God out of the equation, the idol failed them.

Do we do the same thing today?

Have our great, modern hospitals become sanctuaries where we go to worship the Caduceus idol in the form of a great surgeon, a cutting-edge treatment, or a stellar medical reputation? Do we believe in the power of the physician and the hospital more than the power of God? Are we placing our faith in modern medicine and leaving God out of the equation?

In America, many of our hospitals were founded by Jewish or Christian organizations. When they first started, they looked to God as the source of healing. But over the years, many of our most prestigious medical schools and hospitals have lost touch with their faith-filled roots. That's unfortunate for the patients who are there because medical science works best in conjunction with God's healing.

Recently, I've seen research in the medical literature supporting the conclusion that prayer and faith have a positive effect on physical health and healing. These studies suggest that the disciplines of our faith should be a part of our modern medical treatment plan. Though our medical institutions may not be the faith-filled sanctuaries of healing that they once were, we can still pack a prayer and bring our faith with us to the hospital. When we do, it will be a witness to all that God is the source of our healing, not just a symbol on a pole.

TODAY'S RX

In everything you do, look to the source (God) and not the symbol.

On my roughest days, God, help me to remember that you are almighty and sovereign—that you are the source that makes a way for my healing. Grow my faith in you so that I may always seek you and depend on you first as I walk the road to recovery.

FREED FROM SIN AND BAD CHOICES

Because you belong to him, the power of the life-giving Spirit has freed you from the power of sin that leads to death. ROMANS 8:2

When Adam and Eve chose to disobey God and eat the forbidden fruit, they set the course of free, willful disobedience that all of humankind would then follow. As a result, sin entered the world and death along with it. But we have hope because Jesus came to rescue and redeem us from this broken world. All we have to do is accept him as our Savior and put our trust in him.

But even Jesus won't violate our free will.

Every day, I talk to patients who have a history of making bad choices—whether it's smoking, excessive drinking, overeating, lack of exercise, or illegal drug use. In many cases, these choices have shortened their natural lifespan by months, if not years.

When we turn away from our bad habits and make good choices, sometimes the downward trend of health problems can be slowed and occasionally even reversed. If you're in such a situation, it's worth the pain to change.

But even if we don't change our bad habits, we can still change what happens when we sin. When we turn to the Lord, he will release us from the permanent death that is the wages for our sin. And that's a change worth making!

Though our physical bodies will one day fail us and return to dust, God has promised us eternal, heavenly bodies. These new bodies will be complete and healthy, free of sickness, disease, and weakness.

Jesus came to find me even when I wasn't looking for him. When he did, my life turned around 180 degrees from the way I was living before. Prior to meeting Jesus, I was on a pathway filled with sin, destruction, and death. Turning toward Jesus gave me a new life and lifted my spirit out of those destructive behaviors.

No matter which path you're currently on, I know that Jesus can rescue and redeem you. We were made to live perfectly in paradise, not stumbling sinfully through the world. But we have to choose Jesus if we want to be set back on track.

TODAY'S RX

It's not too late to change. Pick one bad habit today, and with the Lord's help, start making good choices.

Jesus, just as you redeemed this broken world, I thank you for how you'll one day fully redeem my body by making me a new creation in you. Thank you for overcoming sickness, weakness, and death and for continually making me new.

FAITH-BASED MEDICINE

Faith shows the reality of what we hope for; it is the evidence we cannot see.
HEBREWS 11:1

When you visit the doctor and he or she outlines a treatment plan for your illness, you trust that the outcome will be what you expect. If the doctor says that this antibiotic will cure your sore throat, you take the pill and expect your throat to get better. But just as you put your trust in your doctor, doctors put their trust in their medical training and experience. Doctors don't just make up their treatment plans; they recommend a course based on what has been clinically proven to work for other patients.

We call this *evidence-based medicine.* Typically, the results of a study are reported as a percentage of positive results versus a percentage of negative results. Seventy percent positive is considered a great outcome. We'd like to have a 100 percent positive outcome, but that never happens. There are too many things we can't control that can cause treatments to fail. For example, an infection may develop resistance. Or one patient's body may not absorb the medication in the same way that someone else's body does, and thus the treatment won't be effective in all cases.

There's only one physician I know who can predict and produce a 100 percent positive outcome for everything he prescribes—the Great Physician. So why don't we put our trust and faith in the good doctor who guarantees his treatment is 100 percent effective every time?

Some say it's because we can't see him.

That's not a problem for me. I have been at the bedsides of hundreds of dying patients over the years. And I have personally witnessed glimpses of heaven as many of them have crossed to the other side. I've watched God keep his promises. If you haven't personally seen the end result evidence and you wonder if it's prudent to place your trust in something you haven't seen, I remind you that we place our faith and trust in things we can't see all the time. For me, there is enough evidence that God keeps his promises that I will fully trust him until the day I die. I have faith in his faithfulness.

TODAY'S RX

The positive outcome for evidence-based medicine is 70 percent. Evidence-based salvation is 100 percent. If you haven't yet placed your faith in the Great Physician, do it today.

Father, I have faith in you to make me well. Thank you for guaranteeing me a home in heaven.

GOING WITH A SMILE

My heart has heard you say, "Come and talk with me." And my heart responds, "LORD, I am coming." PSALM 27:8

People often think that making rounds at a nursing home would be depressing. But it's not. The veterans of life who live there have insights and wisdom that seem to escape those of us who are still running on the hamster wheel. Their softly leathered faces glow with memories.

Dorothy was well into her eighties when she unpacked her few possessions in the twelve-by-twelve-foot room at the care center. As her family members prepared to say good-bye, they began to cry. It was one of the hardest things they'd ever had to do. But Dorothy uttered a conciliatory sigh. She didn't cry. She had endured much worse.

Over the years, I had heard Dorothy's stories. Her father had lost everything in the Great Depression, and she had learned to see everything she received as a blessing from heaven. She and her husband had raised four children together, and she had helped raise her grandchildren. Despite the various hardships she had seen, she had a smile that lit up the room.

"Dr. Anderson, will you stay and talk to me for a little while?" she asked one day.

"Certainly, Dorothy. What's on your mind?"

"Today was my anniversary. If my husband were still living, it would be sixty-five years!"

I picked up her hand and held it in mine. Her papery skin was warm to the touch.

"You know, I'm ready to go. I have everything in order for when I die."

I nodded. I knew she had a do-not-resuscitate order and a living will.

"After I'm gone, can you do one thing for me?"

"Anything," I said.

"Please tell everyone how much I loved them."

"Of course I will," I said, gently patting her arm.

Two days later, I got an early-morning call from one of the nurses at the care center.

"I'm sorry to wake you, Dr. Anderson, but I've just been in to see Dorothy, and she wasn't breathing. But when I saw her, she had a smile on her face."

I love today's verse, because it is such a beautiful reminder to me of Dorothy. She heard God's voice, and she went to him with a smile on her face.

TODAY'S RX

Are you ready? Only God knows the day or the hour, but we want to be ready when he calls us home.

Father, Psalm 139 says that every day of my life is recorded in your book. What reassurance I have knowing you hear every beat of my heart and know every breath I take. Thank you for being in control.

CAREER-SAVING STRENGTH FROM GOD

Strengthen those who have tired hands, and encourage those who have weak knees.
ISAIAH 35:3

I was committed to serving the poor, not only because of my obligation to repay the National Health Service Corps for my medical school scholarship, but also because I believed it was what God wanted me to do. However, three years into my four-year obligation, I almost gave up on both.

At the time, there were only two doctors in our county who were on call, and we were both working off our obligations to the NHSC. But the other doctor's four-year service ended a year before mine. When we discussed what he planned to do when his obligation ended, he said he was going to leave at the end of the year.

If that happened, I would go from being on call every other night and weekend to being on call every night and weekend for at least a year, unless we could find more help.

I immediately notified everyone I knew that we were looking for another doctor. But I also began looking at other options. I was exhausted from the current schedule, and Karen was frustrated that I was never home. If I had to put in a full year of being on call twenty-four hours a day, seven days a week, my health would be at risk, and my family would be irreparably harmed. But if I couldn't transfer to another location within the NHSC, I would have no choice but to repay the remaining balance on my loan and start over somewhere else.

Karen and I still felt as if God had called us here and that we shouldn't leave unless God clearly directed us to. But what if I physically and emotionally couldn't work under the new conditions? We both began to pray.

My former residency director picked up my distress signal and told me he had two graduates who had not yet decided where to go. We ended up hiring both of them! With this news, the other doctor decided to give it another year or two. Within a few days, I went from bearing the full load myself to sharing it with three other doctors!

God not only answered our prayers, but he also confirmed that he wanted us to stay right where we were.

TODAY'S RX

If you are weak and tired, look up. Your strength comes from above.

Lord, when I leave my concerns with you, rather than trying to handle them myself, you answer in ways I have not foreseen. Thank you for showering me with your abundant love and for caring for me so faithfully.

PRAYERS FOR A VOTE TO GO OUR WAY

The council then threatened them further, but they finally let them go because they didn't know how to punish them without starting a riot. For everyone was praising God for this miraculous sign—the healing of a man who had been lame for more than forty years. ACTS 4:21-22

Often when Jesus healed someone, he told the person not to tell anyone. He knew that the religious leaders would respond negatively. So it was no surprise when the disciples also were threatened for performing miracles in Jesus' name. Unfortunately, that kind of backlash still happens today.

One year, on a medical missions trip, we took a van full of supplies into the Andes Mountains of Ecuador and set up a small clinic in a mud hut. God was with us as we treated more than 150 patients with various medical and dental ailments, and the Quechua people invited us into their homes and hearts. It was beautiful to witness so many prayers being answered.

Each night, we showed the *JESUS* film, and the tiny village of fewer than seventy-five people would swell in population to four times that size. Everyone wanted to see the film and learn more about Jesus.

Then, with only a few days left on our trip, the local clergyman called upon the leaders of the tribe to ban us from the area. Apparently, he was uncomfortable with the message that Jesus could be a personal and ever-present Savior. He believed that everyone who wanted to know God must go through him. He didn't like it that we taught the tribe that miracles could still happen in Jesus' name.

From inside the mud hut where we were staying, I heard the voices outside growing louder and becoming more animated. I peered out to catch a glimpse of what was happening. The clergyman was holding a machete and threatening the local leaders, but apparently many of the locals didn't want us to leave. It was finally decided that there would be a vote.

I watched as the clergyman with the machete angrily waved it in the air as people voted. If we lost the vote, we might also lose our lives. Fortunately, God heard our silent but desperate prayers. In the end, the vote was 176 to 92 in our favor.

TODAY'S RX

When you face persecution, know that God is with you and will reveal himself in your time of need.

God, be with the missionaries across the world who are faithfully doing your work. Strengthen them as they face persecution, and protect them from harm. Thank you for their dedication and sacrificial spirits.

PRESENCE IN THE PRESENT MOMENT

Can all your worries add a single moment to your life? MATTHEW 6:27

So many people had come to say good-bye to Paul that they spilled out of his room and into the hallway. When I stopped by, there were family, friends, and neighbors leaning against the wall and standing around his bed. They obviously cared for him deeply. But their faces were lined with worry.

Paul had fought a long and very hard battle with cancer. He'd lived well beyond any medical professional's expectations. And he had been in a lot of pain. Those in the room knew their prayers for healing wouldn't be answered until Paul was on the other side of heaven's veil, and they wanted to be with him on his final journey home.

I watched as his wife held his hand and tearfully prayed for God to intervene. She asked for God's will to be done, and I sensed that she may have added an unspoken request that God's will would be done quickly so that Paul wouldn't continue to suffer.

I took a seat next to Paul's bed and felt the holy presence of God even more than usual. I knew Paul's time would come soon. Each breath was harder for him to take, and his pulse was declining.

"How much longer does he have to struggle?" one of Paul's daughters asked insistently.

"I feel the presence of the Holy One in the room right now, and it won't be long," I reassured her. "But only the Lord knows exactly when that will be."

The worry lines I'd seen earlier softened as the family began to understand that we were on holy ground. A sense of peace that surpasses understanding seemed to fill everyone in the room.

Just as today's verse above says that worry can't add a single moment to our lives, neither can it take a moment away. The transition times of life on earth—our birth and our death—are sacred moments when we can feel God's comfort and presence. At those moments, more than any other, we want to be filled with God's presence, not with our own worry. But sometimes in the midst of our tears and exhaustion, we need fresh eyes to help us see that God is there.

TODAY'S RX

Try not to worry today. Our present and future days are always in God's hands.

Lord, be with those suffering today, and give them your peace.
Show them they are not alone but are enveloped in your love. Help
them through their journey until they are home with you.

ADMITTING THE HARD TRUTH

Even when you are chased by those who seek to kill you, your life is safe in the care of the LORD your God, secure in his treasure pouch! 1 SAMUEL 25:29

Andi arrived in the ER with injuries that didn't match her story—and this wasn't the first time. Over and over, several of us questioned her about the bruises on her face and how and when the "accident" happened.

But her story never added up. She had layers of bruises all over her body, ranging in color from black to green to yellow. Clearly, some of them had been there for a while. There was no way they were all caused by the same incident.

I entered the room with her lab results and X-rays under my arm. "Andi, you don't have any broken bones, but you need to tell me the truth about what happened."

She began sobbing. Through her tears, she told me a story of chronic abuse by an alcoholic husband.

"He's always so remorseful the next day when he sobers up," she said. "But I'm afraid he's going to kill both of us if he doesn't get help." It was the first time she had ever told anyone the truth about what had been happening. I think it was also the first time she recognized the truth herself.

We arranged for Andi to stay in a safe house in Nashville for the night and to receive counseling the next day. The police had already picked up her husband, who had been belligerent with one of the policemen—which assured us that he would remain in jail for a while.

Once Andi was in a safe place, she had time to think and pray. She began to eat better and regained her strength and confidence. The next time she faced her husband, she exhibited her newfound fortitude, insisting that he enroll in treatment for both his alcoholism and his temper.

He didn't want any part of her plan or her. He chose to leave, and a few days later, he filed for divorce. God had intervened in Andi's life to protect her, and now she leaned into him as he led her on a new and safer life journey.

TODAY'S RX

The truth can be hard to admit and even harder to follow. But have courage because it will set you free.

You are my safeguard, Lord. My protector. My Shield. Thank you for watching over me and delivering me from evil.

CROSSING THE RUBICON

Jesus said to him, "Go, for your faith has healed you." Instantly the man could see, and he followed Jesus down the road. MARK 10:52

When Karen and I were in Rome one time, we heard the following story.

Julius Caesar was a general in the Roman army. After great military victories that gave him extraordinary military power, he was ordered by the Roman Senate to resign his command and return home. Some say that the senators began plans for Caesar's assassination then because they feared his popularity with the people.

When Caesar received the orders, he moved his army toward Rome, pausing before the bridge that crossed the Rubicon River into Italy proper. He knew that crossing with his army would be seen as an act of aggression; and yet, if he didn't proceed, he would surely be prosecuted and likely killed.

He hesitated.

Everyone in his army knew the law. If they followed Caesar, they would be considered traitors. Finally, Caesar quoted a line from a play by Menander, "Let the die be cast."

When Caesar crossed the Rubicon River with a legion of men alongside him, he breached an irrevocable point of no return—and hence the phrase, "Crossing the Rubicon." Caesar and his men knew that nothing would ever be the same after that.

In the New Testament story of Bartimaeus, Mark tells us that the blind man faced a similar moment of decision. When Bartimaeus heard that Jesus was nearby, he took off his beggar's garment and asked Jesus to heal him. This symbolic gesture was essentially burning a bridge to his old life. Because of the man's great faith, Jesus healed him. Bartimaeus left his old life, and Mark says he followed Jesus down the road. Bartimaeus had crossed the Rubicon to a new life.

Are we ready to cast our old lives aside and follow Jesus? Will we also go forward with a new vision from Jesus and refuse to look back?

I always want to look forward to my time with the Lord, and I refuse to stay blinded by my past. My prayer is that you will do the same.

TODAY'S RX

The rearview mirror is a tiny reminder of where you have been. Merely glance at it as you keep looking forward, following in the footsteps of Jesus.

God, thank you for the reminder that dwelling in my past does not allow me to move forward. Help me to take action and cross the bridge to what you have planned for me in my future. I desire to be obedient to your call.

WAITING UNTIL THE FOG CLEARS

How do you know what your life will be like tomorrow? Your life is like the morning fog—it's here a little while, then it's gone. What you ought to say is, "If the Lord wants us to, we will live and do this or that." JAMES 4:14-15

"The test results are back. It's colon cancer."

Jeremiah took a deep breath and slumped in his chair. I quietly watched him as he processed the news. After a short pause, he broke the silence with a flood of questions.

"What exactly does this mean? I mean, what do I do tomorrow? Do I just get up and go to work? And more important, what are my chances for a cure?"

"There are a lot of factors that go into answering your questions, and over the next few days and weeks, we'll do our best to sort through them. The first thing we need, though, is to learn what stage the cancer is in."

"What does that mean?"

"That means we will grade it from one to four, with stage four being metastatic—which means it has spread from where it started to another place in your body. That's the worst kind. But let's not worry about that yet. Right now, everything is still unclear. It's like an early morning fog that keeps us from seeing what's on the road ahead. But if you drive the same road at noon, the fog will have dissipated, and we will see clearly. We'll get a better picture in a few days when all of your test results are back. Until then, we'll pray and trust God that the results will show stage one."

"You're right, Dr. Anderson. Worrying won't change the diagnosis. God is in charge of it all, and there's no point in worrying until we know more."

The following week, after all of Jeremiah's test results were in, I called him with the good news. "It is stage one colon cancer, and with surgery, you'll have a good chance of a total cure. So you don't have to worry; you'll have plenty of tomorrows."

"That's great news. After our conversation the other day, I felt peace. I no longer was worried."

TODAY'S RX

We can't worry about tomorrow, but regular checkups and testing can give us information to help clear the fog and provide clarity when something goes wrong.

Pursue me, Lord, as I make my way through the fog of what lies ahead. Be a guiding light so that I may not be consumed by worry, but trust that my future is in your hands. Thank you for your reassuring presence.

PRACTICING SABBATH ALL WEEK LONG

This dear woman, a daughter of Abraham, has been held in bondage by Satan for eighteen years. Isn't it right that she be released, even on the Sabbath? Luke 13:16

I grew up in a community, and in a family, that respected the Sabbath as a day of rest. We went to church and then went home for lunch. After that, we spent the rest of the day taking it easy.

However, on the farm, the animals didn't know it was the Sabbath. For their well-being, we had to keep up some of our daily chores. The time spent caring for them required us to leave our resting mode and work a little, even on Sunday. We also had to take care of any emergencies that came up, such as the birth of a calf.

Jesus recognized that there were times when resting on the Sabbath didn't make much sense. In Luke 14, he asks the Pharisees if the law permits him to heal on the Sabbath. When the Pharisees refuse to answer, Jesus calls them hypocrites. If one of the Pharisees' oxen fell into a pit on the Sabbath, the Pharisee would certainly rescue it.

As farmers, we always looked at our Sunday farm duties as our "ox in the pit." And as a doctor, I understand Jesus' desire to heal the hurting, even if it's on the Sabbath.

I never felt as if I was breaking the Sabbath by doing my job. After all, Jesus never turned away someone in need. Though the Pharisees tried to argue with him or shame him when he performed miracles on the Sabbath, Jesus was there to do his Father's work, regardless.

Has there ever been a time when you were more concerned with getting to church than with loving your fellow man? Church is important. We should worship regularly with other believers. But if we insist on being in church or resting instead of caring for, listening to, or praying for someone in need, we're missing the point of the gospel. When asked what the greatest commandment was, Jesus said, "You must love the Lord your God with all your heart, all your soul, and all your mind. This is the first and greatest commandment. A second is equally important: 'Love your neighbor as yourself'" (Matthew 22:37-39).

TODAY'S RX

Loving others as you love yourself may mean that sometimes you have to sacrifice going to church in order to help.

Thank you, Jesus, that you know my needs and care for me regardless of the day. Help me to have the same compassionate spirit to those in need around me.

THE CRYING CEASES WHEN THE MUSIC COMFORTS

LORD, you know the hopes of the helpless. Surely you will hear their cries and comfort them. PSALM 10:17

When I walked into the nursing home, I could immediately tell what kind of day Phyllis was having by the decibel level of her cries.

Phyllis had cried every day since her stroke. It had taken away her ability to speak, and she was distressed that she could no longer communicate clearly. The staff and I did everything we could. We comforted her, fed her, and kept her clean and dry, but nothing seemed to help. Her crying continued unabated.

Fortunately, her roommate was totally deaf and unaware of Phyllis's plight.

One day, after weeks of Phyllis's crying, a staff member turned on a radio in her room. The soft classical music seemed to immediately affect Phyllis, and the change in volume was obvious to everyone in the home. Phyllis's cries slowed and then stopped. She seemed soothed. For days, she didn't cry at all; she just sat and listened. The days turned into weeks, and the staff started to notice that Phyllis would smile when certain songs played on the radio.

Somehow, as the months passed, the music healed something inside of Phyllis. She no longer looked hopeless, and she no longer cried, unless she was trying to communicate something specific to us.

Phyllis isn't unique. There is something deep within each of us that is touched by music. It resonates in our hearts and souls and heals us from the inside out.

Ever since Phyllis's stroke, people had been praying that she would find comfort, and she did. Now they're praying that she doesn't go deaf like her roommate so the music can continue to comfort her.

TODAY'S RX

God uses music to touch us in places where words can't reach.

I'm grateful, Father, for the healing power of music. Thank you for the calming effect it has on me. May I sing your praises and worship you all the days of my life.

TURN OFF TECHNOLOGY TO TURN OFF ANXIETY

The LORD himself will fight for you. Just stay calm. EXODUS 14:14

Regina came to me with a series of complaints. "I don't know what's going on. My heart is racing, my hands are sweating, and there are times when I can't get a good breath."

I asked her some questions and ordered a few tests. Over the next week, we ruled out a range of possible causes, including problems with her heart or lungs, a stroke, and thyroid disease. Yet her symptoms persisted—which is what eventually confirmed my diagnosis.

"Regina, the tests show you're in great physical shape. All of your results were normal. I'm pretty sure what's causing your symptoms is generalized anxiety disorder, caused by the stress you're under."

Of course, the diagnosis did what I expected it would—it raised her anxiety level.

Anxiety is one of the more common diagnoses in America—some might call it an epidemic. I see it on a daily basis with my patients.

"What do I do about it?" Regina asked. "I'm already stressed enough. I can't keep feeling this way."

"The best thing you can do is avoid the things that cause anxiety. For example, if the news upsets you, stop reading the headlines and watching TV. Take a few hours a day to step away from technology. Put your phone in another room, and turn off the TV and the computer. We were created to live in a garden, not in a world overflowing with bits and bytes. No wonder our brains are screaming for peace and tranquility."

"But am I supposed to just stare at the walls during that time?"

"Use it as a time to reconnect with your friends, family, and God. Go outside and take a walk. Keep a journal about the things you're thinking and feeling. Use the time to pursue things you enjoy."

"That does sound more relaxing, but I'm constantly fighting deadlines at work, and I need my computer."

"Ultimately, if you're not as anxious, you'll make better use of technology. Your brain will work better because you'll be worrying less."

TODAY'S RX

Sometimes, in order to keep calm, we must unplug and just relax.

Lord, I confess that I'm often so distracted by all the day's demands that I do not spend regular quiet time with you. Help me to create space in my day to read your Word and pray. Thank you for the renewal I feel when I invest time with you.

SHE ALWAYS KNEW HE WAS THERE

A demon-possessed man, who was blind and couldn't speak, was brought to Jesus. He healed the man so that he could both speak and see. The crowd was amazed and asked, "Could it be that Jesus is the Son of David, the Messiah?" MATTHEW 12:22-23

By presidential proclamation, today is Helen Keller Day in the United States. This day commemorates her birthday on June 27, 1880.

Helen Keller was a fellow Alabamian. She became blind, deaf, and unable to communicate after a childhood illness. Her early years were extremely difficult, as depicted in the popular play *The Miracle Worker*. When my children participated in this play in high school, Helen Keller's inspiring story of overcoming adversity touched their lives, just as it had mine.

As a small boy, I remember traveling with my family to visit Helen's childhood home in Tuscumbia, Alabama. But I'm not sure I fully understood her life story until several years later, when it was made into a movie.

Without the ability to see or hear, Helen learned to communicate with the help of her tutor, Anne Sullivan. She received an education and became an activist and ambassador for those with disabilities. It is said that clergyman Phillips Brooks (best known as the lyricist of the hymn "O Little Town of Bethlehem") first introduced Helen to the gospel of Jesus Christ. Upon hearing it, Helen is said to have replied that she had always known that Jesus was there, and now she was glad to know his name.

After a tempestuous childhood, Helen's demons were chased away, and a Christ-like spirit followed her the remainder of her days. Her life as a modern-day miracle is similar to that of the man referred to in today's verses. Only God could have accomplished such amazing healing.

TODAY'S RX

Nothing can separate us from the knowledge of God's love—not blindness, deafness, or the inability to communicate.

Thank you, God, that your love has no bounds. You make yourself known to all, reaching people in ways that are vaster than the stars. Thank you for desiring a relationship with me.

JESUS SEES THE SAINT IN THE SINNER'S SMOKE

I have seen what they do, but I will heal them anyway! I will lead them. I will comfort those who mourn. Isaiah 57:18

As I entered the nursing home, nurses scurried past me, waving charts in front of their faces as if trying to shoo away a gnat.

The head nurse saw me and pointed toward the back of the complex. "Your new patient is in the 'break room,' getting some 'fresh air.'"

"Uh, okay. Thanks," I said as I headed toward the back door.

Before I got there, I could smell the smoke, and I knew I'd find Ronny. He had terminal, end-stage metastatic lung cancer. Every treatment had failed, and the nursing notes told the story of why.

While admitted to the hospital, Ronny would leave "against medical advice" a few times a day to "get some fresh air." When the nurses checked on him, they'd find him outside smoking. With his three-pack-a-day habit, which he'd had for more than forty years, I was surprised that he'd made it to the age of sixty.

When I caught up with him at the end of the maintenance hallway—or the "break room," as the nurses had begun calling it—the haze was just lifting from around his face. He smiled a toothless grin at me.

"Look, Ronny, I promised you we'd do everything we could to help you, but the cows are out of the barn. Your time on earth is coming to a close."

"I know," he said, snuffing out a cigarette in one of the cereal bowls he used as an ash tray.

"I have an important question," I said. "It may be the most important question I could ask: Do you know where you're going when you leave this earth?"

"Despite all I've done to myself and others and despite all the misery I've caused, I know that one day soon I'll be with Jesus," he said.

"We may not have anything else to help your cancer, Ronny, but I can promise you that Jesus is the best medicine, by far."

Today's verse seems quite appropriate for Ronny. It's one we should all know because it's a wonderful promise to sinners everywhere—including me.

TODAY'S RX

No matter what you've done, you can't hide behind a smoke screen. Jesus knows everything, and he covers it all with his blood.

Thank you for not giving up on me, Lord, when I continually disobey you. Help me to work past my bad habits and seek you for strength whenever temptation arises. Your promises are healing to my soul.

LAST CHANCE FOR RECOVERY

Return, O Israel, to the LORD your God, for your sins have brought you down. Bring your confessions, and return to the LORD. Say to him, "Forgive all our sins and graciously receive us, so that we may offer you our praises." HOSEA 14:1-2

"I have to confess why I'm here," Micah said before I could even introduce myself. "I've been in five different rehab units, and I've been kicked out of three pain clinics."

My first instinct was to say, "I'm not sure I can help you," but before I could get the words out of my mouth, he continued.

"Please listen. I know this sounds crazy, but I sincerely believe this is my last chance, and I really want to make this work."

Overcoming an addiction to drugs and alcohol is difficult work. Micah had tried eight times, and each time he had failed, but something in his voice told me he was sincere and repentant for the mistakes he'd made in the past. I wanted to be the one to help him move past his failures and see success.

We started by working him through withdrawal. Next, he signed up for a twelve-step program and began attending meetings every day. It was hard work, and there were days when I honestly didn't think he'd make it. But he fought the urges and persisted.

His first sober coin from Alcoholics Anonymous was the hardest for him to earn. Over the next few years, each milestone he achieved was only slightly easier. He obtained each coin by battling his demons in hard-fought victories.

When he received his five-year coin, he came by the office to show it to me. It was the longest sober streak he'd ever had. But unlike the partying he'd done to celebrate in the past, this time "the hard stuff" had a whole new meaning. After five years of hard-won perseverance, he celebrated this milestone with cake, ice cream, and a root beer.

TODAY'S RX

Don't ever give up. It's never too late for God to pull you through.

Father, you are powerful to move mountains. Please move this mountain in me. Only with your help can I make progress toward a healthier life.

THE BLESSINGS OF CHOOSING LIFE

Today I have given you the choice between life and death, between blessings and curses. Now I call on heaven and earth to witness the choice you make. Oh, that you would choose life, so that you and your descendants might live! DEUTERONOMY 30:19

Danny was a child when his mom first brought him to see me. It was shortly after his dad had passed away of acute myocardial infarction. Danny had been a patient of mine ever since.

"So, tell me what's going on," I said.

"Healthwise, I think I'm fine now, but I'm here to discuss my future," he said. "Every man in my family has died of heart disease in his forties. I'm only thirty, but I want to be here for my kids—and, God willing, for my grandkids. My family history shows that some choices will lead to an early grave. I'm hoping to find other choices that will lead to a long life."

Danny's family was genetically predisposed to cholesterol buildup in the arteries. So the first thing we did was some blood work to check Danny's levels. The lab work showed his total cholesterol at 300 with an LDL of 225. That put him at risk.

"If you're serious about avoiding a premature death," I said, "there are some changes you need to start now and stick with for the rest of your life. And it won't be easy."

"I'm all in," Danny said.

We started him on a very strict diet with lots of fruits and leafy vegetables and no processed foods. He also began an exercise program that included jogging for forty-five minutes, three or four times a week. Danny was also a perfect candidate for a new class of cholesterol drugs that had just been released. He agreed to do it all.

Today's verse seems to imply that blessing will follow when we choose life. One of those blessings is living to see our descendants. Danny is a great example of someone who made good choices and reaped the benefits. Twenty years after that initial appointment, he had lost more than one hundred pounds and kept it off. By sticking with the program, he outlived every other male in his family. Part of his reward was being able to hold his first grandchild.

TODAY'S RX

Choose one daily discipline that will enhance your physical life. Then choose a daily discipline to enhance your spiritual life, as well.

May my choices today bring life to myself and to those around me, Lord.
Steer me in the right direction so that all that I say and do is pleasing to you.

JULY CHECKUP

When I was young, summer in South Georgia was revival season. Traveling pastors came to town and preached on sin and salvation for a week. In the days before indoor air conditioning, they used the oppressive July heat as an excuse to preach on hell. We believed everything they said in their sermons because we were already burning up!

One of the symbols used for the Holy Spirit is fire. Even now we say, "He's really on fire!" when we hear someone who is excited about Jesus. This summer, as you travel to see friends and family or visit a church in a new place while you vacation, give some thought to what it means to be on fire. Consider reading Acts to see how the apostles were transformed after they received the Holy Spirit. Look at how Christianity spread like wildfire in those early days, and invite the Holy Spirit to light a renewed fire inside you.

Summer is a great time to start a casual, short-term Bible study in your neighborhood. Ask the neighbors you know, and some that you don't, if they'd be interested in gathering together for a few weeks to read and discuss a specific book. With film-based studies available, you could create a movie premiere atmosphere for several families to come together to watch a Christian film and discuss it over popcorn and Milk Duds. Neighborhood parties, or hosting a barbecue at your house, can be a great time to get to know people in your community. Share your faith as God leads you, and perhaps you'll see the love of Christ spread like fire through your neighborhood.

On July Fourth, we celebrate Independence Day. Though the day will be filled with fireworks, parades, and picnics, it's important to remember that our nation was founded by a small group of Christians who were committed to freedom of religion. However, as our country has grown, many fear that we're moving toward freedom *from* religion. As you listen to politicians and political speeches this July, whether they are speaking at your local fair or on the Sunday morning news shows, ponder what they're saying about our freedom. And realize that Jesus bought us our true freedom—freedom from our sin.

July Booster Shot: July Fourth is a time of celebration and fireworks. Enjoy, but be cautious. Don't hold onto a lit firecracker.

POWER OVER LIFE AND DEATH

Soon afterward Jesus went with his disciples to the village of Nain, and a large crowd followed him. A funeral procession was coming out as he approached the village gate. The young man who had died was a widow's only son, and a large crowd from the village was with her. When the Lord saw her, his heart overflowed with compassion. "Don't cry!" he said. Then he walked over to the coffin and touched it, and the bearers stopped. "Young man," he said, "I tell you, get up." Then the dead boy sat up and began to talk! And Jesus gave him back to his mother. LUKE 7:11-15

The young man from Nain wasn't the only person that Jesus raised from the dead. Jesus repeatedly demonstrated his power over life and death—power that surpasses any medical miracle that might be used to explain it away.

I have been at the bedsides of many patients who were dead for a few minutes while we resuscitated them with CPR. Usually, after thirty minutes of CPR without getting a heartbeat, we will call the code. On rare occasions when we have seen some sign of life even without a heartbeat, we might continue for a bit longer. But two hours of CPR is the maximum. If a patient's heartbeat hasn't returned by then, it's not going to.

I've had only one patient who came back from the dead after two hours of CPR. But when she awoke and told us about where she'd been, she regretted that we'd worked so hard to bring her back. She spent the rest of her life telling people about heaven, and she couldn't wait to go back to stay.

The fact that the boy in Nain was being carried to his funeral means he had been dead for some time—possibly as long as three days. Moreover, he hadn't received any treatment, such as CPR, that might have kept him alive. He was in his coffin, en route to his final resting place.

Yet, at precisely this moment when it seemed as if nothing could be reversed, Jesus brought him back to life. The boy immediately sat up and began to talk as if he'd just been taking a nap. This miracle demonstrates the true power over life and death of our Almighty God.

TODAY'S RX

If you've been told that your death is imminent, ask Jesus for a second opinion.

Jesus, you've raised me to new life by allowing me to be born again. Thank you for calling out to me when I was spiritually dead and for opening my eyes to the beauty of life with you.

A MARRIAGE RESTORED

O Lord my God, I cried to you for help, and you restored my health. Psalm 30:2

When Kevin came to my office, before I could ask about his symptoms, he blurted out, "I have a confession to make. I left my family."

To all appearances, Kevin and his wife had a great family life with their two kids. They attended church together, never missed one of their kids' games, and appeared to be doing well financially.

"I saw your wife a while back, and I knew something was up. Why did you leave?"

"I travel a lot for work. On one of my regular trips, I met someone. We'd have dinner, and she would listen to me when I talked. I felt like she understood me better than my wife did.

"But you appeared to be living the American dream."

"I felt trapped, and I wanted my freedom. I told my wife I needed some time alone."

"Well, now that you're alone, you don't seem very happy."

"I thought moving out would give me some room. But now this woman is pressuring me to go through with a divorce and move to California. That means leaving my kids behind, and I'm not even sure I like this woman that much."

Kevin had built a web of deceit, and now he was all tangled up in it. Realizing the destruction that loomed ahead, he wanted to turn back.

"If you want out of this mess, you have to confess everything to your wife. I'm sure she's willing to work on your marriage. It will be hard, and it will take time, but it'll be worth it. And I know God will bless you if you turn back to him."

Kevin thought about it for a minute. "They offer marriage help at our church. Maybe we could try that. I guess I'd rather make my first marriage better than take a chance on a second marriage that doesn't feel right."

I encouraged Kevin, and we prayed together before he left.

It wasn't easy, and it didn't happen overnight, but Kevin and his wife worked hard to restore their marriage. The turning point came when they decided to put God at the center of their relationship. Three years after Kevin's change of heart, God blessed them with a third child.

TODAY'S RX

Sometimes when we cry out to God, we must confess our sin before he can restore our mental, emotional, and spiritual health.

Father, please be the center of my life. I want to depend on you alone for direction in my relationships and my career. I know that when I place my life in your hands, I'm bound to prosper.

DYING TO SELF AS CHRIST DIED FOR US

When we died with Christ we were set free from the power of sin. ROMANS 6:7

In July 1980, I stopped running from Jesus. I'd been changed from an atheist to a believer in an instant when Jesus spoke to me in a dream while I was camping in the wilderness. Looking back on that experience, I realize I had a funeral and a rebirth at the same time.

The dream I had of heaven confirmed to me that I was a new creature in Christ. In my dream, Jesus told me that I would marry Karen, we would have four children, and I would practice medicine in Tennessee. If you knew my life in Birmingham and my relationship with Karen at that time, you would know how astounding all of that sounded to me. But I heard God's voice, and I wanted to follow wherever he led me.

The next day, I celebrated my conversion by baptizing myself in the waters of Virgin Falls, Tennessee.

After my time in the woods, I often thought about the old life that had died on that trail and how it was washed away in the overflowing waters of the falls. If my old self hadn't died on that solo camping trip, it was destined to die sooner or later. I had been on a path of self-destruction, and nothing else could have saved me from myself.

Instead, I blazed a new trail, following in the steps of our Lord. That new path led me to Karen, my four kids, and my practice in Tennessee.

Christ died so that I might live a new forever life in him, but my old self had to die for me to follow him.

TODAY'S RX

There is no CPR for a life lived apart from God. Without Jesus, we are all destined to die spiritually.

Set me on a new path today, Lord. Replant my feet on your firm foundation.
Help me to let go of the sin that still remains in my heart, and wash me anew.

A MAP THAT IS NEVER OUTDATED

You will show me the way of life, granting me the joy of your presence and the pleasures of living with you forever. Psalm 16:11

We joke about men who won't follow directions or read a map. I was one of those men until July 4, 1980, when Jesus said to me, "Why are you running from me? Your friends are here with me in paradise."

On the day of my conversion from self-proclaimed atheism, Jesus told me that if I would stop running and start listening to him, he would show me the way home. Then he gave me a glimpse of my forever home in heaven, and it was more amazing and real than anything I'd ever experienced.

As a scientist and an atheist, I had been wandering in the desert, searching for the meaning of life. I didn't know that I had the directions in front of me the whole time.

Even though I was an atheist at the time, my mother had sent me a Bible while I was in college. My family had been praying for their prodigal son to return to the faith I'd had as a child. The Bible they gave me was a reminder that God's love would follow me no matter where I went.

I used the Bible often—but not for the purpose for which it was designed. Over the years, it had served as a nice bookend, a place mat, a coaster, and even a doorstop. Not until the evening of July 4, 1980, when I opened its pages and the promises of God poured out over me, did I realize it was the path I had been seeking.

Everything I wanted to know about life was contained in those sixty-six books, bound into a single volume. That night, and every day that followed, God promised to show me the way if I would just open his book. Now, thirty-five years later, God continues to direct my path every time I open his Word.

TODAY'S RX

Take a minute today to read God's Word, trusting that he will use it to guide you, just as he did for me.

God, your Word is like a breath of fresh air, revitalizing my spirit and giving me strength. May I breathe in your wisdom and promises every day of my life.

APPROACHING THE THRONE OF THE OMNIPOTENT

If you need wisdom, ask our generous God, and he will give it to you. He will not rebuke you for asking. James 1:5

Recently, Karen and I caught a local production of *The Wizard of Oz*. I was struck by something I hadn't thought about before—each character in the show is broken. The Cowardly Lion needs courage. The Tin Man needs a heart, and the Scarecrow needs a brain. But without Dorothy to escort them to the Emerald City, they would have remained forever stuck right where they were. They needed Dorothy to approach the great wizard on their behalf. They needed her to intercede for them.

Going to the doctor's office can feel like a trip to see the wizard. Most patients aren't really sure what doctors do, why we do it, or how it's done. They're afraid we'll cause them pain or that we'll discover something embarrassing about them. At such moments, having a personal advocate, a Dorothy, can give them the courage to ask for what they need.

I see patients every day who are accompanied by a Dorothy. Whether it is a parent, friend, son, or daughter-in-law, a Dorothy advocates on the patient's behalf. He or she will coax the patient to speak by saying, "Tell the doctor what you were telling me," or "Do you have any questions you want to ask?" A Dorothy can make sure that both the patient and the doctor have all the necessary information to help the patient get well.

Are you ever afraid to ask your doctor important questions?

Do you ever wish you had a Dorothy with you at your appointments?

What about in your spiritual life? Do you ever feel as if you need an advocate to represent you at the throne of God?

The good news is that we have better than a Dorothy standing with us; we have God's own Son interceding on our behalf before the Father. Because Jesus is our advocate, we can submit our requests to the all-powerful God of the universe with confidence.

Unlike the characters in *The Wizard of Oz*, we never need to worry or be afraid because our advocate—Jesus—is always right beside us.

TODAY'S RX

When it's time to return to our forever home, Jesus is the one who will guide us to where the yellow brick road turns to streets of pure gold.

Jesus, I'm broken and in need of you. Thank you for walking beside me, interceding for me, and restoring all that has failed in my life. I know that, with you, I can be made whole.

PEACE COMES FROM FORGIVENESS

Jesus said to the woman, "Your faith has saved you; go in peace." LUKE 7:50

Sometimes the medicine I prescribe doesn't come from a pharmacy; it comes from a book. That was the case with Suzy.

When I make my rounds at the nursing home, I often hear the TV going in the background. Usually my patients and I are oblivious to the noise, but one morning a familiar voice caught my ear. I stopped what I was doing, looked over at the TV, and there on the screen was Suzy, a young patient of mine, being interviewed on a national talk show.

With her bright blue hair and over-the-top personality, Suzy was easy to recognize. The program was investigating the backgrounds of people from the adult entertainment industry, and Suzy was one of several guests. As her doctor, I knew she was a dancer at a men's club, but she had never said anything about her childhood.

As I caught snippets of the conversation, Suzy spoke of growing up in an abusive household and being bullied at school. She said she'd always been timid and shy as a little girl and that working in adult entertainment had made her feel powerful. But by running from her past, she had ended up in a very dark place. The interviewer wrapped up the show by reflecting on how our past can so often dictate our future.

A few weeks later, Suzy made an appointment to see me. When I entered my office and sat down behind my desk, she began to cry. Gone was the over-the-top personality I'd seen on TV. Before me sat a sad and remorseful little girl.

"Ever since I made my confession on TV," she said, "my world has come crashing down."

She looked at me and wiped away the tears.

"I'm not dancing for money anymore. I opened the door of my heart to Jesus and let him in. But I still can't forgive myself for all the bad and stupid things I've done in my life."

Suzy didn't need a medical prescription; she needed reassurance. I gave her today's verse and told her to read it four times a day. When Jesus says that we're saved by faith, it means we're saved from our past, as well. Suzy just needed to embed this truth in her heart.

TODAY'S RX

If God has forgiven us, we must also forgive ourselves.

Help me to remember, Jesus, that when I don't forgive myself, I make light of your sacrifice. You endured a torturous death to atone for my sin, and I never want to forget that. Thank you for forgiving me and washing me white as snow.

SECRETS TO HEALTH

Keep the commandments and keep your life; despising them leads to death.
PROVERBS 19:16

"That's quite a list of diseases," Elmer said. "I'm a little overwhelmed."

"Let's go over them one by one," I said, pulling up a chair. "You have hypertension; that means your blood pressure is too high. Overeating and a lack of exercise cause this. Diabetes and hyperlipidemia are also related to your diet. You need to eat more fruits and vegetables—the multicolored kind—and less white food such as bread, pasta, rice, and potatoes. You should have only one serving of meat, and it should be lean, like fish or poultry. As for exercise, you need to walk three to five times a week for about thirty minutes each time. You don't need to worry about speed, just keep moving."

"That's a lot to do," Elmer said.

"You also need to give up smoking. We can try a nicotine patch or gum, and if that fails, there's a prescription. But the old-fashioned way is just to throw your cigarettes out."

"That's a long list of rules and regulations. It's like you're giving me the Ten Commandments of Health and telling me I'll die if I don't do them."

"That's not far from the truth. If you don't work on these problems, the first thing you can expect is a heart attack or a cardiovascular event. Having all your problems together increases your risk exponentially. The good news, however, is that it's been shown that those who lose weight, eat a balanced diet, and exercise regularly improve their health and live longer lives. So just like the Ten Commandments in the Old Testament, these rules can help you."

Many of my patients come to me hoping to learn the secret to effective weight loss or how to implement quick health fixes. They're looking for an easy answer to a longer and healthier life. But the secret solution they're looking for is really no secret at all.

"Proper nutrition, regular exercise, and quitting smoking are the secrets to saving your life, Elmer. Frankly, they're better than any medication I could give you. If you follow these rules, you'll find they don't have to be a negative; they can be a positive that helps you extend and enjoy your life here on earth."

TODAY'S RX

The secret to good health is to actually do the things you already know are good for you. Start today.

Father, I am weak when it comes to being disciplined. As Romans 7:19 says, "I want to do what is good, but I don't. I don't want to do what is wrong, but I do it anyway." Help me to make good choices so that I may live a long and healthy life.

BE LIKE THE OLIVE TREE

I am like an olive tree, thriving in the house of God. I will always trust in God's unfailing love. PSALM 52:8

Have you ever had the privilege of sitting under an olive tree? If you ever have the chance, I encourage you to soak up the experience.

When Karen and I visited the California wine country, we sat on a bench under an olive tree and had a picnic. It was a sunny afternoon, and the breeze that gently filtered through the branches cooled us. I watched as the sun's rays glistened on Karen's golden hair, making her look more radiant than ever. Sitting under the olive tree with my wife felt like a brief taste of heaven on earth.

As I breathed in the scent of olives all around me, I reflected on how important the olive tree has been to humanity. Throughout the centuries, the tree's branches have represented peace. After the Flood, the dove brought an olive branch back to Noah as the first evidence that man was once again reconciled with God.

The fruit of the olive tree has special healing properties that were well known in the ancient world and are being rediscovered in our day and age. We are beginning to realize that including olive oil in our diets can help prevent heart disease and hardening of the arteries. Some say that olive oil is one of the healthiest oils to cook with.

From the Old Testament, we learn how olive oil was used to fuel the lampstands in the tabernacle. Jacob poured it on the stone pillar that he'd set up to mark the place where God had spoken to him. Olive oil was also used to anoint the sick, bake bread, and sanctify grain offerings.

No wonder the psalmist uses the olive tree as an image for thriving. The olive tree represents peace and calm, but also purpose and meaning. To live in the house of God as an olive tree would be an honor and a blessing that could be passed down for many generations. I pray for this for you as well as for myself.

TODAY'S RX

Whenever you use olive oil, remember its health benefits, along with how it was used in Old Testament times to glorify God.

Lord, help me to stand fruitful and pure, like an olive tree, in your sight. Use me to bring good news and light to others so that you may be glorified.

LONGEVITY AND THE LOVE OF THE LORD

Moses said this about the tribe of Benjamin: "The people of Benjamin are loved by the Lord *and live in safety beside him. He surrounds them continuously and preserves them from every harm."* Deuteronomy 33:12

Amos sat in his wheelchair, clapping his hands as the nurses brought the cake to him. They lit three candles—a zero between two ones—to commemorate Amos's 101st birthday. As he blew out the candles, I marveled at what a feat it was for him to still be alive.

Not many Southern men live as long as Amos. We Southerners have a lot of unhealthy habits. We think white meat refers to the fat back cut of a pig, so we always ask for seconds. And for many Southerners, tobacco isn't merely a cash crop; it is also a pack-a-day habit that's tough to shake.

Amos's generational longevity astounded those who knew his family. His mama had died when she was ninety-eight, and his daddy died at ninety-five. Most of Amos's kin had spent their entire lives working the farm, doing what their fathers before them had done—tilling the soil and raising a few cows and hogs.

Many of Amos's family members had worked well into their eighties before retiring and letting the next generation take over. Yet, despite all their hard work, along with their fatty diets and tobacco addictions, they have defied the odds, living decades beyond their life expectancies.

I watched as Amos handed out plates of cake to everyone. When it was my turn, I wished him a happy birthday.

"Do you want some ice cream with that cake, Doc?"

I thought of my diet and shook my head. Then I saw Amos's plate—a big fat slice of cake with two heaping scoops of ice cream.

"Amos, why do you think you've lived so long?" I asked.

"I believe the good Lord above gave me this much time on earth so I could share his love with others. But I'm willing to go when my master calls me home."

"Amen!" I said.

Then I asked for a scoop of ice cream.

TODAY'S RX

Every day we're here is a good day to show the love of God to others.

Father, every day in this life is a gift. Whether I have many years ahead of me or not, let me use each day well, valuing what you value and loving as you love.

DAYBREAK'S FRESH START

The faithful love of the LORD never ends! His mercies never cease. Great is his faithfulness; his mercies begin afresh each morning. LAMENTATIONS 3:22-23

Growing up on a farm, I learned that the early morning was the best time to get things done, before all the distractions of the day began to clamor for attention. As a doctor, I have continued that habit. For many years, I got up at 5:00 a.m. and drove twenty miles toward the eastern horizon, watching the sunrise and reflecting on how God's mercies are new every morning.

At the big city hospital, I was usually one of the first doctors on the floor making rounds. This allowed me to get reports from the night shift nurses and greet the oncoming day shift. And because it was early in the morning, I also had the opportunity to speak with my patients as they woke up to hear about their dreams and how they had slept.

Medically speaking, the early hours of the morning are the most common time of day for a heart attack, stroke, or pulmonary embolism. This is due in part to low cortisol levels during the night and a sudden rise in blood pressure when the patient first awakens.

The greatest stories of God's mercy often came during the night, and I was first on the scene to get the full picture. Even though morning is a critical time of day, it is also a time of joy, with the opening of new opportunities. The sunrise sheds light on the darkness of the night. Daybreak brings renewed hope of another day of healing.

TODAY'S RX

Watch tomorrow's sunrise; it's the sweet spot of the day.

God, thank you for each new day, for every breath that fills my lungs, and for every sunrise that reminds me of the hope I have in you.

RESCUED FROM FAMINE

The LORD watches over those who fear him, those who rely on his unfailing love. He rescues them from death and keeps them alive in times of famine. PSALM 33:18-19

Caroline came into my office for a follow-up visit, but her cough hadn't gotten any better.

"You look like you've lost weight," I said.

"With the fever, I haven't been hungry," she said.

"You know the saying, 'Feed a cold, starve a fever'?" I said. "That's wrong. It should be 'Feed a cold, feed a fever.'"

"Okay, I'll try to eat more," she said.

"Did you take what I prescribed for the bronchitis?" I asked.

"Every day, just like you said."

A fever can help our bodies beat an infection, but after several courses of antibiotics, Caroline's fever was past that point.

"I'm going to order a chest X-ray. Your cough should be better by now."

When the results came back, I noticed a spot in the region of the chest cavity that contains all the chest organs except the lungs. Further testing confirmed our worst fear: Caroline had lung cancer. Unfortunately, it was located in a spot that surgery couldn't get to. Her only hope was chemotherapy. With her already depressed immune system, I knew it would be a difficult journey—and the chemo beat her up pretty badly. She lost even more weight, and her once-beautiful hair fell out.

Three months after the chemo ended, Caroline arrived for a follow-up visit, sporting a baseball cap. Tests showed that the tumor had shrunk by 70 percent, but it was now at a standstill, and there was nothing more we could do. Caroline and I agreed that we would continue to pray for remission.

Then I noticed something else in her chart. "Have you gained five pounds?" I said. No one gains weight while on chemo.

Caroline grinned. "Yes, Dr. Anderson. I figured if eating could help me beat a cold, it might also help me beat this cancer!"

Caroline experienced a famine on a personal level, and yet God had kept her alive. Her story is a reminder to me of how God's ancient promises are still applicable today.

TODAY'S RX

Keep eating and drinking when you're sick. Proper nutrition and hydration help your body fight disease.

God, rescue me from all that plagues my mind and body. Nourish me with your promises, and strengthen my spirit with your Word.

STAY CALM AND CARRY ON WORSHIPPING

Moses told the people, "Don't be afraid. Just stand still and watch the LORD *rescue you today. The Egyptians you see today will never be seen again. The* LORD *himself will fight for you. Just stay calm."* EXODUS 14:13-14

The first Ebola cases arrived in the United States amid a great deal of concern. One might even say *panic*. The Centers for Disease Control in Atlanta sent out bulletins and instructions on what people should do if they came in contact with someone who had Ebola. Protocols were implemented to prevent the spread of the disease, which had a death rate of 50 to 90 percent and no known cure.

In cities where health-care workers or visitors to the US were found to have the disease, abatement crews dressed in white hazmat suits evacuated those who lived nearby and professionally cleaned the premises and parking lots. After a death at a Texas hospital, the buildings became a ghost town. In other countries, planes were grounded and borders were closed.

As a doctor, I watched with interest as the American public seemed gripped by fear about a disease that wasn't likely to spread or kill many people in the United States. We have an abundant supply of resources, knowledge, and one of the best health-care systems in the world. In fact, I knew that the flu, which claims thousands of lives each year, was likely to kill more people than Ebola.

Though I agree that it's prudent to take precautions, I fear that all the media coverage of the Ebola crisis did more to cause panic than it did to save lives. We would all do well to heed the advice of Moses by standing still and watching the Lord rescue us, rather than panicking.

God has promised to protect us. That protection can come from CDC bulletins, hazmat suits, or cautious behavior. But, in every case, it comes from God. When we acknowledge that he is our protector, we won't panic; we'll worship.

TODAY'S RX

There will always be plagues, wars, and rumors of wars, but the Word of the Lord will stand forever.

Lord, you are and always have been mighty to save. Thank you for protecting me each day and helping me to cast my worries aside. I trust that you are in control.

NOTHING WILL SEPARATE US FROM HIS LOVE

I am convinced that nothing can ever separate us from God's love. Neither death nor life, neither angels nor demons, neither our fears for today nor our worries about tomorrow—not even the powers of hell can separate us from God's love. No power in the sky above or in the earth below—indeed, nothing in all creation will ever be able to separate us from the love of God that is revealed in Christ Jesus our Lord. ROMANS 8:38-39

One of the first books I studied as a young Christian who hadn't yet matured in his faith was the book of Romans. When Satan tried to attack me or discourage me from the battle, Paul's letter provided comfort. Romans gave me the strength to press on when times were trying.

A few years ago, Karen and I visited Italy. While we were in Rome, we heard stories of the early Christians and the struggles they endured for their faith. These Christians were at war with the political and religious leaders of their day. Many were tortured or put to death in the cruelest of ways.

Rome was also where Paul was imprisoned. It was from a prison in Rome that he wrote so many of the letters that give us such great comfort today. Walking through the city, Karen and I were deeply moved at the thought of what Paul and the early Christians suffered as they kept their faith alive despite the persecution they endured.

These Christians knew that hundreds, perhaps thousands or tens of thousands, of their brothers and sisters would die for the faith. Though they didn't yet have Paul's written words, they held the promise of Jesus in their hearts, knowing that not even death by evil leaders would separate them from God.

When I am with patients who are facing uncertain health outcomes, the verses I most often refer them to are found in Romans. Though my patients' battles are different from the brutality the ancient Christians faced, they are nonetheless in a battle for their lives. To press on, these patients need the same reassurances of God's promises that the early Christians did.

We're blessed to have Paul's words in written form so that whenever we have doubts, his words can remind us of God's love for us.

TODAY'S RX

Do not be anxious or fearful. Nothing can separate us from the love of God.

Thank you for the promise, Lord, that nothing can separate me from you—
not even the hardships and difficulties I face. Remind me of this always
so that I may not be quick to despair, but steadfast in trusting you.

ANSWERING THE BIG QUESTIONS

My child, never forget the things I have taught you. Store my commands in your heart. If you do this, you will live many years, and your life will be satisfying. PROVERBS 3:1-2

Not long after I opened my practice, Jeff brought his newborn son to me. You might say that Benjamin and I grew up together.

It was a joy to watch him develop. He not only met every milestone; he exceeded them. He was a special child gifted by God with a keen intellect. I looked forward to his visits because there was always something new going on in Benjamin's mind.

Jeff and his wife were both educators, and they never missed an opportunity to teach their son. When Benjamin came in for appointments, he'd always have a list of questions about biology and medicine. I would take a few minutes to teach him about the nervous system or how the bones in our feet work together.

Benjamin's most intriguing questions were the ones he started asking as a teenager.

"Dr. Reggie, how do you integrate science with the faith that you've learned at church? Sometimes I have trouble when they're in such opposition to each other."

I explained how both science and faith set out to answer many of the same questions. How did we get here? Why are we the way we are? What makes us different from others? But science and religion use different approaches to get answers. Science looks at observable data, things that can be measured and replicated. God, on the other hand, can't be directly observed. What we know about him we learn from Scripture, tradition, and personal experience.

"Science can't create art or beauty. It can't fill our souls with meaning and purpose. And though humans can sometimes get religion wrong, God himself is never wrong."

I explained that Jesus didn't die on the cross to reconcile us to a scientific theory; he died to reconcile us with our creator. Christian faith was completed on the cross, and it is our identity in Christ that gives us purpose and meaning.

When Benjamin grew up, he became a doctor, and he told me that his career choice was influenced by our early conversations.

"You're the one who told me there are no conflicts in Christ," he said.

TODAY'S RX

When we teach the next generation, we can help them avoid the mistakes of the past.

Father, thank you for filling my life with meaning and purpose. I take comfort in knowing that you so intricately made me with gifts, abilities, and interests that I can use and develop as I pursue your plan for my life.

CONVERSATIONS WITH A FRIEND

Take delight in the LORD, and he will give you your heart's desires. PSALM 37:4

Have you ever prayed for something that your heart intensely desired?

Sometimes, it can seem selfish to pray for our requests when we look around and see illness, poverty, and hunger. How do we ask for the things we want when so many single moms, orphans, and war refugees have more important needs?

Yet, in today's verse, God invites us to embrace his love and take delight in him. He wants us to know him so intimately that his desires will be ours as well.

Many times I haven't felt worthy of asking God for my desires. I would tell myself he's too busy to be bothered. But that's not what he says.

He says we should take delight in becoming closer to him. He says that he will know our desires—those things that are unique to us and those things that are buried deep in our souls. God knows them, even if we've never put words to them, because God know us intimately.

I know what God has done for me. There is nothing I have to do to earn his favor. All I have to do is delight in him, and he knew the desires of my heart without me whispering a word.

God wants that kind of closeness and intimacy with all of his children. He wants that with you.

Take a moment today to delight in him. Start by telling him three things you love and adore about him and listen closely as he responds to you. You and I are both worthy because we are sons and daughters of the King. And that is something we can all delight in!

TODAY'S RX

Be still and know that your heavenly Father is also your closest and most intimate friend—the kind of friend who knows what you want before you even say it.

Jesus, you are the King of kings enthroned in heaven, and yet you bow down to listen to my prayers, to know me intimately, and to give me the desires of my heart. I can't help but delight in you. I'm completely unworthy, but you count me as righteous. Thank you.

SNAKEBIT

These miraculous signs will accompany those who believe: They will cast out demons in my name, and they will speak in new languages. They will be able to handle snakes with safety, and if they drink anything poisonous, it won't hurt them. They will be able to place their hands on the sick, and they will be healed. MARK 16:17-18

It was well past midnight in the emergency room when a new patient arrived. As I walked into the exam room, it was obvious that Bobby and his drinking buddy had spent the night in a smoky bar. They reeked of alcohol and cigarettes.

Bobby held up his right hand. It was swollen to twice the size of his left.

"Got bit by a copperhead," he said. "But we caught him. I got him in a feed sack in the back of the truck."

I took a look at his hand, which revealed two tiny puncture marks consistent with a snakebite. He was telling the truth. From the swelling, I could tell the venom was spreading. If he wasn't so intoxicated, he'd be experiencing severe pain.

"What were you doing with a poisonous snake at midnight?" I asked.

"My buddy and I were driving down Possum Swallow Road near the creek. The snake was smack-dab in the middle of the road."

"Okay, but how'd you get bit?"

"I got out of my truck and tried to catch it right behind the eyes. But I guess he had too much wiggle room."

As I began to treat his snakebite, I silently prayed two prayers.

Father, help me to do your healing work on this snakebite. And help Bobby to make the changes in his life that will give him a better future.

By the next morning, the antivenin had proven effective, and the booze had worn off. Though Bobby was likely to have some pain for a while, he was fortunate. We can all thank the Lord for saving us, even when we're not using our God-given sense.

Today's verse says that "miraculous signs will accompany those who believe." My prayer for Bobby's healing had been answered, but only time would tell if my prayer for his future would also be answered. But I believe in a God of miracles and second chances.

TODAY'S RX

Do you ever feel snakebit in life? Make a list of the miraculous things you've witnessed, and use it as a reminder of God's faithfulness and power.

God, make yourself known to me today. Place your hand of healing on my tired body. May your promises be a balm to my heart, and may your presence soothe me.

OUR GOD IS LARGE AND IN CHARGE

Why are you scheming against the L*ORD? He will destroy you with one blow; he won't need to strike twice!* NAHUM 1:9

Recently, I had to say farewell to one of my long-standing patients.

"Are you ready to be with Jesus?" I asked him when I knew his time was near.

His answer was an enthusiastic, "Yes! Yes! Yes!"

But his children were saying, "No, no, no. Lord, please don't take him," as they cried and mourned the loss that we all saw coming.

Once the patient had passed away and the family's tears slowed, they began to see his death with new eyes. They knew that one day in the future, their father would welcome them to their eternal home with great rejoicing. And on that day, their reunion would be complete.

Before the Fall, God's plan was for us to live with him in Eden, where we would never know disease or pain. But when sin entered the world, our physical lives were changed forever. Illness and sickness are God's enemies. And sometimes, they can seem like mighty enemies, scheming against us with pain and suffering.

God sent his son, Jesus, to reestablish the covenant, and it is through our belief in Jesus that we know there is more to life than the physical life we see. Though Satan tries to destroy us, no plot or scheme of his can succeed against us. God promised us long ago that he will prevail and destroy the enemy with one blow.

When someone is sick, we pray for healing, and sometimes the Lord answers our prayers with a miraculous healing. But sometimes he doesn't. In such circumstances, we can feel as if the enemy has won. But God still heals us in death, as was the case with my patient. In death, God heals us with new bodies.

The glory of heaven can be hard to fully comprehend for those of us who are left behind. But what I can tell you from my experience sitting at the bedsides of so many dying saints is that both types of healing are answers to our prayers. And both are in God's sovereign will.

TODAY'S RX

Whether God heals us here and now or then and there, his answer to our prayer for healing is always "yes!"

Lord, let my heart be at peace with your will. However you choose to provide healing, may you ultimately be glorified.

GOD'S FOOD

By his divine power, God has given us everything we need for living a godly life. We have received all of this by coming to know him, the one who called us to himself by means of his marvelous glory and excellence. 2 PETER 1:3

Seth pinched his stomach, and he could pinch a lot more than an inch. "Dr. Anderson, I need to lose this gut. What's the best way to do that?"

"Tell me about your diet."

"Not every day, but I usually get a muffin or croissant with my latte for breakfast. For lunch, I'm usually busy, so I hit whatever fast food joint is close. If I'm running late at night, which is often, I'll grab a pizza or Chinese takeout on my way home."

"Do you snack?"

"Sometimes I'll grab a candy bar or chips out of the vending machine if I'm hungry."

As I listened to Seth describe what he ate, I thought about how much things have changed. Growing up on the farm, I understood firsthand that our food came from God. He gave us the rain and the sun. Some years, he blessed us with bumper crops; but even in the lean years, we knew that our needs were in his hands.

With the rise of fast food, things are certainly more convenient, but they're also disconnected from God's divine purpose. If my patients understood more about where their food came from, I knew they'd be more likely to choose foods that were healthy, not just convenient.

I gave Seth a few simple rules to help him lose weight.

"First, eat food the way God made it. If you can pick it and eat it without doing much else to it, it will be healthier for you. That's not always the fastest way to get a meal, but it's the best way. God's food is simple. But when we highly process it, we change those simple foods into something that isn't good for our bodies. If you want results, eat more fruits and vegetables and avoid the drive-through windows and vending machines."

When Seth came in a year later, I immediately noticed the change in his weight. He had dropped forty pounds.

"What did you do with it all?" I asked.

"I left it at the drive-through window."

TODAY'S RX

What's convenient for your schedule may be catastrophic for your health. For best results, choose foods according to God's plan.

Father, it can be a struggle to eat healthy foods. Help me to give up what's quick and convenient for what is nourishing. Enrich both my body and my life with food that you've designed to bring me energy and physical strength.

NETTIE'S TIME

[Paul] said, "Why all this weeping? You are breaking my heart! I am ready not only to be jailed at Jerusalem but even to die for the sake of the Lord Jesus." When it was clear that we couldn't persuade him, we gave up and said, "The Lord's will be done."
Acts 21:13-14

Nettie was the nursing home's sentry. She posted herself in an overstuffed armchair in the center of the foyer. From her command post, she made sure that no one came in the front door without a proper greeting or left without a friendly good-bye. So when I walked in one day and she wasn't at her post, I was concerned.

"Where's Nettie today?" I asked the head nurse. "She isn't in her chair."

"She didn't get up for breakfast this morning. She asked to have a tray delivered instead," the nurse said.

This wasn't like Nettie. She was usually first in line for breakfast so she would be available to help the other residents take their trays back to the kitchen when they were finished.

"I'm not scheduled to see her today, but I'd like to stop in before I do the rest of my rounds."

I followed the nurse to Nettie's room, not knowing what to expect. But there she sat with her trademark smile, resting in bed just as eager to greet me as if she were seated in her armchair near the front door.

I made small talk with her while I checked her vitals and reviewed her recent lab work. Soon, the talk turned serious.

"I know my time is coming," she said. "My body is wearing out, and my job here on earth is finished. I'm just waiting for the Lord to come get me."

"But, Nettie, your vitals are all stable; and there's nothing remarkable in your lab results. You're just as healthy today as you were last week. Why do you think you're going home soon? Are you having pain?"

"I'm not having any pain. But I've lived eighty-eight great years, and that's well beyond what I thought I would live. I just know my time is near."

Three days later, Nettie passed through the veil that separates this world from the next. When her time came, she was ready to go.

TODAY'S RX

We won't pass through the veil until the Lord says it's time, but it's good to be ready for him when he calls.

God, I hope I have as much peace as Nettie had when it comes time for you to call me home. Don't let me despair the end of my earthly life, but infuse my heart with great hope for what awaits me in heaven.

SURPRISING WORDS

Stretch out your hand with healing power; may miraculous signs and wonders be done through the name of your holy servant Jesus. Acts 4:30

During an overnight shift in the ER, I was summoned to see a young boy who had fallen and hit his head.

"I heard that throwing up after hitting your head is a bad thing, so I brought him in," his mother said.

Though it was 1:30 in the morning, the mother was fully dressed and completely made up. *If she had time to get ready, how serious could it be?* I wondered as I started my exam.

The boy's pupils were equal and reactive. He was attentive and easily followed my directions. "Where did you hurt your head?" I asked. He pointed to the spot, and I felt it.

It was a normal neural exam. He was a normal kid who'd gotten a bump on the head. But as I turned to ask the nurse to give the mother a head injury instruction sheet, I heard myself say instead, "Well, his exam looks good, but I think we should send him to Vanderbilt to get a CT scan."

I had no idea why I'd said that. The words just slipped out of my mouth. The nurse looked at me like I was a lunatic, and the mother seemed confused. Without knowing why, I sensed that something more was going on.

It was no small thing to find a neurosurgeon in the middle of the night. Moreover, the nurse had to order an ambulance to take the boy, and there was a ton of paperwork involved.

Though I had no objective data to back up my referral, I had a sense that something was happening that only God could explain.

Four hours later, the neurosurgeon phoned and surprised me with these words: "I'm glad you sent him over. I just got out of surgery. We evacuated a hematoma from his brain. If you hadn't gotten him here in time, he would have died."

I'm convinced that it was God who spoke the words to send that boy to Vanderbilt; he simply used my mouth to do it.

TODAY'S RX

When you hear a still, small voice, be open to it. You just might witness a miracle.

Father, I invite you to speak through me today, offering kindness and counsel to those around me who are in need. May my words be pleasing to you and a comfort those who are hurting.

HEART AND MIND MATTERS

Because of your anger, my whole body is sick; my health is broken because of my sins.
Psalm 38:3

Our physical, emotional, and spiritual health are all connected. You don't have to go to medical school or even live in the modern world to know that. Looking at today's verse from Psalm 38, we can see that even King David made the connection.

A number of years ago, during my residency in family medicine, I was the medical director of a small psychiatric hospital. There, I was responsible for the physical care of approximately thirty patients who were suffering from various types of mental illness. That year, I saw example after example of the very same point that David made thousands of years ago. If you are suffering emotionally or spiritually, your physical health will suffer as well.

David suffered great physical pain due to his sin. He was unable to stand and had wounds that didn't heal. He suffered from fever, blurred vision, exhaustion, and pain. Though illness isn't necessarily caused by sin, David knew that he had to get his spiritual health back before he could restore his physical health. That is often true for us, too. Once our spiritual and emotional health is back on track, often our physical symptoms will improve as well.

TODAY'S RX

If you're feeling anxious, depressed, or angry, find a qualified Christian counselor to guide you to the Lord for emotional healing. Your physical symptoms may soon lessen or disappear.

Lord, I see how stress takes its toll on my body. Please lighten my heart and remove all anxiousness and worry. Help me to get on track toward a more joyful, healthy way of living.

COMPASSIONATE ANGER

A man with leprosy came and knelt in front of Jesus, begging to be healed. "If you are willing, you can heal me and make me clean," he said. Moved with compassion, Jesus reached out and touched him. "I am willing," he said. "Be healed!" Instantly the leprosy disappeared, and the man was healed. MARK 1:40-42

While doing research on today's verses, I learned that in some translations Jesus is said to be *indignant*, while others say he was moved with compassion. These seem like such contradictory emotions. Compassion is the desire to lend a helping hand, whereas indignation triggers a fighting response. How could the Bible scholars who translated these verses choose such opposing words to describe Jesus at that same moment?

Actually, I understand completely, because I have experienced these same emotions myself. In the world of medicine, those contradictory feelings often occur simultaneously. I remember one patient's diagnosis that made me feel both compassion and anger with equal intensity.

Mia was a quiet, petite woman who had a childlike innocence about her. She'd recently experienced some flu-like symptoms and a lot of fatigue. She'd lost some weight and seemed much frailer than I recalled the last time I'd seen her.

We ran some tests, and the results were shocking. This mother of two had HIV! But *how*? Usually, HIV is related to promiscuity or IV drug use. Was she secretly using drugs? There were no tracks on her arms and no evidence of drugs in her blood or urine.

I gave Mia the bad news in my office, and then I asked her, "Have you ever had a blood transfusion?"

"No, but I know how I got the HIV, if that's what you're asking."

With a mixture of resignation and resolve, Mia told me that her ex-husband had contracted the virus during one of his many affairs. And then he'd passed it along to his unsuspecting wife. At that moment, I felt overwhelming compassion for Mia and what she would now have to endure, and extreme anger at her ex-husband.

When Jesus met the leper, his heart went out to the man even as his anger was kindled by the destructiveness of the disease and the social stigma attached to it. Yes, compassion and anger can work together, but compassion should always come first.

TODAY'S RX

Direct your compassion toward other people and your anger toward the evil one who oppresses them.

God, it angers me to see how lives are ravaged by disease—how people suffer and families are broken—and yet it is in these times that your love is so greatly shown through compassionate acts of mercy. Speak to all who are suffering today and surround them with your love.

PATIENT EXPECTATION

All glory to God, who is able, through his mighty power at work within us, to accomplish infinitely more than we might ask or think. Glory to him in the church and in Christ Jesus through all generations forever and ever! Amen. EPHESIANS 3:20-21

Do you often feel as if you're in the waiting room of life? Does it seem like you've been waiting forever for the Great Physician to emerge from the operating room to give you the news you long to hear?

In those moments when we're waiting for an answer to prayer, the results of a medical test, or the end of therapy to see if our strength has returned, we can change our view from one of passive waiting to one of patient expectation. When we open our Bibles, we see God's plan and purpose through his words, which provide us with the comfort we need to know that all will soon be well because God can accomplish infinitely more than we might ask or imagine.

Too often when we pray for healing, we stop short of asking for all we want. With our weak logic and feeble faith, we think that if we ask for just a little bit of healing, God is more apt to answer than if we were to ask for complete healing. But today's verses remind us that God's mighty power at work within us can do more than we think.

I have seen many medical miracles that can only be explained by God's "mighty power at work." Many of these miracles are documented in this devotional and in my first book, *Appointments with Heaven*. In addition to the healings I've witnessed, I have also seen God's power at the bedsides of those who are about to meet Jesus face-to-face.

Both physical and spiritual healing are part of God's plan. We are often shielded from all the reasons he does what he does, but today's verses remind us that he is all-powerful and that all glory belongs to him—even when we're in the waiting room of life.

TODAY'S RX

The next time you're waiting, rather than pacing and wondering, read God's Word and know that he is able to do everything that is within his will.

Jesus, thank you for this reminder that you are capable of more than I can even imagine. I boldly ask for complete healing and a clean bill of health in your name.

A CHILD BY FAITH

It was by faith that even Sarah was able to have a child, though she was barren and was too old. She believed that God would keep his promise. HEBREWS 11:11

Melissa was forty-three, and her husband was approaching fifty. They had a good marriage and had tried to have children but had been unsuccessful. Over the years, the constant reminder of not having children took its toll on both of them. Being childless for life seemed too much to bear.

One desperate day, they both poured their hearts out to God in prayer. Afterward, they believed that God had chosen a different path for them—adoption. They started to investigate. With help from their family and aid from a charity, the cost was within their means. Though it would take a little longer than nine months, they proceeded as if they were expecting.

When the time came, they traveled to the other side of the world to meet their precious baby girl. Conditions were not great in their new daughter's home country, and traveling with an infant was grueling. Melissa was exhausted by the time she returned home.

A few days later, I met Melissa when she brought Lily to my office for an initial checkup. After I examined Lily, Melissa said, "Do you have time to work me in too? I'm not feeling well after this trip. I want to get up with Lily at night, but I'm so exhausted I can't seem to get out of bed. I don't know if the trip took all my strength or if I caught something while I was traveling."

A physical exam didn't reveal anything abnormal, so I did a blood workup to see what that would reveal.

I called Melissa the next day at home. "It looks like Lily is going to have a little brother or sister. Congratulations! You're pregnant!"

Melissa and her husband thought Melissa's time to have a baby had passed, but they stepped out in faith to the calling that God set before them. It turns out that God didn't think Melissa's time had passed; he thought it was a great time to give Lily a little sister.

TODAY'S RX

Be faithful to respond to God's call today. He may surprise you with a double blessing.

Thank you for listening to my most earnest cries, Lord. You know what I long for, and I ask that you will provide for all my needs in your way and your time.

JUNGLE SACRIFICES

Jesus traveled through all the towns and villages of that area, teaching in the synagogues and announcing the Good News about the Kingdom. And he healed every kind of disease and illness. MATTHEW 9:35

One of my trips to Ecuador took me to the jungle lowlands, where life is very different from life in Tennessee. Before I left Nashville, my missionary friend reminded me to get all my shots.

The heat in this part of Ecuador reminded me of South Georgia in July. Gnats and mosquitoes big enough to carry off a small child swarmed and splattered on the windshield as our mobile medical caravan bumped along the dirt roads.

At night, we slept under the jungle canopy, looking up through mosquito nets to catch a glimpse of the stars. We had to be wary of nocturnal animals, some of which could inflict serious injury if we weren't careful.

We stayed in the shallow part of the river for bathing, and no swimming was allowed. That was fine with me. A waterfall provided a cleansing shower. Our drinking water was boiled and used in coffee or strong tea to keep us from getting intestinal parasites. This was not the living water that Jesus promised!

While we were concerned about our own health and safety, none of our problems compared to those of the patients we treated each day. During daylight hours, we saw between 100 and 150 patients—many of whom had never seen a doctor before. Meanwhile, an additional 300 or 400 villagers sat patiently watching the *JESUS* film and listening to the pastor's healing message.

I'm not saying, "Look at all the sacrifices we made to help so many people!" because nothing would be further from the truth. God's Word—spoken through the pastor and portrayed in the *JESUS* film—healed many more people than our hands did. And the people we treated medically had a tremendous impact on healing us spiritually—even more so than our healing them physically.

The New Testament is filled with stories of Jesus traveling through back roads, small towns, and large urban areas to attend to hurting people. He willingly gave up the comforts of life to meet the needs of humanity. Having had just a taste of that has transformed the way I read the Bible.

TODAY'S RX

Jesus did so much to heal us. All he asks in return is that we place our trust in him.

Jesus, use me as a model of your compassion and love. Help me to forsake my own comforts for what's important—sharing your Good News. Thank you for all you've done to spread your love to the edges of the earth.

CHOOSING YOUR MASTER

O LORD, I am your servant; yes, I am your servant, born into your household; you have freed me from my chains. I will offer you a sacrifice of thanksgiving and call on the name of the LORD. PSALM 116:16-17

Perhaps you're preoccupied with work to the exclusion of time with God. Or maybe you're involved in a destructive relationship. It could also be that an addiction or an obsession stands between you and your heavenly Father.

Satan will attempt to enslave us in any way he can. And often we won't realize we're in bondage to something until it's too late. Do a quick inventory:

Is there something unhealthy that consumes your mind and body?
Are you working too much to try to prove yourself worthy?
Are you seeking fame and fortune while neglecting your physical, emotional, or spiritual health?
Are you in a relationship that takes you away from God, your family, or friends?
Are you addicted to anything? Common addictions include food, sex, pornography, tobacco, alcohol, and drugs.

You don't have to answer *yes* to every question to know you're in a bad position—answering *maybe* to just a single question could be enough to suggest that you're being mastered by something that is stealing your life.

The good news is that God sent his Son, and then his Holy Spirit, to free us from our chains. We don't have to be a slave to anyone other than Christ. The life you dream of is possible. You can have peace, comfort, and a deep joy that can't be taken from you by circumstances. All you have to do is reach out to God. He holds the key that will unlock the chains that tie you down.

Take the first step to your new life now. I have patients who have received their twenty-year coin, signifying two decades of freedom from their old life of addiction. They tell me they keep it in their pockets as a reminder of the life they left and the freedom they have found in Jesus. Have faith that Jesus will help you leave behind your old ways. He has already assured us that it's possible.

TODAY'S RX

We all must choose which master we will serve. Choose wisely; choose God.

God, help me to choose you over all else. I long to be obedient to you.

THE TRIP THAT COULDN'T WAIT

If you are presenting a sacrifice at the altar in the Temple and you suddenly remember that someone has something against you, leave your sacrifice there at the altar. Go and be reconciled to that person. Then come and offer your sacrifice to God.
MATTHEW 5:23-24

Jim had lived a full life, and he had the belly to prove it. Eating and drinking had gotten him to well over 300 pounds. The side effects of his unhealthy habits included hypertension, hyperlipidemia, and high blood pressure.

For years, I had warned him that nothing good would come of his lifestyle, but he refused to listen. So it wasn't much of a surprise when he ended up in the ER with a 90 percent blockage in his left anterior descending coronary artery. This was serious; the LAD isn't called the widowmaker for nothing.

We admitted Jim to the cardiac floor, and the cardiologist planned surgery for the next morning. But when I stopped by on rounds, Jim had left the hospital against medical advice. I was stunned. Had I not made it clear to him how life-threatening his situation was? I couldn't imagine what he thought was so important that he had to leave the hospital. I just prayed it was worth it.

Two weeks later, I was in my office when I heard someone huffing and puffing his way down the hall. I saw it was Jim coming toward me.

"I wasn't sure I'd ever see you alive again," I said.

"I have a daughter," Jim said, resting his back against the wall as he tried to catch his breath. "Haven't seen her in years. Divorced from her mom. They moved out of state. I had to see her again before I died."

A nurse brought him a chair, and I grabbed my stethoscope. He was still breathing hard as we sat him down.

"I just didn't want to die on the table without fixing our relationship. Now that we're good, I'm ready for surgery. Can you get me back into the hospital?"

I've seen lots of patients try to get things right with God before undergoing surgery, but Jim was the first I'd seen go to such lengths to set things right with his daughter. Somehow, I think that pleased God, as well.

TODAY'S RX

Getting your relationships in order is good for your heart and your soul.

Father, loosen my grip on stubbornness and pride, and help me to seek forgiveness for those I've hurt. I see now that I have been in the wrong. May I honor you with my attitude and conduct from this day forward.

TEENAGE TEARS

Let your unfailing love comfort me, just as you promised me, your servant. Surround me with your tender mercies so I may live, for your instructions are my delight.
Psalm 119:76-77

"Courtney has lost a lot of weight," her mom said, "and I am worried about her. Can you run some tests to see what's wrong?"

Courtney sat on the exam table picking at her nails, looking down the entire time her mother spoke. I'd taken care of Courtney since she was an infant. I'd watched her grow into a kind and generous young woman. But something wasn't right. She wasn't her usual bubbly self.

"May I speak with Courtney privately?" I said.

Her mother agreed to give us some space and stepped out of the room.

I knew this would be a hard conversation to have with a seventeen-year-old, but I hoped she knew me well enough to feel comfortable telling me what was really going on.

"Courtney, the last time I saw you, you weighed 150 pounds, and now you're down to 120. Why do you think you're losing weight?"

"I guess it's because I'm not eating very well. I hide it. I tell my family that I've already eaten or that I'm going to go out to eat with friends, but then I never do."

"Why is that?"

"I don't know. I guess I'm not hungry."

"How are you sleeping?"

"Not good. Ever since I broke up with my boyfriend, I can't fall asleep. I wake up in the middle of the night and just lie there thinking or crying."

"Tell me about that."

"I thought Josh and I were going to get married when we graduated. But now . . . I don't know what I'm going to do."

If anyone you know is having trouble with sleep or appetite, look to see if there's an emotional cause. This can often point the way to a diagnosis. Fortunately, for Courtney, things got better. A few months after our appointment, she had regained her confidence. And not long after that, another boy asked her to the homecoming dance.

As parents, our job is to guide our teens and encourage them to seek Jesus as their source of confidence.

TODAY'S RX

Tears and the teen years commonly go together. But if the tears reach flood stage, look for professional help.

Father, may I be a source of encouragement and light to the teens in my life. Help me to plant seeds of faith in their lives and show them that they have worth.

A HEALING SACRIFICE

There is no greater love than to lay down one's life for one's friends. JOHN 15:13

Hayes was forty-five years old and in perfect health. He came in to see me one day and said, "I'm feeling tired and achy all over. I think I have the flu."

"It's the middle of summer, not flu season," I said, "but let's run some tests and see what's up."

His urine sample was dark, and I immediately knew that something was wrong. Blood tests confirmed what I feared—Hayes was in renal failure and needed immediate dialysis.

"What happened to my kidneys?" he said. "I don't get it. I've taken good care of myself. I don't smoke or drink, and I get plenty of exercise and sleep. I'm not under any stress at home or work, and until I came down with these symptoms, I felt great."

I had to agree with Hayes. He was the picture of health and had nothing in his family history that would suggest kidney failure.

"By chance did you take any medication that isn't in your chart?" I asked.

He looked puzzled. "No. I've only taken what you've prescribed for me, so it should all be in there," he said. Then I saw a flash of recognition cross his face. "I took some leg cramp medication from my brother a couple of weeks ago. That wouldn't cause this, would it?"

That one dose of quinine started a chain reaction that resulted in Hayes's renal failure. The mystery was solved, but the consequences were severe. The journey ahead would not be easy.

We started Hayes immediately on dialysis while beginning the search for a suitable transplant donor. After six months, a donor was found, and Hayes received a new kidney. When I spoke with him in the hospital after his successful surgery, he said, "I feel better physically than I have in months, but it's hard knowing that someone else had to die for me to live."

"If you think about it, Hayes," I said, "Jesus was the first person to offer up his physical body so that others could live. We are healed because of the wounds he suffered."

"I never thought about it that way," Hayes said. "I guess that whoever left me this kidney was following in the steps of Jesus."

TODAY'S RX

Never take medication prescribed for someone else. The effects could be deadly.

Lord, your Word tells us that it was Christ's suffering that brought us life. He had to be pierced and crushed for us to have healing. Thank you for the heart-wrenching sacrifice you made so that we could be made whole.

EXPECT A MIRACLE, TELL THE STORY

If God is for us, who can ever be against us? Romans 8:31

If you saw Norm sitting in my waiting room, he wouldn't look any different from any of the other blue-collar workers waiting to see me. He wore flannel work shirts and dungarees and drove an old Ford pickup, but Norm wasn't part of the crew—he was the guy who owned the company.

I don't know how much money he makes, but I know he has riches beyond this world that he values more than anything.

Norm entered the exam room and sat down in a chair instead of on the examining table. "Dr. Anderson, I've been pretty vocal about my faith for a long time, but after what I've been through recently, I have even more reason to talk about it."

I had always known Norm to be outspoken about his faith. He'd once brought me a sign that said, "Without God, there is no America."

"When I turned seventy, I went in for my screening like you said. Well, the doctor told me I had a triple A, which sounded like a good grade to me but turned out to be bad news—an abdominal aortic aneurysm, which can be really dangerous. I told the surgeon, 'If it's my time to go, I'm going to go.' But he talked me into doing the surgery anyway."

"That's a pretty big operation, even for someone young and healthy," I said.

"I know," he said. "The surgeon said that all was going well, but then my kidneys started to fail and so did my heart. Turns out I nearly died in surgery, and they had to take me to the ICU. But that wasn't the only thing that happened. During that time, I saw Jesus. He turned me around and told me I had to go back, that I had more work to do here on earth. And he wasn't talking about my business; he was talking about doing *his* business. So now that I'm back, I'm telling everyone who will listen."

Norm told me that he'd come home from the hospital and rehab six weeks earlier than anyone expected. "Do you believe in miracles, Doc? Because I sure do!"

TODAY'S RX

Trust in the Lord and expect a miracle. Then, like Norm, tell everyone about it.

Jesus, help me to share my faith with others, offering them the same life-giving hope that you offered me. May their ears be open to your story, and may their lives be changed.

PRAYING FOR A SHOT TO SING

My heart is confident in you, O God; no wonder I can sing your praises with all my heart! PSALM 108:1

Nashville is affectionately called Music City, and it seems there is a venue for live music on nearly every corner. Musicians and wannabes flock to Nashville to work in the industry, or at least to rub shoulders with like-minded individuals.

Many of my patients are in the music business, and those who sing depend on their voices to make a living. Unlike a piano player, for example, when vocalists get sick, they can literally lose their jobs, so it puts a lot of pressure on me when they can't sing.

Toni came to see me in the middle of flu season. It seemed that nearly every patient I saw that week had some sort of upper respiratory ailment.

"I can't talk, much less sing," she whispered. "And I have an audition tomorrow. I've been working on it for months, and I really need the job."

She looked pitiful sitting on the exam table. Her eyes were droopy, and her cheeks were flushed. She could barely speak above a whisper.

I ran some tests, and the results weren't good. She had both strep and mono. Either one would be difficult to cure in time for her audition the next day, but with both, it was next to impossible. But together we would do what we could. I gave her a shot of antibiotics for the strep and a steroid shot to shrink the lymph tissue. That seemed like the best option considering the importance of her audition.

"This will get things started, but I need you to come back and see me next week, so I can make sure you're recovering."

"Of course!" she whispered. "But can you also pray for my audition? I really need this gig . . ."

I took her hands in mine, and we prayed for healing and for God's will to be done at her audition.

The next week, Toni came back to the office. Not only did she feel better, but she was full of thanks and praise to Jesus.

"I got the tour!" she said, her voice as strong as ever. "I think the shots helped, but the prayers helped even more."

TODAY'S RX

Even when it seems like a shot in the dark—pray!

Whenever I'm too lazy to pray, Lord, remind me that it is my lifeblood—that it keeps me hopeful and in communication with you for all that I need. Thank you for never being too lazy to listen.

AUGUST CHECKUP

During August, the ER is often full of heat-related illnesses. Kidney stones, heart attacks, heat strokes, and dehydration are all common. The elderly and the very young are especially at risk and susceptible to heat-related illnesses. Check on your young children and elderly parents and grandparents frequently this time of year. Also, if your children are playing sports, make sure they hydrate well before practices and games, and that the coaches allow adequate water and rest breaks.

On the farm, water means everything. Without enough water, crops wither and die. With too much water, they can't be harvested because the fields are too soggy. Vegetables such as squash, zucchini, tomatoes, and carrots can get too watery and split open. They can also develop fungus or root rot. If you want a good harvest, it's critical to have the proper amount of water during the growing season.

The same is true for us spiritually. Perhaps you've been traveling this summer or doing other things that have kept you away from church, or you stopped reading your Bible because the kids were home. Now is the time to get back into the routine so that you are filling yourself with the "living water" you need to grow and produce fruit.

Jesus invites all who thirst to come to him and drink and never be thirsty again. This is such a beautiful picture of what he offers us—a spring of eternal water that never runs dry. The Bible is full of references to water, both literally and symbolically. Just as water flowed out of Eden, so it will flow from the throne of God and the Lamb on the New Earth. Many of Jesus' miracles took place near or with water. He used water to heal the blind, he was with the Samaritan woman at the well where she gathered water, and his first miracle was turning water into wine.

This month, as you spend time by the pool, drink a glass of ice water at the beach, or use water to make lemonade, consider ways you can incorporate more *living water* into the month of August. Maybe it's saying a prayer each time you take a drink. Maybe it is a study of how water is mentioned in Scripture. Or maybe it's time for you to take a bigger step in your faith journey and consider baptism. Nothing feels better than getting dunked in August!

Spend time with God in a quiet, cool place as you fill your soul with the living water that only Jesus, our Savior, can supply.

August Booster Shot: It's important to remember that, even if you are traveling, you need to take care of your health. Take your medications with you, and carry them on board if you're flying. If your medication needs to be refrigerated, call ahead to make sure there are accommodations where you'll be staying. And always carry a few extra days' worth of medication and supplies in case of an emergency.

WATER FOR LIFE

The LORD will guide you continually, giving you water when you are dry and restoring your strength. You will be like a well-watered garden, like an ever-flowing spring. ISAIAH 58:11

When the woman was brought into the ER, I immediately recognized Charlotte, whom I'd known for many years. She had recently turned eighty and had told me she was ready to go whenever the Lord called her. With how she looked now, I thought she might be going sooner, rather than later.

"Dr. Anderson, Charlotte hasn't eaten in over a week. She has a living will, and she specifically ruled out heroic measures, but is there something we can do?"

When I examined Charlotte, she didn't blink or move. Her mucus membranes were dry, and her skin tented when pinched. There wasn't an extra drop of water in her system.

"I know she said no ventilator or CPR, but I believe she checked the box to receive IV fluids and antibiotics, if needed, for a short while. Let's send her blood work to the lab."

It didn't take long for the test results to confirm my suspicions. Charlotte was severely dehydrated, and her kidneys were shutting down. She also had a urinary tract infection. At her age, this combination is often fatal. I spoke to her family about treatment options, while still honoring her wishes for no heroic measures.

After a short conversation and much prayer, we agreed to give her fluids and antibiotics for the next forty-eight hours. Then we'd reassess. "That allows us to make her more comfortable while giving God time to make his will known."

By the next morning, her lab numbers looked better. Her BUN had dropped from 120 to 80 (normal is 6–20), and her creatinine had dropped from 5.0 to 3.2 (normal is 0.5–1.0). She had turned the corner. God wasn't calling her home just yet.

We kept Charlotte in the hospital until we were sure her infection had cleared up and she was no longer dehydrated. During that time, her mental fog also cleared. We had treated her medically, but more important, the Lord had refreshed her with new life from his living water. Charlotte soon returned home and continued to be a blessing and a joy to her family.

TODAY'S RX

When we're physically dehydrated, we need IV fluids to restore us. If you're spiritually dehydrated, ask God to refresh you with his living water.

Lord, I confess that my faith often goes through dry seasons, being withered by the world around me. Fill me with your wisdom and truth so that my faith may instead be like an ever-flowing spring, bringing glory to you.

A SAVIOR AMID THE CORNSTALKS

He lifted me out of the pit of despair, out of the mud and the mire. He set my feet on solid ground and steadied me as I walked along. Psalm 40:2

I was ten weeks into a twelve-week summer job selling the Volume Library door-to-door in southern Illinois. As I drove past towering cornfields, I rehearsed my next house call, where I hoped to find an eager buyer. Instead of paying attention to the road, I was studying the map and my notes on the passenger seat.

Then it was too late.

An eighteen-wheeler sideswiped my Volkswagen Beetle, tossing my Bug up and onto the grille of the truck, where I became a hood ornament. When the semi finally came to a stop a hundred yards from where we first made contact and once my brain stopped swimming, I looked up to see the truck driver staring at me, white as a ghost.

He jumped out, ran toward me, and managed to pry open my crumpled door, using some kind of superhuman strength.

"Son, I didn't see you. Are you all right?"

His words echoed in my head until I understood what he was asking. "I think so," I said. I felt a little woozy, but otherwise I was fine. A tear rolled down my cheek as I realized I had just been spared a tragic death.

"I'll go get help," the driver said as he staggered back to his rig.

By the time he got back, my mind and heart had settled a bit. Though at the time I professed to be an atheist, somewhere inside I knew that God was the one who had spared my life. He alone knew my past and where my heart was at that moment. Instead of allowing me to die, alone and apart from him, he picked me up and set me back on solid ground. Three years later, when he revealed himself to me in a dream, I was ready to turn back to him.

Today, I look back at the accident and my second chance, and I thank God for being there and caring for me, even when I didn't care to know him. I believe he saved me that day to give me time to come back to him.

TODAY'S RX

God can change the direction of your life at any given moment—but it's less painful if you turn to him first.

God, help me to realize day in and day out how you intervene in my life to keep me from harm's way. May I have a thankful heart, knowing that you are my protector.

HIDDEN HURTS

He heals the brokenhearted and bandages their wounds. Psalm 147:3

When I make rounds, the nurses will update me on any changes with my patients. Typically this means vital signs, inputs and outputs (I/Os), and how many bandage changes on wounds.

More experienced nurses will often give me insight into a patient's anger or depression or tell me about a visitor who was especially upsetting. Many times, the patients themselves will tell me when there's more going on than meets the eye.

Through the years, I've learned a lot about my patients while dressing wounds, casting broken bones, or waiting for X-rays to come back. During those times, patients may open up a bit and share the story behind the story that brought them to the hospital. The physical injury becomes the beginning of an invitation to hear about what's really hurting them.

Amy's ankle injury was not particularly severe, but the story of how the injury occurred brought a whole new level of concern. She had fallen down a set of stairs and twisted her ankle on the landing—but then she told me she'd been pushed down the stairs while being kicked out of her house. Once we got her patched up, she began to cry that she had nowhere to go.

We made a few phone calls and found a women's shelter where she would be safe and have a roof over her head.

Amy's ankle healed slowly, along with her broken heart. Eventually, she found a new home and a job. With independence came a new sense of confidence that transformed the timid, frightened young woman I had first met in the ER.

Though Amy had been injured in her fall down the stairs, I saw it as God's intervention to protect her from greater harm, while he simultaneously pushed open a door that Amy had desperately tried to keep shut—bringing healing to the root of her problem.

Sometimes it can seem as if no one sees or cares about your pain. In those moments, be still and know that God not only cares for your bumps and bruises, he also cares for your banged-up and bruised heart. He has the power and the compassion to heal them both.

TODAY'S RX

Whether others see your pain or not, be assured that the Great Physician sees everything, and he has a treatment plan to restore you to health, inside and out.

Father, thank you for tending to my heart. Even when all seems lost and I feel alone, I have the promise of your presence beside me, caring for me and walking me toward healing.

A BOLD ASK

Let us come boldly to the throne of our gracious God. There we will receive his mercy, and we will find grace to help us when we need it most. Hebrews 4:16

"My baby's back there; you have to let me in! You have to let me in!"

The mother's distraught screams could be heard echoing from the waiting room, through the ER door, and down the hall where we were doing everything we could to stabilize her twenty-five-year-old son's condition. The young man had been in a rollover car accident and had been brought in on a spinal board.

"We need to let her back here," I said. "She's not going to give up, and she needs to be a part of what we're trying to do."

A few moments later, the door swung open, and the woman rushed toward her son. "My baby, my baby, what are we going to do?"

"Right now, we are stabilizing him and arranging for a transfer to the trauma unit. This would also be a good time for us to pray. He will need every prayer—and then some."

"Don't worry too much about praying," the woman said. "I'm his momma. That's my job."

This woman had boldly burst into the emergency room and immediately pressed into what was needed to save her son's life. That's the same kind of boldness that God wants from us when we approach him with our cares, concerns, injuries, and pain. He wants us to boldly let him know our needs and fears and to come to him with hearts of thanksgiving for all he has done and will do for us. As today's verse above says, the throne of God is where we will find his grace and mercy when we need it most.

TODAY'S RX

Cast all your concerns on God, for he cares for you.

Jesus, just as the blind, deaf, and leprous approached you for healing, I come before you now asking for healing. You are my only hope.

LOOKING FORWARD AND BACK

Those who have been ransomed by the LORD will return. They will enter Jerusalem singing, crowned with everlasting joy. Sorrow and mourning will disappear, and they will be filled with joy and gladness. ISAIAH 51:11

I used to look forward to summers in South Georgia, when I would play with my cousins and help with the watermelon harvest. But after my friends were murdered there, everything about the place seemed to have changed. The landscape wasn't as green or as vibrant as I remembered; it seemed flat and gray. No longer did the aroma of ripe watermelons linger in the air; now all I could smell was the stench from the paper mill. As the town grappled with what had happened in their community, it seemed the void was filled with only pain and grief.

I had changed as well. I was no longer the innocent boy who had jumped down eagerly from the watermelon truck each noonday, hungry for lunch after a morning in the fields. I had lost my appetite, and time seemed to have slowed under the hot afternoon sun. Even back home in Alabama, everything seemed different. We were all struggling with if, and how, life would ever seem normal again.

For me, it wasn't until the Lord drew back the curtain and gave me a glimpse of heaven—thereby unlocking the gates of hell I'd been living behind—that my joy was restored and I was able to move into a renewed life with him.

The next summer when I visited South Georgia, it was still just as hot as I remembered. But this time the lilacs and roses were in full bloom. The colors and the scents of heaven were everywhere. Sorrow and mourning had given way to renewed hope and vision.

As today's verse promises, our suffering is only temporary, when seen from an eternal perspective. The leaves of grief will turn after the season is over. Though the memories will last, we will have a renewed life *filled* with joy and gladness.

TODAY'S RX

On those dark stretches along the road of life, keep pressing forward. Our forever home is just around the bend, and our heavenly Father awaits with open arms.

Sometimes it's hard to see the light at the end of the tunnel, Lord, and I struggle to keep on hoping. Please pursue me in these moments and penetrate the fog that I'm wandering through. I know you are there.

ALL IT TAKES IS A GLIMPSE

Always be full of joy in the Lord. I say it again—rejoice! PHILIPPIANS 4:4

When I was on vacation in Venice, Italy, I sat in the Piazza San Marco and watched the tourists entering and leaving St. Mark's Basilica. The cathedral has opulent gold mosaics throughout, which have earned it the nickname Chiesa d'Oro, or Church of Gold.

The tourists I saw all had such joy on their faces! I'm sure they were delighted to catch a glimpse of the basilica's splendor. As I watched, it made me think, *This is how we should live our entire lives—full of joy, wonder, and worship.*

My mind wandered to thoughts of Jesus' disciples—how they had lived their lives and how most were martyred for their faith. *Did they live lives full of joy?*

Eleven of the twelve apostles died by some form of execution. They must have struggled and suffered much more hardship than we, who live in a world of comfort and convenience, could ever imagine.

Yet throughout their days on earth and even at the untimely moment of their deaths, their hearts were filled with joy. I have to believe that, no matter what happened to them, no matter how bad their days were, their eyes were fixed on their forever home in heaven.

When I find I'm having a difficult day, I try to think about eternity in paradise worshipping the Father, Son, and Holy Spirit. As I reflect on the delight I observed on the faces of the tourists who visited the ornate cathedral at St. Mark's, I imagine the freedom and joy we would have in our lives if we focused on our future in eternity.

I pray that God will give you a heavenly glimpse of our Promised Land to help sustain you on your bad days. With each passing day, we know it won't be long before we join him there.

TODAY'S RX

Resolve to live today in joy, knowing that you are one day closer to the joy of your forever home.

Lord, I give this day to you, promising to approach it with a joyful spirit and glad heart.

GIVING ORDERS

The officer said, "Lord, I am not worthy to have you come into my home. Just say the word from where you are, and my servant will be healed. I know this because I am under the authority of my superior officers, and I have authority over my soldiers. I only need to say, 'Go,' and they go, or 'Come,' and they come. And if I say to my slaves, 'Do this,' they do it." When Jesus heard this, he was amazed. Turning to those who were following him, he said, "I tell you the truth, I haven't seen faith like this in all Israel!" MATTHEW 8:8-10

Like the Roman centurion in today's Scripture passage, doctors have the authority to give orders. On a daily basis, we order medications for pain control or antibiotics for infections. We order tests to diagnose cancer and diabetes. We also order procedures such as surgery, radiation, or chemotherapy if we believe they can help cure a patient's disease. But most commonly we give "doctor's orders" to our patients to eat better, exercise more, or go on bed rest during a pregnancy.

When we give these orders, we depend entirely on other people to carry them out. A nurse administers the medications. A lab tech does the tests. A radiologist does the X-ray or applies the radiation treatment. And it's up to the patient to eat better, exercise more, or stay in bed.

But of all the millions of orders that doctors have given over the years, none has come close to what Jesus was asked to do. The Roman officer wanted Jesus to heal his servant—not by using tests to diagnose the problem or medications to fix it, not by coming to his house to see what was wrong with the servant, but by simply saying the word.

This would be equivalent to my getting a call on the weekend from a nurse in the ER about a patient I'd never met. If the nurse said, "He's in a lot of pain, and he's paralyzed from the waist down. We haven't done any tests, but you don't need to come in; just say the word and I'm sure he'll be fine," I would think she was crazy. What an impossible request!

But Jesus didn't think the centurion was crazy—instead, he was amazed at his faith. This Gentile soldier believed that Jesus had control over time, distance, and disease—and he was right! What kind of faith would it take for you to believe that?

No matter how much faith we put in modern medicine or in our doctors, nothing compares to the kinds of healing we see when we put our faith in Jesus.

TODAY'S RX

Follow your doctor's orders, but also have confidence that Jesus heals completely.

Jesus, your name is the one word I need to be healed. May your name be continually on my lips every day of my life.

TRUSTING IS THE BEST MEDICINE FOR UNCERTAINTY

While he was still speaking to her, a messenger arrived from the home of Jairus, the leader of the synagogue. He told him, "Your daughter is dead. There's no use troubling the Teacher now." But when Jesus heard what had happened, he said to Jairus, "Don't be afraid. Just have faith, and she will be healed." When they arrived at the house, Jesus wouldn't let anyone go in with him except Peter, John, James, and the little girl's father and mother. The house was filled with people weeping and wailing, but he said, "Stop the weeping! She isn't dead; she's only asleep." But the crowd laughed at him because they all knew she had died. Then Jesus took her by the hand and said in a loud voice, "My child, get up!" And at that moment her life returned, and she immediately stood up! Then Jesus told them to give her something to eat. Her parents were overwhelmed, but Jesus insisted that they not tell anyone what had happened. LUKE 8:49-56

The medical system can be filled with uncertainty, and uncertainty often brings fear. As a doctor, a large part of my job is reassuring my patients—whether it's about the results of a test, the outcome of a needed surgery, or even their fear of death.

I encourage my patients to pray, trust, and believe that Jesus can heal. Many already do, even without my prompting. But too often, trusting Jesus is our last resort. We turn to our faith when nothing else seems to work.

I've often wondered if we would see more miraculous healings if we relied on our faith *first*, rather than last—if we trusted, rather than feared. When we put our faith on a shelf to be used only in times of emergency, does it lose its potency, like expired medications?

One of Jesus' most common commands is, "Do not be afraid." The opposite of fear is faith. If we fear the outcome of a test or procedure or if we fear death itself, the antidote is placing our faith in the Great Healer. He has already promised to heal us for all eternity.

TODAY'S RX

Make "faith first, not last" your new motto. Trust God with all your fears and frailties.

Whenever fear grabs hold of me, Lord, help me to call on your name. Calm me and show me that you are in control. Give me faith to believe that nothing can keep me from your great love.

BATTLING FOR THE LORD'S VICTORY

The horse is prepared for the day of battle, but the victory belongs to the LORD.
PROVERBS 21:31

Though God is the ultimate physician who heals us, today's verse reminds us that we must also play a part in our health care. Just as the warrior makes sure that his horse is always ready for battle, we must do what we can to make sure we take care of ourselves.

Recently, I had to talk to a patient about his choices. Because he wasn't doing his part, we couldn't do ours.

Richard was an overweight, middle-aged man who suffered from a variety of health concerns, including diabetes and high blood pressure. He was now scheduled to have heart surgery, but we were unable to proceed because of other factors related to his condition.

"I'm sorry to tell you that we can't do your surgery today, Richard."

"Why not? I thought everything was on schedule."

"It was, but the tests showed that your diabetes is out of control, and your blood pressure is too high. We need to get those things taken care of before we can do open heart bypass surgery. If you're healthy, you're more likely to have a better outcome, and your recovery will be smoother."

A few days later, Richard's numbers had come down, and he was back on the docket for surgery. He was now ready physically, but he was also ready emotionally and spiritually in a way I'd never seen from him before.

"Dr. Anderson, would you pray with me before surgery?"

"Of course," I said. "Lord, we know that we have done all we can to prepare for this day. Richard has done all he could do to be as healthy and as ready as he can. We pray this morning for the surgery team that has prepared to operate on him. We ask you to guide every move of their hands and to use them to heal Richard's heart. We know that all things are possible through you. And we trust that your will be done. Amen."

As today's proverb suggests, Richard had done all he could to prepare for the battle, and now the victory was up to the Lord.

TODAY'S RX

Do all you can to prepare, and leave the rest up to God, trusting him for the victory.

Father, prepare the way for me on this healing journey. It is only by your direction that I know the way to go.

PLANS TO PROSPER

"For I know the plans I have for you," says the Lord. *"They are plans for good and not for disaster, to give you a future and a hope."* Jeremiah 29:11

I hadn't seen Bert, or any members of his family, for more than three years. Then he showed up one day with a form for me to sign.

"I need to have a physical for my new job," Bert said. "I'm hoping everything checks out because it's been a while since I was last here."

"It has been a long time, hasn't it?" I said, looking at his chart.

"The downturn in the economy just about did us in. We had to sell our house and rent an apartment in the low-rent section of town. I need this job. I've got to get my kids out of there and move them to a better school district."

"Bert, I know this job is very important to you and to your family. And I know you've tasted bitter waters and survived up to this point, though I'm sure sometimes it didn't seem like you would. But I want you to know that regardless of what this exam shows, I am confident that God has a good plan for you and for the life of your family."

I thought about the above verse in Jeremiah and prayed that God would deliver on that promise for Bert.

During his exam, a couple of small things revealed themselves, but they were minor problems. Frankly, they were the kinds of stress-related, wear-and-tear issues I'd expect to see on anyone who'd been through what he and his family had been through for the past three years.

"There's nothing in this exam that will keep you from getting the job," I said. I happily signed his form.

"I promise once my new insurance kicks in, I will get the kids here for their well visits and their shots. I can't tell you how blessed I am that God carried us through those dark times." Bert was whistling as he walked out the door.

I wish all my patients would believe what Bert already knew to be true. God's plans are never meant to harm or hurt us. His plans are always for our good.

TODAY'S RX

Even in our darkest hours, our heavenly Father shines his light to show us the way to the fulfillment of his promises.

Though my future is unclear, Lord, I know you are in control.
Help me not to rely on my own strength and understanding, but to
depend on you to lead me to pathways of healing and light.

PARENTS OF DISCARDED CHILDREN

God has said, "I will never fail you. I will never abandon you." HEBREWS 13:5

When we think about today's verse, sometimes it's hard to imagine what it means for God to never fail us or abandon us. Most of us have had experiences in life when others have let us down or not lived up to our expectations. We've experienced loneliness, and we know what it feels like to be forgotten.

Bob and Linda's children understand abandonment in ways you or I probably never will—nor would want to. But with Bob and Linda as their adoptive parents now, I know these kids will never feel abandoned again.

When Bob and Linda heard that a large mental health facility was closing, they knew that some wards of the state would have nowhere to go. So, they got involved and decided to adopt two mentally impaired adults and care for them as they would their own children. They asked me to do the adoption physicals, and I was happy to play a small part in the beautiful thing they were doing.

A few months later, Bob and Linda were back in my office.

This time, they had three little boys with them. Each one was malnourished and below the fifth percentile for height and weight for their ages. It was obvious that these boys had been severely neglected their entire lives. Bob and Linda had been foster parenting them for weeks, and now they wanted to adopt them.

"I need to be honest with you," I said. "Your hands are already full with your two adult children. These boys are going to need a lot of time and attention to recover from all they've been through. I'm not trying to scare you; I just want you to know what you're getting into."

Bob and Linda were unfazed. They looked at these boys the same way first-time parents look at their brand-new babies. They were already in love with these new additions to their family.

When I think of God's promise that he will never fail us or abandon us, I think of how Bob and Linda have loved kids that others thought were unlovable. Those kids can now rest easy, knowing that their new parents will never abandon them.

TODAY'S RX

Even when we are unlovely and unwanted, God adopts us into his family and calls us his children.

Thank you for adopting me into your family, Lord, and for showing me unconditional love. Help me to model your kindness and compassion to those who are lost and hurting.

LOOKING THE SAME WAY

Let the peace that comes from Christ rule in your hearts. For as members of one body you are called to live in peace. And always be thankful. COLOSSIANS 3:15

One of the greatest joys that Karen and I experienced on the book tour for *Appointments with Heaven* was the outpouring of love and acceptance from so many different denominations. We were invited to share our stories with messianic Jews, evangelicals, charismatics, Methodists, Presbyterians, and Baptists. If there were theological walls between us, they seemed to crumble when the doors opened and they invited us in.

I distinctly remember the first interview I did. It was a panel discussion on a TV show with two other men, and we were being interviewed about our experiences with heaven. On my left sat a messianic Jewish rabbi; on my right was an African American man who'd had had a near-death experience, during which he'd glimpsed heaven and lived to tell about what he saw. I was a simple country doctor who held the hands of the dying and got a taste of eternity when I walked them to the foyer of heaven.

I enjoyed the interview immensely, and when we finished, I couldn't wait to hear Karen's thoughts. She had been in the green room, watching the show on the monitors. When I found her, she said, "Considering the fact that you all have such different backgrounds, I didn't see any theological differences between the three of you. You all seemed more alike than different."

I hoped that the viewers saw what Karen had seen—that we were alike in our love of God. Moreover, that we all had a God-given purpose to tell our stories of what we'd seen.

I think the reason that Karen didn't see any differences is because, when our focus is on the throne of God and not on ourselves, we begin to look more and more like our heavenly Father. Though the other two men and I went our separate ways after the program, I'm certain I will see them in heaven. But I don't know for sure that we'll recognize each other. By the time we're all in heaven, I think we'll be much more alike than we will be different.

TODAY'S RX

In God's eyes, we are all created equal, with equal possibilities of being conformed to look like him.

Continue to mold my heart so that it matches yours, Father.
I desire to be a reflection of your character and love.

THIS IS MY CHILD

The Spirit of God, who raised Jesus from the dead, lives in you. And just as God raised Christ Jesus from the dead, he will give life to your mortal bodies by this same Spirit living within you. ROMANS 8:11

When Bobby arrived in the ER, his right pupil was blown, he had a skull fracture, and brain tissue leaked from a laceration on his scalp. I'd never known anyone to survive a thirty-foot fall onto a concrete floor, so my first thought wasn't about saving his life—it was about how I would tell his parents that their son was gone.

Our job was to keep Bobby alive until air transport arrived. I immediately began working on his obstructed airway, and as I worked, I prayed silently, *Please, God. Help us help him!*

Amid the hum of the ER, I heard the barest trace of a voice say, *"This is my child."*

For the next twenty-three minutes, as we worked to keep Bobby alive, I heard the whisper over and over again: *"This is my child."*

Suddenly, there was a commotion in the waiting room as Bobby's parents arrived. "Where's my child?" I heard his mother cry. "Is he dead?"

As the nurses tried to calm her down, I was struck by the similarity of her words—"Where is my child?"—with what I'd been hearing: "This is my child."

By God's grace, Bobby survived. The skull fracture had saved his life by enlarging the available space for his brain to swell.

Several weeks later, I visited Bobby at the rehab center, and he greeted me with a left-handed high five. His right arm wasn't functioning as well, but he was working hard in rehab and continuing to make progress. I told him about the whisper I'd heard and its similarity to his mother's words when she had arrived.

"God saved you for a purpose, Bobby, and I look forward to seeing what it is."

Bobby eventually returned to work. Soon he fell in love with a young woman, and they moved out West after they got married. A year and a half later, Bobby's parents stopped by with a photo of their new grandson. On the back, Bobby had written, "This is my child."[7]

TODAY'S RX

You are a child of God and God always cares for his children. Make a list of how he has cared for you.

I am your child, Lord. And you are my Father. I will proudly proclaim that as long as I have breath.

STANDING FIRM

Israel is no stronger than its capital, Samaria, and Samaria is no stronger than its king, Pekah son of Remaliah. Unless your faith is firm, I cannot make you stand firm.
ISAIAH 7:9

Today's verse says that unless we have a firm faith, we won't stand firm. As a Christian doctor, I know that physical and spiritual strength must work together for us to be at our best. That's why I was so worried about Craig.

At the nursing home where Craig was sent following his stroke, most of the patients were in their seventies or eighties. Craig was only fifty, but he looked much older. He was disabled and confused. He also had dysarthria, which means he had speech impairments and trouble understanding language.

It was hard to know how to begin treating a patient like Craig. In order to recover, he needed a lot of help. And I wasn't sure how well he would do. He seemed defeated in body, mind, and spirit.

Craig's stroke was the result of some bad habits: smoking, drinking, and years of poor nutrition. We could correct many of those habits while he was in our long-term care facility, but his mind would take much longer to unlock.

I wrote orders for Craig to receive physical, occupational, and speech therapy. I prescribed antidepressants and recommended that Craig attend counseling. The staff and I also prayed for God to rebuild his spirit. I was hopeful that if Craig could once again talk and eat on his own, we might stand a good chance of helping him overcome his depression, as well.

Because it was a Christian nursing home, pastors often visited and prayed with the patients. The nursing staff knew that Craig had not been a churchgoer in the past, but they gently and quietly urged him to open up and consider God as a resource for life renewal.

It didn't happen immediately, but as the weeks turned into months and the nurses continued to pray for Craig, eventually he began to pray for himself as well. By the time he was ready to go home, he was fifty pounds lighter, no longer smoked, and instead of drinking spirits, he was filled with the Holy Spirit. He now stood firmly on his feet and in his faith.

TODAY'S RX

If your body isn't healing as fast as you'd like, consider whether your spirit may also need healing.

However shaky the world becomes, God, help me to always stand firm in my faith. Do not let me gravitate toward or fall victim to Satan's ways; instead, keep my eyes focused on heaven and the glory that awaits me there.

REKINDLE YOUR COMMITMENT

You will be blessed above all the nations of the earth. None of your men or women will be childless, and all your livestock will bear young. And the LORD will protect you from all sickness. He will not let you suffer from the terrible diseases you knew in Egypt, but he will inflict them on all your enemies! DEUTERONOMY 7:14-15

One can only imagine the conditions in Egypt, where the Israelites were held in bondage. They likely lived in close quarters with little food and without clean water. And as with so many other groups kept in slavery, disease was likely to be rampant under those conditions.

When God freed them, he gave them healthy food, fresh water, and a Sabbath rest for renewal. All of these were new blessings to the Israelites. However, it wasn't long before they lost patience in waiting for the Promised Land and wanted to return to the lives they had known in Egypt.

Perhaps there has been a time in your life when you felt as if you were held in bondage to an unhealthy lifestyle. You ate and drank foods that weren't good for you, or you ate and drank in excessive amounts. At some point, you realized that you needed to be free from this bondage, and you or your doctor put together a set of healthy guidelines and restrictions. The good news was that, when you followed the new plan, you lost weight and gained control over other ailments, such as diabetes or hypertension, that had plagued you for years.

But then you started thinking that perhaps you could ease up on some of the new restrictions. You wanted to dabble in your old way of life, even if just for a little bit. But suddenly, those old diseases flared up again.

When we're focused on living healthy, holy lives, we strive to do what's good for us. Sometimes we slip and fall, but we can always get back up and recommit ourselves.

TODAY'S RX

Rekindle your commitment to healthy living, and enjoy the renewed life that God has promised.

Lord, I confess that I'm often swayed by what's easy and convenient, rather than committed to what takes time and energy. I don't want to be lazy when it comes to my health, so please help me establish healthy guidelines for my life and ultimately glorify you with my body.

FEAR NOT, GOD HEALS IN SURPRISING WAYS

The Lord stands at your right hand to protect you. He will strike down many kings when his anger erupts. Psalm 110:5

When I entered the hospital room and saw the empty bed, it took me a second to locate Becky, who was cowering in the corner with her face to the wall. She didn't respond to my greeting.

"She's been like this for twenty minutes," whispered the nurse.

"Why are you crying?" I asked. Becky's rocking increased, and she refused to look at me.

"Is there anything I can do to help?"

"No."

"Do you want to talk about it?"

"Nothin' to say."

Her answers to my questions were short, to the point, and noncommittal. But her face told me something was wrong. The flow of tears was slowed only by the occasional swipe of her sleeve across her face. Looking at her closely, I could see the fear in her eyes. Becky was terrified. She was in the midst of a full-blown panic attack.

"Becky," I said softly, "What are you afraid of?"

"I don't know?"

The questioning tone of her answer confirmed my hunch. Though Becky didn't have an answer for calming her fears, fortunately I did, thanks to some good research on mood disorders from Dr. Rick Shelton, a psychiatrist at the University of Alabama at Birmingham. From Dr. Shelton's work, I knew that panic disorders affected many people, but also that there were some helpful treatment guidelines to follow.

When confronted with a patient like Becky, whose fear was overwhelming, the first thing I did was pray that God would reveal his protective nature and help alleviate her symptoms. I'm pretty sure that Dr. Shelton would recommend the same course of action because during the years when he was a professor at Vanderbilt, he was also my Sunday school teacher.

God protects and heals us in surprising ways—including using our brothers and sisters in Christ.

TODAY'S RX

When fear claws at your heart, remember that God is the greatest heart surgeon, and he is always on call.

Jesus, lift me from the strongholds of panic and distress. Help my heart to be still. Embrace me and reassure me of your love.

STRENGTH FOR THE FIGHT, PEACE FOR THE FUTURE

The LORD gives his people strength. The LORD blesses them with peace. PSALM 29:11

"I just don't have the strength or will to go one more day," Harvey said. "I'm battle worn. My 'get up and go' done 'got up and went.' I just want to step away from the front lines and have permanent R&R."

Harvey's battle vocabulary was familiar. We often heard similar descriptions from the patients who were referred to our nursing home by the Veteran's Administration. These brave souls had seen the worst of the worst and lived to tell about it. They had post-traumatic stress disorder long before it was even recognized as a syndrome.

Many of the older vets fought in wars that today's teens don't even remember. They fought battles that literally were won in the trenches. In those days, they didn't call it PTSD; they called it shell shock, or combat fatigue, but it's the same thing.

PTSD is an emotional disorder that takes away a soldier's peace and emotional resolve. Recovery takes time and therapy and requires a team of providers coordinating all areas of the veteran's health care. But sometimes even the best medical science and practice can't put all the mental and emotional jigsaw pieces back together again. Only Jesus can.

Most of us have not been in combat, but we've figuratively dodged a few stray bullets in life. Maybe your battle is your marriage, cancer, a friendship, a job, or financial concerns. The effects of the stress can be the same. The constant barrage of stress, fear, and uncertainty wears us out physically, emotionally, and spiritually.

Remember, we were created to live in a garden; yet here we are smack-dab in the middle of the most epic battle ever fought—the battle between good and evil. We continually hear the sirens of jealousy, anger, crime, and disease warning us to take shelter. While the battle with the enemy of our souls rages on, we place our confidence in our holy Commander-in-Chief, who gives us strength when we need it most. We rest in the knowledge that he has already defeated the enemy. The victory is his, and it's also ours for eternity.

TODAY'S RX

Rest in and renew your strength in God's faithful promises. He has defeated the enemy, and the victory is ours.

God, the battles I face on a daily basis are wearing me down. I'm wounded and under attack. Please remind me of the hope I have in you—and your victory over death—to help me through.

LEARNING TO WALK IN CHRIST

O Lord, I give my life to you. I trust in you, my God! Do not let me be disgraced, or let my enemies rejoice in my defeat. . . . Show me the right path, O Lord; point out the road for me to follow. Lead me by your truth and teach me, for you are the God who saves me. All day long I put my hope in you. Psalm 25:1-2, 4-5

After my campsite conversion from atheism, I returned to Birmingham a new man in Christ. But I was still a neophyte when it came to matters of faith. I didn't know the lingo, and at the Bible study I attended, I was always the last one to locate the passage we were reading. Whenever I was asked a question, I stumbled and stammered, trying to figure out what to say.

I became very insecure because I wasn't used to learning from other people. I'd spent most of my life being the top dog who taught others.

One day an old friend said, "Where have you been, Reggie? We haven't seen you at the bar in weeks. Come hang out with us tonight."

"I'm sorry," I said, "but I can't. I'm attending a Bible study."

He started chuckling. "A what?"

"A Bible study."

He broke out in a full belly laugh. "You're going to a Bible study? That's a good one!"

"Gotta run. I'll catch you later," I said.

As I walked away, I could still hear him laughing, and his ridicule stung.

I tried to chase away my feelings of embarrassment by reciting Romans 6:23, the verse I had memorized for the study that night: "For the wages of sin is death, but the free gift of God is eternal life through Christ Jesus our Lord."

As I thought about the meaning of the verse, God spoke to me through it, reminding me that my insecurity and the ridicule I had endured were all temporary. The decision I'd made to accept God's gift of salvation was something I would have for eternity.

Looking back at those days, the beauty of my ignorance was that I had to live every day by faith, trusting God that I wouldn't get lost in this brave new world. As I learned more about God from his Word, I came to trust him completely.

TODAY'S RX

Be humble in your new life with Christ. Every baby crawls before learning to walk.

Father, when I'm discouraged about my walk of faith, help me to remember that it is not a race, but a journey. Help me to savor the season I'm in, gaining knowledge and insights from your Word.

WARRIORS FOR THE KING

My health may fail, and my spirit may grow weak, but God remains the strength of my heart; he is mine forever. PSALM 73:26

One of my greatest joys in life is visiting a nursing home. When I review the medical records of my patients, I can see how age and disease have made them a shadow of the person they once were. But the stories they tell are often uplifting and inspirational. They defy the weariness of the storyteller's aging mind and body.

When I listen to older people talk about their life and faith, I realize how much more I receive from these quiet souls than I give. I'm also reminded that growing old is not for the faint of heart. These seniors wear their silver hair with pride as if it were a shiny metal star given to a great warrior at the end of a battle.

In many ways, that's what these saints are—aging warriors who have given their all for the King of kings. And though their minds are not as sharp as they once were, and though their eyes and ears have begun to fail them in this world, their vision of what awaits them in heaven is clear. Like the psalmist, they know they will soon be in the presence of their King forever.

TODAY'S RX

We all age, so let us do it with grace and humility, forever looking to our God as the strength of our hearts.

God, may I always have a grateful heart for every day I'm given. My life is a gift, and I praise you for all the joys and experiences you've given me.

CONFESSING THE STRUGGLE FOR HEALING

Confess your sins to each other and pray for each other so that you may be healed. The earnest prayer of a righteous person has great power and produces wonderful results.
James 5:16

Max was a longtime patient of mine, and I knew him very well. Some of his gravest sins had been committed against his own body. Unfortunately, his body was now paying him back.

Max was a smoker who never heeded my yearly urgings to quit. Eventually, he developed a chronic cough and then chronic bronchitis, followed by a diagnosis of COPD—chronic obstructive pulmonary disease. Though I did everything I could to persuade him to quit, Max was determined to go his own way.

Then everything worsened. Over just a few months, Max was hospitalized multiple times for pneumonia, and each episode was more difficult. I watched the pain envelop him as he struggled to breathe.

One day, I went to Max's room and sat down on his bed. I looked him in the eye and said, "Max, if you insist on continuing to smoke, there's nothing I can do to keep you out of the hospital. At some point, you'll end up in the ICU on a ventilator."

"You're right. But I can't do it on my own. I need help from you and God. Otherwise, I don't think I can do it at all."

Tobacco is a hard habit to quit. It is very similar to morphine in that both stimulate the area of the brain associated with pleasure. I started Max on Chantix and talked about what he could do to lessen the cravings, but I knew his recovery wouldn't be easy.

To my surprise, he quit smoking!

I think one of the reasons he was finally able to quit was because, for the first time, he *decided* he was going to do it, instead of just nodding in agreement during our conversation. Second, he confessed that he couldn't do it on his own. He needed help to curb his desire and to make the necessary life changes. It has been five years since Max last smoked, and he now has a healthy outlook on the future.

On our own we are powerless over sin, but when we confess to one another, we find the power we need.

TODAY'S RX

Confess your struggles to someone who will pray for you, and pray together for God's power.

Lord, place on my heart today the name of a person to whom I can be accountable and pray with to help me get past my struggles. Grow me as a result of this relationship, and allow me to break free of my sin.

THE HEALER WHO STILL DRAWS CROWDS

That evening after sunset, many sick and demon-possessed people were brought to Jesus. The whole town gathered at the door to watch. So Jesus healed many people who were sick with various diseases, and he cast out many demons. But because the demons knew who he was, he did not allow them to speak. MARK 1:32-34

Everywhere Jesus walked, he could always draw a crowd. Amid the masses, there were always those who needed healing and those who sought spiritual understanding. Not much has changed in two thousand years.

A missionary friend of mine from Ecuador called after he received a copy of the *JESUS* movie in Spanish. For some time, he had been praying for an evangelical tool he could use in the villages where his medical caravan went to heal the sick. He was delighted to discover that the movie presented the gospel concisely in a way the villagers could understand. He asked me to come see the impact for myself the next time I could make it to Ecuador.

The weeks leading up to that trip were full of preparations. What I needed to pack depended on where we were going, so I waited for my friend's call.

"We've been invited to go to a remote village at 14,000 feet, so prepare for snow and ice," he said.

"Really?" I asked, confused. "Snow and ice at the equator?"

A few days later, we set up camp and a makeshift clinic in the main mud hut of a mountain village. At night, the whole town came out to watch the *JESUS* film. Most had never seen a movie, and they were amazed by the modern technology. They came out of curiosity, but they left with a fuller understanding of who Jesus is.

There was a great outpouring of the Holy Spirit through this film project. Many were spiritually saved, and some were physically healed. I was astonished and amazed to see ancient scenes of the Bible come alive right before my eyes. Crowds still gather to see Jesus, and he still has the power to render us speechless.

TODAY'S RX

Run to Jesus. He still heals.

Jesus, I have no doubt about your power. You continue to make yourself known in remarkable ways across the world, bringing new life to people of all backgrounds. Thank you for loving your children so well.

CONTAMINATED AND CLEANSED

You must distinguish between what is sacred and what is common, between what is ceremonially unclean and what is clean. Leviticus 10:10

Today's verse was written for the priestly sons of Aaron as they made offerings in the temple, but the same wisdom has other applications as well.

Doctors make decisions every day—sometimes hourly—about what is sterile and what is contaminated. And we must take the necessary precautions to protect our patients and ourselves.

Back in the 1980s, when I began my career in medicine, a new disease sprang up that confounded the medical community. At first, we thought it was an uncommon type of pneumonia (*Pneumocystis carinii*), but when we saw reports of Kaposi's sarcoma, a rare cancer, in the same group of people, it seemed strange that a rare infection and a rare cancer would occur closely within the same population. Something was disrupting their immune system, and it seemed to be highly contagious.

It was soon identified as a brand-new infection or a previously unknown virus. And it was spreading quickly. I first saw it in an IV drug abuser who had lived in a large city. He was the first patient we diagnosed with HIV.

The unknown risk factors gave me pause. We knew it was a blood-borne illness, but how much contact with contaminated blood would put someone at risk? I was working as a resident at the time and was regularly placing IVs in patients for dialysis. Would I contract this seemingly untreatable disease?

The same concerns apply to us spiritually. We may think that a "little bit of sin" can't hurt us, but how much does it take before we're contaminated? In a hospital, sometimes one microscopic drop is enough. When it comes to our sins, once we've been exposed, how do we become clean?

An AIDS conference in San Francisco reassured me that most health-care providers would be safe, as long as we were careful to distinguish between things that were sterile or contaminated. Universal precautions were put in place to help us know the difference.

The same is true spiritually. If we know the difference between what is good for us and what is not, we can avoid being contaminated by sin. But when we succumb, we have the assurance that Jesus died so we could be cleansed and have eternal life.

TODAY'S RX

Use precautions to avoid spiritual contamination. But if you're exposed, turn to Jesus for cleansing and renewal.

Father, help me to choose what is sacred over what is common. This world is temporary, but you are holy and eternal, and I desire to please you with my life.

LIFE-CHANGING ACCIDENT

You have shown me the way of life, and you will fill me with the joy of your presence.
ACTS 2:28

"The car wreck banged me up pretty good," Todd said as he tried to sit up in his hospital bed.

"Don't sit up," I said as I eased him back down. "You're lucky to be alive!"

Todd had an open right tibia/fibular fracture, a fractured left wrist, and road rash on most of the left side of his body. Though it would be a long recovery, at least his life had been spared. The drunk driver who hit him had died at the scene.

"What's so scary is that my family could have been with me. I had just dropped them off before heading in to work an extra late shift."

"It's clear to me that God stood with you *and* your family."

"Without a doubt. But it bothers me that someone else died. We're praying every day for his family. I can't get them out of my mind."

"That's not unusual, Todd. It will take time and therapy to heal your broken bones, but also your heart and mind. Though we can't see those injuries, they're just as real as the physical ones."

A few days later, Todd was moved to a rehab facility to continue his recovery. With the help of a caring group of nurses and a therapist who was able to help him make sense of what had happened, the results were nothing short of miraculous. Six weeks after the accident, Todd walked out of the unit and went back home to his family.

A year later, Todd stopped by my office with a letter of gratitude for the team that had surrounded him and his family during those dark days.

"So, I assume you're back to your old self, and you've resumed your previous level of activity?" I asked.

"Actually, no. The accident made me realize that I needed to make some changes. If I had been with my family that night, I might never have gotten in the accident. For me, it was a wake-up call that I needed to spend more time with the people I love. All that recovery time showed me what really matters and what really brings joy to my life. That's how I want to spend the rest of my life."

TODAY'S RX

Even when the path is difficult, God will sustain you with his presence.

Lord, when everything shatters before me, please help me to pick up the pieces. Show me how to start again, and give me new clarity as to what's important in my life.

CALLED TO HEAL

The Pharisees called a meeting to plot how to kill Jesus. But Jesus knew what they were planning. So he left that area, and many people followed him. He healed all the sick among them. MATTHEW 12:14-15

One night, our local emergency room received a report from a nearby city that there had been an incident in their ER, and we should be on alert.

Apparently, a man had come into the hospital seeking help for back pain. Specifically, he wanted a prescription for narcotics. When the physician who was working in the ER that night refused to write the prescription, the man pulled a gun and shot the doctor. The ER doctor died in the same trauma room where he had saved countless lives.

Because we're in a small town, we typically feel safe from the kind of crime found in larger cities. Nevertheless, we took extra precaution, hiring a security guard and asking the local police to patrol more often on the graveyard shift.

Just when things seemed back to normal, thieves broke into a local pharmacy looking for the same strong narcotics that had cost the city doctor his life.

At that point, we had to change the way we did business. We posted a sign telling patients that certain kinds of medications would no longer be available in our hospital or written as a prescription. We hoped that would keep the drug lords away. But in the back of our minds, the potential threat still existed.

In those rare moments when I feel fear about a potential threat, I think about Jesus. Even though he had a bounty on his head, he didn't let that stop him from healing the sick. Jesus often did the sensible thing—change locations—but he didn't stop doing the work his Father had sent him to do. By removing narcotics and prescription-writing from the ER, we've tried to do the sensible thing. But God called me to heal the sick and minister to the hurting, and I want to be like Jesus. Despite the threats, I will continue to do what he's called me to do.

TODAY'S RX

Fear not! Nothing can stop Jesus from healing the sick.

Father, give me the courage to face my fears today and to honor you with all I do and say. Do not let me back down, but trust wholeheartedly in you.

SOCIAL SERVICES

God will generously provide all you need. Then you will always have everything you need and plenty left over to share with others. 2 CORINTHIANS 9:8

When I was growing up in Plantersville, Alabama, our doors were never locked. In fact, the only door that was ever closed was the screen door, and that was only to keep out the flies.

Screen doors really aren't doors at all. They are invitations to come inside, especially if the smell of freshly baked bread or apple pie is wafting from within. In Plantersville, everyone shared what they had with anyone who in need or who came by. There always seemed to be plenty, and no one was left out.

This was back before government programs were enlisted to take care of the poor and needy. We were taught to help others because that's just what folks did back then. We helped others and knew they would help us. When a family suffered a tragedy, neighbors near and far fixed meals to feed the family for weeks, months, or however long it took them to get back on their feet.

If a house burned down or a barn was demolished in a storm, the men in town gathered with whatever materials and supplies they had to help rebuild. This was simply our way of life.

But times have changed. Social programs have replaced social neighbors. Doors are no longer open; they are closed and locked to protect the material goods that people have amassed. And even that isn't enough to protect our stuff. Now, we install alarms and cameras to keep thieves and the needy away. Our world seems less interested in sharing our stuff and more interested in sharing our opinions on social media.

We used to depend on God to supply all our needs. Today's verse says that he will provide so generously that we will always have more than enough to share with others. But, somehow, we've left that promise behind a locked door. Perhaps we've left God behind too.

We need to remember that God doesn't want—or need—to be locked up and protected. He beckons us from the screen door with a pie in the oven. His invitation is always open for all who care to enter.

TODAY'S RX

Open hands lead to open hearts. The more we share, the better our world will be.

God, help me to have more of a servant's heart and provide for those in need. You are glorified in these kind acts, and I desire to reflect your loving nature.

SLOW AND STEADY WINS THE HEALING RACE

I wait quietly before God, for my victory comes from him. He alone is my rock and my salvation, my fortress where I will never be shaken. PSALM 62:1-2

Sharon had seen multiple specialists and had a variety of tests, and all the results had come back negative. But still her symptoms persisted. Mostly, she seemed weak and unable to eat or keep much down.

With no indication that anything was physically wrong, Sharon had been admitted to our rehab hospital to help her regain her strength and feel better.

"I know they think I'm crazy," she said, turning toward me. "All the tests came back negative, so I *must* be crazy."

I sat down on the bed next to her. "Sharon, you've been through a lot lately. You've had three deaths in your family this year—your mother, your father, and then your husband. That's pretty hard to take. And now your daughter is heading off to college, leaving you with an empty house. That's another big adjustment. Any one of those things alone could sap your strength, steal your appetite, and make you feel sick."

"Yeah, I guess you're right," Sharon said. "I just feel as if I am crashing and burning."

"Life is like a three-legged stool. When everything is balanced, we're stable, but when one leg is taken away, our lives begin to teeter, and we risk losing control. You've had all three legs kicked out from under you. No wonder you're in a downward spiral."

"I guess you're right," she said. "I think my failure to thrive is a physical symptom of a spiritual problem. I know that my parents and husband are in heaven with Jesus, and I look forward to being reunited someday. But in the meantime, I've failed to listen to God because I've been so focused on my losses. But I think I'm ready to get back on track."

Sharon had a kaleidoscope of needs, and we tried to help her in every way we could, with good nutrition, physical therapy, and compassionate listening. In just a few weeks, her worst symptoms completely vanished. She had learned how to pick herself up off the floor and trust in God's ability to guide her life.

TODAY'S RX

If you've been knocked down, trust the Lord to set you back on your feet and give you renewed strength to run the race of life.

Father, there are days when my strength is sapped and my walls begin to crumble. I'm vulnerable to what the world tells me, and I do not hear your voice. Please be with me in these moments, encouraging me and strengthening me so that I may stand upright again.

THE THIRST FOR KNOWLEDGE IS REAL

I pray for you constantly, asking God, the glorious Father of our Lord Jesus Christ, to give you spiritual wisdom and insight so that you might grow in your knowledge of God.
EPHESIANS 1:16-17

The reason that Eve ate from the tree of the knowledge of good and evil was that she knew she didn't know everything that God knew, and she wanted to. One of our basic human needs is to understand things. We have a thirst for knowledge. That's how we were created.

When I lived as an atheist, I believed that if I learned everything I could about science, literature, math, and the arts, it would eventually fill all of the emptiness inside of me. So I ran toward the false god of knowledge, trying to accumulate as much of it as I could. But knowledge didn't satisfy. And it didn't fill the void.

I didn't know it at the time, but when I was feeding on the tree of knowledge, I was like a stranded sailor who drinks seawater. At first, it appears to quench his thirst, but eventually the salt water will cause his kidneys to fail as the poisonous salt dries up his system. What he thinks will save his life leads instead to total organ failure and death.

Spiritually, it is only by drinking the living water of Christ that our thirst will be satisfied and we will have eternal life. Fortunately, before it was too late, I discovered that knowing and experiencing Christ is the only way to quench our thirst for knowledge and fill our emotional emptiness.

TODAY'S RX

Stop chasing false gods. Though we may hunger and thirst for things that satisfy us temporarily, only faith in Jesus will ensure that we get exactly what we need for fullness of life.

Help me to strive after you, Lord, instead of striving after this world. May I give up my distractions and dedicate time to you today, learning more about you and your ways.

IMITATION IS THE SINCEREST FORM OF LEARNING

I tell you the truth, the Son can do nothing by himself. He does only what he sees the Father doing. Whatever the Father does, the Son also does. For the Father loves the Son and shows him everything he is doing. In fact, the Father will show him how to do even greater works than healing this man. Then you will truly be astonished. JOHN 5:19-20

In medical school, the attending physician is considered a god by the residents, interns, and medical students. More than just a mentor, the attending physician teaches what it means to be a doctor—how to behave in various situations and even how to have fun. I remember trying to absorb as much wisdom and knowledge as I could from the attending physician during my time in medical school at the University of Alabama at Birmingham.

One day when I was leaving class, an older doctor came tottering down the hallway, and the students who greeted him did so in an almost reverential way.

"Who's that?" I asked an older student.

"He was Dr. Harrison's protégé."

We all knew who Dr. Harrison was. He had retired shortly before I began my medical school studies at UAB and had died not long after that, but Dr. Harrison's legacy lived on through the doctors he had mentored. He also continued to influence thousands of young doctors as the author of one of our textbooks, *Harrison's Principles of Internal Medicine.*

While at UAB, he guided the young medical school students as if they were his own children. He was not only a teacher, but also an advocate for patients.

But as accomplished as Dr. Harrison was, he had also been mentored by someone. In his case, it was his father, a country doctor who also practiced in Alabama. The elder Dr. Harrison had studied under Dr. Osler, whose famous quote was, "Listen to your patient, he is telling you the diagnosis."

Those of us who are Christian doctors have another mentor as well. By reading the Bible, we can see how Jesus cared for those who were sick and hurting. He's the best teacher for us to model our lives and our practices after.

TODAY'S RX

See one, do one, teach one is a model followed in the medical profession, but we can all do the same thing. Whom have you watched to get better? How can you do what they did? And how can you help someone else get better?

Father, thank you for teaching me through your Word and through the work of your Son, Jesus Christ. May I always look to you for wisdom and direction.

DEMANDING DOESN'T RESULT IN FAVORABLE RESULTS

One day the Pharisees and Sadducees came to test Jesus, demanding that he show them a miraculous sign from heaven to prove his authority. He replied, . . . "Only an evil, adulterous generation would demand a miraculous sign, but the only sign I will give them is the sign of the prophet Jonah." Then Jesus left them and went away. MATTHEW 16:1-2, 4

We all know people who demand instead of ask. They bully their way through everything. When my schedule is completely booked and patients can't get an appointment, they show up at the registration desk and demand to be seen.

This behavior may work the first or second time they try it, but soon other people catch on. Their overbearing behavior wears thin very quickly, and the next time they try to push their way through the same door, they may find it locked.

We don't like that kind of pushy behavior from others, but how often do we act that way toward God? In our prayer lives, do we demand rather than request? Do we make a list and ask God to supply us with prosperity, health, a great job, and a new relationship?

God is not a genie in a bottle who gives us three wishes on command. Our prayers should always be humble ones. We should pray for God's will, not our own. He wants to bless us, but not necessarily on our terms.

Sometimes, when we're so focused on what we want, we can be ignorant of what a blessing even looks like. We ask for something, and God says, "I have something better for you."

He wants all things to work together for the good of those who love him, within his perfect will, and that should be our prayer as well. Continue to persistently knock on his door in prayer, but rather than pushing through, wait for the Lord to open it and give you his answer.

TODAY'S RX

Demanding treatment we think we deserve could mean missing out on the blessings that God desires to give us.

Lord, help me to approach you out of reverence and respect. After all, you are the Lord of lords and King of kings. May I be patient in lifting my prayer requests up to you, waiting to hear from you in your perfect timing.

A PRAYER FOR OUR CHILDREN

Those who fear the LORD are secure; he will be a refuge for their children.
PROVERBS 14:26

When I was still an atheist, Karen challenged me to pray a simple prayer: "God, if you are real, reveal yourself and show me your ways."

That prayer was answered in spectacular fashion when I married Karen and we later had four children. As soon as our children were born, and every day since, we have prayed for them. We have asked God to use them for his glory in the uttermost parts of the world. And in the spirit of that first simple prayer that I prayed, we've also asked God to make himself known in very personal ways in their daily lives.

With Kristen living in Ireland, Ashley in Los Angeles, David in Birmingham, and Julia nearby—but working with an organization that helps orphans all over the world—we are amazed at God's faithfulness. God has been with each one of our kids, and they are all committed to following him.

To this day, we continue to pray for their protection and well-being. But we also recognize that the safety net God has placed around them is greater than any protection Karen and I could ever supply.

Now, with two grandkids on the way, we spend even more time in prayer. For this next generation, we continue to pray a variation of the prayer that Karen first challenged me with: "God, reveal yourself to these grandbabies and show them your ways."

Because of our confidence in God and his faithfulness, we can wake up every morning without worrying about the news headlines. Though our kids' and grandkids' paths through life may not be easy, we now have generations of evidence to prove that God not only protects his own, but he also promises never to leave them or forsake them.

TODAY'S RX

The same God who protects you and blesses you will also protect and bless succeeding generations.

What a comfort this promise is, Father. You shepherd your sheep, keeping a watchful eye over every one of them. Be with my family today, and protect them from harm. Use me and my family members for your glory.

TRUSTING HEARTS

The LORD is my strength and shield. I trust him with all my heart. He helps me, and my heart is filled with joy. I burst out in songs of thanksgiving. PSALM 28:7

Even at our small hospital, we're aware of the latest medications and protocols. But implementing them can sometimes be an act of faith.

"My heart! My heart! Help me! Please help me!"

We heard the man enter the ER before we saw him. We immediately attended to him and could see that all his symptoms indicated an acute myocardial infarction. He was having a heart attack. A quick medical history revealed that he had high cholesterol, diabetes, hypertension, and a family history of heart disease. The EKG and blood work confirmed our diagnosis.

Tissue plasminogen activator antigen, or tPA, had just been approved as a treatment to bust up blood clots blocking the coronary arteries. But it came with the risk of causing immediate death from bleeding. And with the shot costing more than $2,000, any decision to use it would not be taken lightly.

This man seemed to be the perfect candidate, but he would also be the first person to receive this lifesaving drug in our small hospital. The cardiologist gave us the green light over the phone.

As we mixed the medication and began infusing it through his IV, I prayed that we were doing the right thing. The assembled medical staff collectively held our breath as we waited to see what would happen.

Within a few minutes, the man's chest pain stopped, and we all began to breathe easier—including the patient. We repeated the EKG and could see improvement in blood flow. The treatment had worked. We celebrated with high fives.

Three days later, the cardiologist called back with his report. The patient had a 99 percent blockage of the left main artery. If we had sent him from our rural hospital to the main cardiology center in Nashville, he probably would have died on the way. According to the cardiologist, the tPA had saved this man's life.

Remembering my prayers that night, I knew that God was the one who had truly saved the patient's life. It brought me great joy to give the Great Physician a holy high five.

TODAY'S RX

Are there any blockages in your life that are choking out the living water? God has just the right answer at just the right time.

God, help me to seek you when it comes to making decisions. May I trust your judgment above my own and walk faithfully according to your will.

SEPTEMBER CHECKUP

September was harvest time on our farm. Watermelon was our cash crop, but that was just to hold us over until we could harvest our real crop: peanuts. Depending on the harvest each year, we'd either make most of our money from the peanut crop, or we'd end up working for peanuts. Appropriately, we started harvesting on Labor Day, and we continued throughout the glorious month of September. I remember watching the rich soil being turned over to reveal the fruit of the peanut vines. It was a sign that we would have enough harvest to sustain us through the winter ahead. We also used this time to set aside seed for the following year's crop. As farmers, we depended on God for the growing conditions—the sunshine and rain that we couldn't control—but we took responsibility for the things we could, like harvesting at the right time and setting aside seeds to prepare for the next year.

In our spiritual lives, if we want to yield good fruit, we must put down roots into the rich soil of God's Word. Though we can't control the circumstances of our lives, we can cultivate our hearts and allow God to plant good seeds of wisdom, faith, and guidance there.

This month, as you read the Scriptures, look for the promises that God has made to us. Write down verses that are meaningful to you at this time in your life, and put them someplace where you will see them and read them often—on the refrigerator, the bathroom mirror, or your desk at work. These verses are roots that anchor you to the Word of God and bring nourishment to your soul. When trouble comes and you need to call on these promises, you'll harvest the fruit of your labors. Now is a good time to prepare and set aside nourishment for the winter ahead.

In the medical field, September is when we start encouraging our patients to get flu shots. We want them to be as prepared as possible for a flu outbreak that may happen over the winter. In the same way, inoculating yourself by storing God's Word in your heart now can help you avoid sin and suffering later. It will also sustain you through the coming dark and cold winter months that will soon be here.

September Booster Shot: September is also the beginning of football season and other events that involve large, gathered crowds. People will start spending more time indoors, making germs easier to spread. Cough into the crook of your elbow when you feel a tickle coming on, but open your mouth to spread the love of Christ through your speech.

THREE IN ONE

You know that God anointed Jesus of Nazareth with the Holy Spirit and with power.
Acts 10:38

Long before I studied medicine, I studied chemistry. In class, we used mathematical equations to explain the properties of elements. Depending on the environment the element was in, the properties could be very different.

For example, we studied how water boils at 212 degrees Fahrenheit or 100 degrees Celsius when it is at sea level. But in the same location with a different temperature—say 32 degrees Fahrenheit (or zero degrees Celsius)—the water becomes solid ice.

Just as water can exist in three different forms—liquid, solid, and gas—we have a God whose essence doesn't change, but who reveals himself to us in the form of three distinct persons—Father, Son, and Holy Spirit. Today's verse refers to how God the Father anointed Jesus the Son with power from the Holy Spirit. This gives us a picture of the three persons of the triune God we worship. They are one and the same yet different.

Just as water has different functions in its various forms—ice preserves, water replenishes, and steam purifies—we depend on the differing functions of the three persons of the Trinity.

In what ways do the different expressions of the triune God preserve, replenish, or purify us? I believe it's like physical chemistry: It depends on the specific environment—physical, mental, emotional, or spiritual. In the end, regardless of the environment, we need all three aspects of God's presence for our complete spiritual health.

TODAY'S RX

Does your faith feel stale? Consider how each person of the Trinity could help to preserve, replenish, or purify your soul and spirit.

Thank you, Father, for how you have preserved your Word in my heart and whisper it to me in just the right moments, for how you have replenished me with hope from the Holy Spirit for the days ahead, and for how you have purified me from my sin through the shedding of your Son's blood. I am forever grateful.

FREEDOM THAT MONEY CAN'T BUY

Peter said, "I don't have any silver or gold for you. But I'll give you what I have. In the name of Jesus Christ the Nazarene, get up and walk!" Then Peter took the lame man by the right hand and helped him up. And as he did, the man's feet and ankles were instantly healed and strengthened. He jumped up, stood on his feet, and began to walk! Then, walking, leaping, and praising God, he went into the Temple with them. ACTS 3:6-8

Art's situation was like many I've seen over the years. He developed debilitating arthritis at a young age. When it got so bad that he could barely walk, he was put on disability. He saw specialists in orthopedics and rheumatology but was unable to qualify for surgery because he didn't have insurance.

I began seeing Art on a regular basis as he came in for pain medication and to get a signature on his disability forms to validate what was obvious to anyone who saw him—he was physically unable to work.

One day, he came in with some good news. After nearly two years on disability, he qualified for government insurance and was now able to have the surgery he needed to replace both knee joints. Six weeks later, he was out of a wheelchair and walking. After additional rehab, he threw away his crutches.

The next time I saw him, Art had a big grin on his face.

"No disability papers this time, Dr. Anderson," he said. "Instead, I need a physical for my new job."

"That's great news, Art!"

"All the praise goes to God for removing the chains of bureaucracy and for the miracle of surgery to rid me of this disability."

I think of Art whenever I hear the story of the lame man whom God healed through Peter. For the first time in this man's life, he could walk, run, and leap for joy. I can only imagine the response inside the Temple when he walked in with Peter and John, praising God in front of the same people who had been tossing coins at him for years. Now he had a freedom that money couldn't buy.

It's exciting to know that this miracle happened after Jesus ascended into heaven—that, even today, miracles can still happen in his name.

TODAY'S RX

Don't settle for mere silver and gold. Ask God to heal you and set you free.

Lord, remind me daily that all good gifts come from you—and that nothing this world has to offer compares to your power and strength. May you alone receive praise and glory for restoring the health and strengthening the spirits of those in need.

THE ULTIMATE SACRIFICE

He personally carried our sins in his body on the cross so that we can be dead to sin and live for what is right. By his wounds you are healed. 1 PETER 2:24

When I read today's verse, I think about the fact that Jesus carried our sins in his body. As an emergency room doctor accustomed to seeing trauma, I understand how much Jesus suffered in the twenty-four hours prior to his death. The extent of his injuries would have caused an unbearable amount of pain, yet he bore it. Thinking about it makes me shudder—and also makes me profoundly grateful.

When the weight of all our sins—past, present, and future, for all humanity—is added up, only Jesus could carry that overwhelming burden.

If we trust that our entire debt was paid on the cross that day, then we know that every barrier that would keep us from a full and healthy life has been knocked down. Christ died so we can be dead to sin and alive for all eternity. Every day we have of life and health is because of what Jesus did for us on the cross. He healed us once and for all.

Our freedom from sin was purchased by the ultimate sacrifice on the cross. By his wounds we are healed.

TODAY'S RX

Have you put your trust in Jesus as the ultimate sacrifice for your sins? If not, don't wait any longer. Surrender your life to him today.

Jesus, thank you for taking on my sin and enduring the cross. I put all of my trust in you, knowing that it is only by your blood that I have life—and life to the full.

DAD'S BIRTH INTO ETERNITY

I know the LORD is always with me. I will not be shaken, for he is right beside me. No wonder my heart is glad, and I rejoice. My body rests in safety. PSALM 16:8-9

The family had gathered in my father's hospital room. Mom was there, along with my sister and brother, my wife, Karen, and three of our four kids. Mom was quiet. I reached for her hand and took it in mine.

"Dad's not dying," I said. "He's getting ready to be born into another world." I reminded her that when babies are born into this world, they do so kicking and screaming. But believers, who know where they are going, are peacefully born into the next world. Mom smiled at the thought.

"Look around," I said, pointing at my siblings. "When the doctor first saw the tops of our heads, he said, 'The baby is crowning.'"

She nodded.

"Now we're witnessing Dad's crowning into heaven. A crown will be placed on his head as he is delivered into eternity."

"I like the thought of that," Mom said.

Dad was resting, and the family was talking quietly when my sister spoke up and said, "Can we sing for Dad?"

Someone started singing a hymn, and the rest of us joined in. We sang through all the classic hymns that Dad liked. The kids harmonized when they knew the tune and improvised when they didn't know the words. The musically challenged adults, like me, did our best to follow along. It became a sacred celebration, and Dad was the guest of honor, not a patient who was about to die.

When Dad's breathing became more erratic and labored, we all placed our hands on him to let him know we were there. As we sang a final song, Dad took his last breath on earth and was born into the next world. As the last bit of life left his body, I felt the warmth of his spirit drain away and a fresh breeze waft into the room. When his spirit passed my cheek, it felt light and youthful, as if he had traded his old body for one more vibrant than ever.

The tears we shed that afternoon were tears of joy as we celebrated Dad's birth into heaven.[8]

TODAY'S RX

Our final breath on earth will be our first breath in heaven as we inhale the sweet atmosphere of eternity.

You are a God of peace, Father. Thank you for your gentle presence and comforting embrace. I look forward to the day when I am welcomed home.

HIGH-POWERED JOY

[The Lord] said, "My grace is all you need. My power works best in weakness." So now I am glad to boast about my weaknesses, so that the power of Christ can work through me. 2 Corinthians 12:9

I pulled into the parking lot and saw a special transport van parked outside my office. It was unusual to see it there so early, but I didn't give it much thought. But when my nurse met me at the door, I should have known that my day was going to be unusual.

"You have two new patients," she said. "So don't look shocked when you go in."

I wasn't worried. I've seen just about everything in my thirty years as a doctor. I walked in expecting to see two kids, possibly with some kind of disfigurement. Instead, I found two grown men in wheelchairs—and then I saw what the nurse had warned me about.

Instead of quietly waiting for their appointment, the brothers were racing each other up and down the hallway in their wheelchairs, trying to jump the half-inch molding in the doorway that separated one area from another. The whole time, they were laughing and teasing each other.

My nurse beckoned them down the hallway to the exam room and then jumped out of the way as they raced toward the open door.

The men had Becker muscular dystrophy, a spectrum of muscle diseases that typically strikes males in the prime of life. So, from a medical standpoint, it wasn't surprising that two brothers close in age had come down with the disease at nearly the same time.

"How did you deal with the news when you were first diagnosed?" I asked.

"Oh, we knew it would happen," the first one said. "The disease runs in our family. An uncle and a cousin both have it as well."

"But we know that God is good, and he's in control of our lives," the second one added.

I now understood why they seemed to be faring so well despite the severity of their disease, which has no known cure and will keep them in wheelchairs for the rest of their lives. Their keen sense of humor, large personalities, and love of life had certainly influenced their health in positive ways. But even more so, they had discovered the truth of Nehemiah 8:10: "The joy of the Lord is your strength!"

TODAY'S RX

God's glory shines brightest when the weak are made strong.

God, if my weaknesses are what bring you glory, then I pray you will use them today. Fill my heart with joy. Thank you for your grace and for your all-sufficient power.

INSIDE-OUT PEACE

"Daughter," he said to her, "your faith has made you well. Go in peace." Luke 8:48

"My life is in pieces. I don't even know where to start," Angie said.

"Let's start with what substances you've taken recently," I said.

She responded with a list of drugs that would put most people to sleep for a week. But Angie's addiction was so out of control that the massive quantities barely affected her.

"I want to get my life back on track, but I don't know how. Can you help me?"

"Are you ready and willing to change your lifestyle?"

"Yes!" she said emphatically. "That's why I'm here. I've had three overdoses, and yet I keep craving more. But if I don't stop, I know it will kill me."

"Okay. We need to run some tests. Then we'll start the detox process."

I admitted her to the medical ward for treatment and then to the psych ward for rehab. As she was waiting to be transferred, I seized the opportunity to talk with her.

"When you first came in, you said that you felt as if your spirit had died. What did you mean?"

That simple question opened the floodgates, and Angie poured out her story. A victim of abuse, she had used drugs to numb the pain and help her forget. But it only made her susceptible to more abuse. It was a vicious cycle, and she didn't know how to escape it. As she talked, her story felt more like a confession, and I felt more like her priest than her doctor. I told her that Jesus forgave her and that he could heal her spiritually as well as physically.

In rehab, Angie slowly healed the open wounds in her soul, and gradually she became strong enough to go home. In retrospect, I realized that her confession to me was something she desperately needed. She had to unload all the shame of her former life before she could take positive steps toward a new life.

She was discharged into the care of a halfway house but still came in regularly to monitor her Hepatitis C—a battle scar that was eventually resolved with new treatment. During this time, God began to reveal himself to her, and she finally found peace as he healed her soul.

TODAY'S RX

Don't wait for physical healing to find peace with God. Seek him first, and healing will follow.

God, heal the scars on my heart, and make me new. Be a balm to the painful memories that still lie in wait within me. I desire to surrender everything to you.

GOD HEALS COMPLETELY

Let all that I am praise the LORD; may I never forget the good things he does for me. He forgives all my sins and heals all my diseases. PSALM 103:2-3

Reading, and applying, Psalm 103 is a great way to begin the healing process. We should always look to the Lord first. And we should praise him with every fiber of our being—body, soul, and spirit.

If we do this even in the midst of our greatest suffering, we can be confident that whatever happens is in God's hands, and our healing will always be complete.

Often we think that our bodies must be healed in order for our prayers to be answered. But if we look to God's perfect will and trust his perfect wisdom, we will begin to grasp—and feel—how much he loves us, and we will begin to understand, and accept, that sometimes his plan looks different from ours. Can you praise him even though you haven't yet seen the healing you desire?

God is omniscient. He sees beyond the here and now, and he gives us glimpses of eternity. In our forever life with him, we will see that he not only forgives our sins, but he also heals all our diseases. There is always hope for the future with the knowledge that one day we will be healed and whole—mind, soul, and body.

TODAY'S RX

Praise God for your healing, even if it is yet to come.

I stand in awe of you, Father, knowing you are good.
You've seen my sin and still call me worthy. Thank you for providing healing in your perfect way and timing.

NOT JUST SEIZURE FREE—BUT HEALED COMPLETELY

A man in the crowd called out to him, "Teacher, I beg you to look at my son, my only child. An evil spirit keeps seizing him, making him scream. It throws him into convulsions so that he foams at the mouth. It batters him and hardly ever leaves him alone. I begged your disciples to cast out the spirit, but they couldn't do it." Jesus said, "You faithless and corrupt people! How long must I be with you and put up with you?" Then he said to the man, "Bring your son here." As the boy came forward, the demon knocked him to the ground and threw him into a violent convulsion. But Jesus rebuked the evil spirit and healed the boy. Then he gave him back to his father. Awe gripped the people as they saw this majestic display of God's power. LUKE 9:38-43

Epilepsy has been around for as long as recorded history. Unfortunately, for many years it was thought to be the result of demonic possession. We now understand it as a life-threatening and life-altering disease that can affect anyone.

Patients with epilepsy and active seizures face a lot of restrictions. They can't work with machinery or drive, and they aren't able to obtain a pilot's license. They're also advised to avoid jobs that require balance, such as climbing a ladder, because they could potentially injure themselves or someone else.

Modern medicine has developed medications that work for about 70 percent of epileptic patients, but there is still not a complete cure for the disease.

Even today, epileptics can be stigmatized and judged by people who aren't familiar with the disease. We all want to be in control of how we act, especially in public, but epilepsy steals that control. A violent convulsion can throw a person to the ground and cause a loss of bowel and bladder control. It's a vulnerable and embarrassing condition.

When Jesus healed the young boy, he didn't just stop the seizures. He healed him completely—physically, mentally, and spiritually. I believe that Jesus also healed the hardened hearts of those who had judged the boy. Luke records that those who witnessed the miracle were gripped with awe. They had never seen anyone with those symptoms healed so quickly and completely.

TODAY'S RX

If you have an illness with social implications, pray that you can be a source of understanding for those you encounter in public.

Jesus, soften my heart for those in my life who are sick and physically impaired. Help me to see them through your eyes, and provide for them in ways that give them joy and hope.

MOVING MOUNTAINS BETWEEN NEIGHBORS

"The mountains may move and the hills disappear, but even then my faithful love for you will remain. My covenant of blessing will never be broken," says the LORD, *who has mercy on you.* ISAIAH 54:10

When we moved to Middle Tennessee from West Tennessee, it took a while to adjust to the new terrain. We were now surrounded by mountains and hills, and for the first time, our next-door neighbors were not just a wave away. The hills and hollows that separated us physically also seemed to separate us spiritually and emotionally.

That sense of separateness was fueled by a question that came up from time to time. "You're not from around here, are you?" the locals would ask. The rural community we'd moved to was similar to the one I grew up in. It was a place where most folks were kin or married to kin. We were neither.

I believe that the famous feud between the Hatfields and McCoys persisted because neither side was familiar with the other. If familiarity breeds contempt, lack of familiarity can give rise to even greater alienation. Anytime people feel isolated or separated, their default emotion seems to be suspicion.

Fortunately, that sense of alienation didn't last long after our move. Day by day, we met our neighbors, and God broke down the barriers that separated us from our new community. His loving grace began to smooth out our differences, and trust began to spring forth, flowing like the mighty Cumberland River that sustains life in the region.

God led us to this rural area, and he was the one who knocked down the mountains to allow his healing touch to bring life and health to our new home.

TODAY'S RX

If you're isolated or alone, trust that God can move mountains. His covenant of blessing will never be broken.

Father, show me how I may reach out to the lonely and build friendships with those who are different from me. Whether it's visiting those in a nursing home or simply getting to know my neighbors, please place that desire on my heart and lead the way.

HEALING WORDS

Some people make cutting remarks, but the words of the wise bring healing.
PROVERBS 12:18

Thirteen-year-old Carly was a good student, excelling in all her classes. Her mother spent her days as Carly's full-time academic coach, doing everything she could to help her daughter gain entry into an elite university. Though admission to college was still years away, Carly's mother talked about it so much during her appointment that I became concerned that she wasn't taking time to just enjoy being Carly's mom.

During one of Carly's annual exams, when her mother stepped out of the exam room to take a phone call, Carly looked at me and said, "Can I talk to you while my mom is out of the room?"

"Absolutely," I said, sitting down next to her.

As my young patient struggled to put her feelings into words, I sensed that something was wrong. After a long silence, Carly blurted, "My mother thinks everything has to be perfect. If it's not, she snaps at me."

Once Carly had worked up the courage to speak, the words came tumbling out.

With tears pooling in her eyes, she described how her mother's controlling behavior and occasional outbursts made Carly feel helpless and out of control. The pressure to live up to her mother's high standards was immense. I noticed that Carly's nails were bitten to the quick, and she was slightly underweight for her height.

"Tell me about your weight," I said.

"I know, I'm so fat," Carly said. "When I look in the mirror, all I see is a big blob."

I decided that an intervention was necessary. I referred Carly to a pediatric psychiatrist at Vanderbilt Medical Center who specialized in eating disorders.

Over the next few months, God intervened as well.

Both Carly and her mother began the long process of redemptive healing. They attended counseling separately and together and followed their counselor's advice. Carly started eating regular meals and worked to have a balanced lifestyle.

Year after year, I followed their progress as the two women became emotionally healthy. Eventually, they celebrated Carly's admission to an Ivy League school. By her own choice, Carly had surpassed every goal her mother had set for her. She's now in medical school, studying to become a psychiatrist.

TODAY'S RX

Before you speak, remember the wise words of Bambi's friend Thumper: "If you can't say something nice, don't say anything at all."

Lord, let my words build others up today, not bring them down. Help me to reflect the kindness of your Spirit and be a source of encouragement and light to them.

THE BATTLE AGAINST CANCER

We are human, but we don't wage war as humans do. We use God's mighty weapons, not worldly weapons, to knock down the strongholds of human reasoning and to destroy false arguments. We destroy every proud obstacle that keeps people from knowing God. We capture their rebellious thoughts and teach them to obey Christ. 2 Corinthians 10:3-5

"Ruthie, it's been a while since I've seen you," I said to one of my longtime patients.

"I know. I haven't been in for my regular checkups because I just didn't have the money for the appointment or all the tests."

"What brings you in today?" I asked.

"I just qualified for Medicare."

"So how are you feeling?"

"Well . . ." she began, and I sensed some anxiety in her voice. "I lost some weight, and I don't know how, but my tummy is bigger than ever."

A quick look revealed she had temple wasting—a concave depression near her temples—making her forehead seem larger than normal. That can be a sign of rapid weight loss or malnutrition.

"Hold out your arms," I said. They seemed slighter than what I remembered. I said a silent prayer as I deduced what had caused her weight loss.

Next I examined her abdomen, and I was alarmed by what I felt. "I'm going to need to order a few tests," I said.

Ruthie commented again about how glad she was to have Medicare.

A week later, I had the results of her CT scan and lab work. Her CA125 test was positive for ovarian cancer.

Ruthie came into my office ready to receive the bad news. "You know, you helped me through my mom's death a number of years ago. And then again when my husband went to be with the Lord," She was a strong woman of faith, and she would need to rely on God for the road ahead. "I know this will be a battle, but with the Lord, we will fight it."

When I read today's verse, I'm reminded of Ruthie's resolve to fight. Though we did everything we could for her medically, she knew that God's mighty weapons would help her the most.

TODAY'S RX

Arm yourself with the strength of God, and he will knock down the strongholds in your life.

As you say in your Word, Father, help me to put on the peace of the Good News and the salvation I have received as armor against the battles I face. Protect me along the way, and help me to stand firm.

A JOY WORTH PROTECTING

With every bone in my body I will praise him: "LORD, who can compare with you? Who else rescues the helpless from the strong? Who else protects the helpless and poor from those who rob them?" PSALM 35:10

Before choosing family practice, I entertained the idea of specializing in obstetrics. I had great memories of being a medical student and delivering my first set of twins and how doubly excited everyone was at their birth. There is nothing like the joy that fills the room when new parents hear their baby's healthy first cry. It's an intoxicating feeling, too, for someone who typically deals with people who aren't feeling well.

Around that same time, *Roe v. Wade* became law. That landmark decision allowed abortions up until the third trimester. The thought of that sickened me. As I researched residency programs in obstetrics, I saw that many of them offered training in these techniques. I realized that my personal values would be in conflict with the prevailing public opinion.

At the time, I didn't think I had the strength or courage to spend the rest of my career fighting those battles. So, I set my sights on helping rural and poor families maintain their health and found peace as a country doctor. In my own little practice, away from the city, I thought I would be far from the abortion fight. At the time, I didn't realize that the battle would spill into every corner of our nation.

Even after all these years, I still don't believe the war is lost. Many of our Christian friends are working to protect the rights of the unborn, the weak, and the unprotected. Each baby who is saved, either through counseling with the mother or adoption, is a victory for life—for that child's life. Slowly, the tide is turning. More and more people are coming to understand what I learned early in my training—there is no greater joy than the first cry of a newborn baby.

TODAY'S RX

God will continue the war against evil, even when we don't have the will or strength to join him. He is our strength and deliverer, and he rescues and protects the helpless.

Lord, continue to fight this fight and protect the lives of the unborn. May we not be careless with your creation, but work together to provide for the needs of mothers and their babies. Instill your peace and provision into all of those who need to hear from you today.

GUIDANCE COUNSELOR

The LORD says, "I will guide you along the best pathway for your life. I will advise you and watch over you." PSALM 32:8

"What do you mean I failed the test? I've never failed a test in my life!" I said, protesting much more than the moment called for.

"It was only an eye test," the doctor said, "you'll get past it."

What he didn't know was that failing the eye exam was the only thing preventing me from becoming an Air Force pilot. I was eighteen years old and poor. Becoming a pilot was the only way I knew to get off the farm and fly away from the memories of my past.

I went to see my college professor and told him what had happened. "You could get another job in the military," he suggested.

"If I can't fly, I don't want another job in the military!"

"Then what do you want to do?"

"I don't know."

"You would make a good dentist," he said.

I returned a month later, even more upset than I'd been the first time. "I failed that test, too, because I couldn't see the pictures!"

"Ahh," he said. "You should take the MCAT to get into medical school. It doesn't have all of that visual perception stuff on it. You would make a fine doctor."

So, for the third time in three months, I went to take a test that would determine the direction of my life. I didn't have a lot of hope.

A few weeks later, the results came in the mail. I had passed! Apparently, being able to see well is not a requirement for becoming a doctor.

Looking back, it's easy for me to see how God guided me toward the path he had for my life, even though I had other plans and was an atheist at the time. God nudged me through open doors and nudged me past closed doors and even squeezed me through a window or two. I didn't know he was guiding me, until much later when he and I became reacquainted.

To this day, he continues to guide me through life, and he will until I reach the other side of the veil and see him face-to-face.

TODAY'S RX

If you are surrounded by confusion and closed doors, look to God for guidance.

Give me peace, Lord, when my plans do not always align with yours. Show me the path to take, and restore my hope when doors seem to continually shut in front of me. You know the way, and I will follow after you.

LEARNING LESSON

Even though Jesus was God's Son, he learned obedience from the things he suffered. HEBREWS 5:8

Pain is a great teacher. I can still remember how the hot stove felt when I touched it for the first time as a child. The burn was so painful that I never made that mistake again.

Many of life's lessons come through suffering. When we're learning to drive, it may be a ticket that teaches us that speed limits are laws, not suggestions. If we forget to wear sunscreen at the beach, the painful sunburn will remind us for next time. Some people, though, need more than one encounter with the hot stove or the traffic cop to learn their lesson. But the more times they push their luck, the more dangerous the consequences become.

Bubba was a great hunting and fishing partner, unless he brought along the bottle. Whenever he got together with the sour mash, he focused more on his next drink than on the things that really mattered—like his wife and kids.

Bubba's wife, Trish, always worried when Bubba spent the weekend fishing on the Tennessee River. She knew he consumed unhealthy amounts of alcohol there. Later, she became concerned when his weekend vice spilled over into Monday through Friday. She asked me to speak to him about it the next time he came in.

A week or so later, when Bubba stumbled through the door. I didn't have to guess what he'd been up to; I could smell it. His eyes looked a little jaundiced, so I asked him to sit on the table so I could take a closer look.

It was clear that his drinking had become a serious problem, and I ordered some tests. When the results came back, his liver enzymes were sky-high, and his bilirubin reading was twice the normal level. All indications showed hepatic (liver) failure from alcoholism.

"Bubba, all your suffering is self-inflicted. Your only chance of long-term survival is complete abstinence from alcohol." He had touched the hot stove one too many times, and now the scars would be permanent.

Bubba's family stood by him as he went through detox and rehab. It was a long road, but he came through. On the seventh anniversary of his sobriety, Bubba threw a party—not at the fishing camp where he used to celebrate but at his church.

TODAY'S RX

Turn away from temptation, and seek the Lord for your fulfillment.

Jesus, you are the great Teacher, and I thank you for teaching me much over my lifetime. You've taught me valuable lessons through both joyful and painful experiences, and I pray that I may share those experiences with other to help show them the way.

TOO SICK TO SPEAK

The Holy Spirit helps us in our weakness. For example, we don't know what God wants us to pray for. But the Holy Spirit prays for us with groanings that cannot be expressed in words. ROMANS 8:26

Walking down the hall, I heard the sounds of distress coming from Stacy's room. It didn't sound like screams or cries, but something more like moans and grunts. I quickened my pace.

When I entered the room, the moaning grew louder, and I saw Stacy writhing in pain.

"Stacy, it's Dr. Anderson. Can you tell me what's wrong?" Her answer contained no words, just more moaning. "Can you tell me where it hurts?" She began to vomit. "Can you tell me how long this has been going on?" Her only response was more vomiting and moaning. Clearly, she was too sick to speak, and she needed me to intercede and help her.

As today's verse suggests, there are times when we are too weak or sick to pray or we don't know how to pray as we should. But in those moments, the Holy Spirit intercedes for us. When language fails us, God still hears our souls' deepest cries.

I asked God to help me figure out what was causing Stacy's pain. I could see that she was jaundiced, and when I touched the upper right quadrant of her abdomen, her moaning grew more intense. Though she was too sick to speak, all the signs and symptoms pointed to gallstones. I suspected she had a stone lodged in her bile duct, blocking the outflow from her liver and pancreas. A CT scan and liver function test confirmed the diagnosis.

We scheduled an endoscopic retrograde cholangiopancreatography procedure (ERCP) to pluck the stone away. When I saw Stacy the next morning on rounds, she was no longer writhing and moaning. She looked a whole lot better, and she could talk. We chatted briefly, and I told her how blessed she was, because only a few years ago, this disease would have been life-threatening.

Even though she hadn't been able to speak at the height of her suffering, we both agreed that God had heard her prayers and that the Holy Spirit had interceded to help me diagnose her problem.

TODAY'S RX

If you don't know what to say or you're too weak or tired to pray, allow the Holy Spirit to intercede with groanings that are beyond words.

Holy Spirit, speak for me in times of distress and despair when I simply don't have the words. Lift me out of the fog of worry, and comfort me with your perfect peace.

EIGHTIES LADIES

Everyone tried to touch him, because healing power went out from him, and he healed everyone. Luke 6:19

On Wednesday afternoons, I visit my patients at the local nursing home. They range in age from eighty to ninety years old, and there are three times as many women as men. Several years ago, I affectionately began calling them my Eighties Ladies.

The nurses told me that on the days I was expected to visit, the Eighties Ladies would quickly finish breakfast so they could dress up—"because Dr. Anderson is coming today!" They put a fresh coat of paint on the old barn and adorned themselves with jewelry. By the time I arrived, they would be decked out in their most colorful scarves and beads, and their smiles were framed with fresh lipstick.

Typically, nothing had changed medically since I'd seen them the previous week, but holding their hands and talking with them did wonders to brighten their spirits.

When I finished my appointed rounds at the home, I often stood at the nurses' station to update the medical charts. Soon a group of Eighties Ladies would see me and gather around. Some would suddenly develop new complaints so they could spend time talking to me. Others would ask me endless questions just so they could engage me in conversation. The hardest part was answering questions from the patients with dementia. They would ask the same question over and over. At moments like that, I wished I had the Lord's patience.

When the geriatric gatherings grew a little too rowdy, the nurses would go into crowd control mode and start wheeling them back to their rooms. When that happened, I felt guilty. I wished I had more time to spend with each of them.

I know that God will eventually heal all of my Eighties Ladies, if not here and now, then when they cross over to their forever home.

TODAY'S RX

No matter how old or sick we are, our souls long for the healing touch of Jesus. Today, you can be his hands and feet by touching someone's life who needs to feel his presence.

Jesus, thank you that I can always come to you with my concerns and pleas for help. I praise you for never growing tired of hearing from me and for always waiting expectantly to spend time together. I'm grateful for your vast love.

THRIVING LIFE

Fear of the LORD leads to life, bringing security and protection from harm.
PROVERBS 19:23

My dad taught the agriculture classes at the high school I attended as a teenager. I took one class from him in which I learned the names of all the woodworking tools, and I built a set of bookcases for our home as a final project.

Two other students worked together to build a greenhouse, and it was quite impressive. Walking through the plastic veil was like walking into another world. On the inside, they had created their own miniature Garden of Eden.

Inside the security and protection of the greenhouse, the plants grew perfectly. Because of the barriers to the outside, there didn't appear to be any bugs. They could control the temperature, the amount of food, and the water each plant received. Disease, if it existed, was limited. Inside the greenhouse, the plants did more than just survive; they thrived.

It wasn't surprising to me that all the farmers in Plantersville wanted one. Those students kept building until they had filled our tiny town with more than one hundred greenhouses!

Today's verse says that fear of the Lord leads to life. In Hebrew, the word for "life," *chay*, means to be alive, green, and overflowing like a waterfall. When we call upon God, he wraps a protective barrier of safety and security around us, and he gives us just the right amount of love and nourishment to lead us to abundant life. As our love for him grows, we are perfected in much the same way as plants in a greenhouse. Though intruders and disease may enter our world, they can't devour us because God is in control.

TODAY'S RX

If you're trying to survive on your own, turn to the Lord and you will thrive.

Father, put up the necessary barriers in my life to protect me from harm. Allow me to thrive in your presence. I desire to grow and mature as a believer and to be a beautiful creation in you.

ORDINARY FAITH HEALING

I have pleaded in prayer for you, Simon, that your faith should not fail. LUKE 22:32

When Anthony received a diagnosis of renal cell carcinoma, he called me for advice.

"What do you think about my going to the Mayo Clinic for treatment?" he asked.

"Half the success of any treatment is the patient's belief that it's the right plan. If you want to go to the Mayo Clinic, you should go."

I knew his only real chance for long-term survival was a complete and clean surgical removal of the cancer, and Mayo would do a great job.

A few weeks later, I saw Anthony sitting in his truck with a big grin on his face. "Hey, Dr. Anderson!" he called out. "They got it all. I just wanted you to know."

"That's great to hear," I said.

A year later, Anthony went back for a checkup and found the cancer had returned. The doctors removed three lymph nodes.

"We'll just keep praying for God's will," I said, knowing the news wasn't good.

"But I need to tell you something else," he said. One night, around two o'clock in the morning, I woke up and started praying real hard, asking God to heal me. Suddenly, a man and a woman stood at the foot of my bed. They said to me, 'How do you know you haven't already been healed?' And then—I know this is going to sound weird, but—"

"Tell me," I said. "I've experienced a few weird things of my own."

"As they left, the wall suddenly opened up right next to them, and for about two minutes, I got a glimpse of heaven."

"What did you see?"

"It was the most beautiful garden with vibrantly colored flowers. I felt as if I could reach out and touch it, but then it was gone."

"Anthony, that sounds a lot like what I experienced in a dream one time."

"No matter what happens to this body, my faith has been strengthened, I know I've been healed, and I don't have any more fear."

"I know what you're talking about. God gave you a glimpse of home."

"But, why me?" Anthony asked. "I'm just an ordinary guy. I don't even know Scripture that well."

"I don't know, but I know that the disciples were just ordinary guys until they met Jesus too."

TODAY'S RX

In his wisdom, God may give you a glimpse of your forever healing.

Thank you for revealing yourself in unexpected ways, Lord. You never fail to astound me by showing me glimpses of your glory. I long to experience more of you.

STRENGTH FOR YOUR BATTLE

They did not conquer the land with their swords; it was not their own strong arm that gave them victory. It was your right hand and strong arm and the blinding light from your face that helped them, for you loved them. . . . Only by your power can we push back our enemies; only in your name can we trample our foes. I do not trust in my bow; I do not count on my sword to save me. PSALM 44:3, 5-6

When Kellee was diagnosed with ovarian cancer, she knew it wasn't a battle she could fight on her own. Though the available treatments for the disease had progressed enough over the past few years to give Kellee hope for recovery, the battle still would not be easy. The survival rate for the kind of cancer she had was fifty-fifty at best.

"I'm tired. I'm not sure I have the strength to push through," Kellee confided to me one day.

"I understand. This treatment isn't easy. But I believe the Lord will be your strength when you can't muster it on your own," I said. I reminded her that God had gotten her through the first phase, and I was confident he would see her through the next one as well. I told her that God would be with her every step of the way.

During Kellee's treatment, her white blood count dropped dangerously low. So did her red blood count and platelets. She had to be placed into reverse isolation to protect her from the outside world. During this time, she did not rely on weapons of war or medicine to vanquish her cancerous foe. Instead, she found power in the presence of God.

The battle was long and hard, but it paid off. Weeks later, the final round of chemo was finished. With jubilation in her heart and joy in her eyes, she embraced her family. Together they celebrated her recovery and God's victory.

TODAY'S RX

When the battle seems long and hard, fear not. God's strong arm and the blinding light from his face will help you.

God, I long to be strengthened and revitalized—to celebrate recovery from all that I have faced. Give me the endurance I need to make it through and stand victorious in your sight.

THE BEST MEDICINE

The thief's purpose is to steal and kill and destroy. My purpose is to give them a rich and satisfying life. JOHN 10:10

"Is this right?" I asked the officer as I pointed to the crime report.

"Yeah, the only thing they took was her medicine."

"They took my medicine? Don't they know I need it?" Gertie was clearly upset, and she had a right to be. She was eighty years old and had come to the ER after being the victim of a break-in.

"Doctor, did they take everything? They must know I can't live without my medicine."

Gertie was a brittle diabetic with severe hypertension. She had survived two strokes, but they had left her in severe and chronic pain. We had tried everything to control it, but in the end, we had no choice but to prescribe narcotics.

Though unhurt during the break-in, she was obviously upset by the situation. I pulled up a chair to talk to her. "Gertie, this sort of thing is happening everywhere. There's a group of people who will do anything they can to get their hands on these medications. But you mustn't worry. God is ultimately in control, and he will protect you. Now, we've already called the pharmacy, and they have all of your medications ready to be picked up. I've also asked the officers to step up the patrols in your neighborhood and keep an extra eye on you."

"Thank you for getting my medicine, Dr. Anderson. I couldn't live without it, you know."

Talking with Gertie that night reminded me of today's verse. Without God, our lives would be a mess. But with him, we can have a rich and satisfying life. I can't imagine anything worse than a thief who would try to take that security away, yet we know there is an evil one who wants to do exactly that. Just as Gertie was focused on her medication and not on the thieves who tried to take it, we need to keep our focus on God, with the confidence that he can protect us from anyone or anything who tries to harm us.

TODAY'S RX

Turn to the Lord daily, and put your trust in him. Truly, we cannot go a day without him.

It's only by your grace and power, Father, that I have life. Thank you for each new day. Help me to focus on you today, lifting my prayers to you and reading your Word for the wisdom I need.

TRUST YOUR PROVIDER

For the word of the L*ORD holds true, and we can trust everything he does.* Psalm 33:4

I have often seen medical treatments prescribed to patients that should work, but for some reason, they don't. I've also seen treatments that shouldn't work because they had no scientific basis, and yet they work; the patients thrived and got well.

Why does the same treatment plan or medication work for one person and not for another?

What's the difference between treatments that work and those that don't?

I believe it has to do with whether the patient trusts the treatment plan and the doctor who prescribed it.

Nearly every medical study—whether testing a new treatment or a new drug—is tested against a placebo (no medical treatment). Though a placebo doesn't have any medical value, it always results in a positive response for some people. In other words, doing nothing works just as effectively as the medicine or treatment that is being tested. This is called the placebo effect. The reason we see the placebo effect work positively is because patients who don't know they are receiving the placebo believe that whatever they are taking works. In some cases, the response rate to the placebo can be as high as 30 percent.

That's the kind of faith God wants us to place in him and his words. When it seems as if nothing is happening and there is no proof that we are receiving what we think we need, he wants us to trust his Word. If we believe in God's Word, he is faithful to keep the promises he has made to us, and he's proved this over and over again, not only in the Bible but in our lives.

As today's verse says, the word of the Lord holds true. If faith in a placebo works 30 percent of the time, imagine what 100 percent faith in God can do!

TODAY'S RX

Trust God. He still keeps his word.

God, you are faithful, and your Word always proves true. I know I can go to it for the answers I need. Help me to seek your truth above all else and come to you first for counsel.

FAITH WITHOUT DOUBT

Jesus told them, "I tell you the truth, if you have faith and don't doubt, you can do things like this and much more. You can even say to this mountain, 'May you be lifted up and thrown into the sea,' and it will happen." MATTHEW 21:21

"I've been having pains in my right side on and off for about six months," Bill said. "But recently it's gotten worse. I think it might be a gallbladder attack."

"Why don't you lie back and let me take a look," I said.

Bill reclined on the exam table as I examined his abdominal area. He had moderate to severe pain with bloating and cramping in the upper right quadrant. But when I felt his abdomen, I knew it was more than what we first expected. His liver was approximately two centimeters below the ridge of his ribs, and it felt a bit firm.

Bill had never been a drinker or an IV drug user. He had four healthy children, and there had never been any family history of liver disease.

"I'd like for you to have an ultrasound, but the tech isn't in today, so I'm going to order a CT scan instead."

"I'm sure it's just my gallbladder acting up," Bill said, but he agreed to the scan.

When the results came back, they confirmed my suspicions and Bill's worst fear. He had liver cancer. I sat down with him to go over the results.

"How much time do I have left?" he asked. He was a Bible-believing Christian, and he respected my opinion.

"The textbooks say six months to a year, but we both know that with God anything is possible."

Today's verse reminds us that not only can God do incredible things, but we can do those same things and much more if we have faith and don't doubt. Bill lived for another four and a half years before God called him home to his complete healing in heaven. I consider those extra four years to be a mountain moved.

TODAY'S RX

Remove the barriers of doubt, and God will move mountains.

Help me to put my full confidence in you, Father, knowing you are capable of all things. Do not let me doubt your goodness, but remember how you've always been faithful to me.

LOST AND FOUND

I will search for my lost ones who strayed away, and I will bring them safely home again. I will bandage the injured and strengthen the weak. But I will destroy those who are fat and powerful. I will feed them, yes—feed them justice! EZEKIEL 34:16

Have you ever gotten lost? It can be a frightening experience. That's why today's verse is so reassuring. God searches for the lost ones who stray and brings them safely home again. What a beautiful promise!

With GPS on our smartphones, most of us don't get lost as often as we may have in the past. As soon as we take a wrong turn, the GPS voice scolds us, automatically recalculating the route to our destination or telling us to turn around.

But there are some places where GPS doesn't work or where the nearest cell tower may be out of range. That happened to me in Ireland when my smartphone wasn't smart enough to communicate with the local system. Technically, I was off the grid.

In an effort to see something new, I had strayed just far enough away from where we were staying that I didn't recognize any landmarks. In addition, driving on the opposite side of the road disrupted my usual sense of direction. Soon, I had to admit that I was lost and confused. I needed to turn around and get back on the main road to the City Centre.

The right thing to do would have been to stop and ask directions, but I was in a foreign land, and I wasn't sure if it was safe. So I just kept driving. Eventually, my random turns led me to a sign that pointed toward Newcastle. From there, I knew how to get back.

Have you ever felt so lost that all you could do was go around in circles? Life sometimes becomes a big roundabout going in the wrong direction. That's what happened to me spiritually when I was an atheist. Fortunately, what worked for me in Ireland also worked to get my life back on track: I looked up, and a sign from God pointed me in the direction I should go.

TODAY'S RX

When you get lost, stop and pray, and be ready to follow the signs that point the way home.

Father, I confess that I'm often distracted by things of this world and lose sight of you. Thank you for not giving up on me, but going to great lengths to steer me back and point me in the right direction.

THE HURT BENEATH THE PAIN

I said to myself, "I will watch what I do and not sin in what I say. I will hold my tongue when the ungodly are around me." PSALM 39:1

As a country doctor, I've known many of my patients for years. When I see them, I often sit down and ask them how things are going. Sometimes they'll complain about their latest ailment. Whether it's a headache, insomnia, irritable bowel syndrome, or anxiety, they give me all the details.

I start by asking them the symptoms they're experiencing, and then I ask them when the symptoms started. One thing I've noticed is that often the start of a physical ailment is triggered by a breakdown in a relationship with a loved one. The headaches start after a fight with a daughter-in-law. The insomnia happens the day a loved one takes away the car keys. The irritable bowel syndrome gets worse after harsh words with a neighbor.

As they tell me their symptoms and when they started, they move from describing their physical pain to unmasking their emotional pain. They'll tell me about their fear, anger, or bitterness. They'll even go so far as to give me the personal and intimate details of conversations that happened—or should have happened. As gently as possible, I try to point out the connection between their physical ailments and their emotional anguish.

Has someone ever said something that cut right through your soul? If so, realize that it can affect you and your health in many ways. When it happens, it's important to pray through the issues.

Seek to resolve it like Jesus would.

This may mean having a confrontation with some honest words about how the other person hurt you. It may mean you need to ask for forgiveness for something you said or offer forgiveness for something the other person said. It may mean that you both need to agree to disagree so you can move past your past. These kinds of encounters can be hard, so I encourage you to seek wise counsel from a friend, a pastor, or a therapist to give you the courage to do what you need to do.

As much as I'd like to cure all of my patients' physical symptoms, nothing I try will be a permanent fix unless they treat the underlying relationship problems as well.

TODAY'S RX

Don't bury your pain; bring it to the Lord in prayer.

Lord, help me to release the pain and bitterness I feel from broken relationships. Ease my anger and lighten my heart, allowing me to forgive and move past what has weighed heavily on me for so long.

PASSING ON THE BLESSING

After Jesus left the synagogue with James and John, they went to Simon and Andrew's home. Now Simon's mother-in-law was sick in bed with a high fever. They told Jesus about her right away. So he went to her bedside, took her by the hand, and helped her sit up. Then the fever left her, and she prepared a meal for them. MARK 1:29-31

Simon's mother-in-law was lying in bed with a high fever, and Simon was very concerned about her. I'm sure the other disciples were, too, but let's face it, they were probably a little disappointed. They had planned to spend the night at Simon's. They were expecting an evening meal and a place to sleep. But with Simon's mother-in-law in bed, their choices became limited; they couldn't have a pizza delivered or order Chinese takeout. In addition, they had to be worried about catching whatever it was she had.

When I receive a call from the hospital or nursing home staff, the first thing I do is ask about the patient's temperature. God created our bodies to heal themselves when something goes wrong; and in its simplest form, a fever is often a sign that the patient is fighting an infection.

But in the ancient world, before aspirin and antibiotics, a fever could signal a life-threatening illness. In fact, the fever itself could be life-threatening.

That's why it was so important for Jesus to go directly to the bedside of Simon's mother-in-law. There, he took her hand and helped her to sit up. Immediately the fever was gone, and she was able to get up.

Think about how complete this healing was. Most of us, when we've been sick, will still be fatigued and in need of rest, even after the fever is gone. But Simon's mother-in-law felt good enough immediately to get out of bed and begin preparing a meal for everyone.

I believe she did exactly what Jesus wants all of us to do. When he blesses us, whether financially, with good health, or in some other way, he wants us to pass that blessing along to someone else.

TODAY'S RX

For your own good health, pass along a blessing to someone else.

God, you've shown me your great love through the kind acts of others when I've been sick. Please help me to do the same, shining your light and love on those in need.

OUR WONDERFULLY CREATIVE GOD

Look! I am creating new heavens and a new earth, and no one will even think about the old ones anymore. Isaiah 65:17

The breathtaking evidence of God's creation is all around us, if only we would take the time to look. I remember watching with Karen—before she and I were even dating—the most incredible sunset I'd ever seen. I knew she felt the beauty, too, because we were both very quiet as the baby blue sky turned to pinks and yellows and then deepened into an almost indescribable rose hue as the final rays of sunlight faded into the horizon.

Karen told me later that at that moment she realized just how creative God could be. This was during a time when she was still uncertain about the sincerity of my newfound faith, and she had been resisting my attempts to build a closer relationship with her. But when she saw that sunset, she realized that if God could use colors and light to paint the sky with such splendor, perhaps he could also bring an agnostic to faith through our evenings of memorizing Scripture together. She felt as if she needed to be faithful to whatever God's call was on her life, even if it meant stepping outside of her set expectations to consider a relationship that, until then, she hadn't been open to.

Another time when I felt completely in awe of God's creativity was when I dissected a human cadaver in medical school. It was so obvious to me that there was something different about humanity. How could we have possibly come into being by accident or random chance? I was intrigued, fascinated, and confused all at the same time. But mostly I was curious. That curiosity took me onto a path that led me back to God.

God is the source of all creativity. There is no limit to what he can do. I can hardly wait to get to heaven to see the fullness of all he has done.

TODAY'S RX

List some examples of God's creativity that you've observed. If God's creation on earth is that marvelous, can you imagine what heaven must be like?

God, I praise you for making the earth and the sky and the sea, and everything that has life; for the heavens and all the planets, moons, and stars. But no matter how glorious things appear here on earth, I know they are but a dim shadow of what awaits us in heaven with you.

LOOK ON THE SUNNY SIDE FOR HEALTH

A cheerful look brings joy to the heart; good news makes for good health.
PROVERBS 15:30

Have you ever sat in a doctor's office waiting for test results to come back? Did you dread getting bad news? Or were you optimistic that everything would be okay?

Every day, I see patients who fear the worst, but they are hoping and praying that I have good news for them. Most of the time I do. But on those occasions when a test comes back positive for cancer or an unwanted diagnosis is confirmed, I find that patients accept their condition better if I deliver the bad news with a dose of optimism.

Whether you're ill or someone you know is sick, you can do the same thing—think positively. Looking at the glass as half-full rather than half-empty will invariably lead to a better outcome. Science backs this up. Studies have shown that patients who have a positive outlook on life, even if it is shortened by disease, will live longer and more comfortably than those who don't.

When I walk the last mile with terminal cancer patients, I don't avoid talking about cancer. But I try to help them embrace the journey, even if it's a tough row to hoe.

TODAY'S RX

No matter how hard it might be, pray that the Lord will bring joy, cheer, and lightness to your burden.

Lord, fill me with your presence as I walk the road to recovery.
Help me not to despair, but to keep a positive outlook on all
I face, knowing that with you I have reason for hope.

SAYING GOOD-BYE

Whoever has the Son has life; whoever does not have God's Son does not have life.
1 JOHN 5:12

"Hey, Dr. Anderson," George said. "You know how you've been encouraging me to seek God through all this? I want you to know, I got baptized last Sunday."

I was happy to hear the news, but from the smell of alcohol on George's jacket, I had concerns about the true condition of his life. George's son had died in a car accident four years earlier, and the aftermath had been painful for George and his family.

Alcoholism can sneak up on a person, and I saw the danger signs with George. He had started out having a nightcap to help him fall asleep, but it didn't quite help. So he tried two drinks before bed. But the more he drank, the worse things got—strengthening rather than eliminating his feelings of sorrow.

When I asked how many drinks he had each day, he said four or five, but when we got the results of his liver function test, they revealed that he was drinking far more than he would admit. I decided to tackle it head-on.

"George, I'm happy you were baptized and that you have a closer relationship with Jesus. But I know you're drinking more than you've said. I also know that, with God's help and the resources I can provide, you can stop drinking and conquer the demons that keep you awake at night."

George hung his head. "You're right. My drinking is out of control. Sometimes at night, I wake up with the shakes. I don't want to do this anymore. How can I quit?"

"You've already taken the first step on the road to recovery by admitting to yourself that you have a problem. The good news is that Jesus will also be a friend you can lean on as you quit drinking. I'll help you get through the delirium tremens, and I can also prescribe medication to stop your urge to drink."

George did as he was told, leaning on Jesus when things got hard. Six months later, he earned his six-month token from AA, and his health was restored to what it had been before his son's accident. As he got healthier, he was able to say good-bye to his son and begin to live his life for Jesus, the Son of God.

TODAY'S RX

Jesus is a faithful friend in all kinds of adversity.

Jesus, I lean on you today for the strength I need. You are more than just my Savior; you're a faithful friend. I pray for your support to keep me upright in the midst of my pain.

WHO GETS THE CREDIT?

When the Pharisees heard about the miracle, they said, "No wonder he can cast out demons. He gets his power from Satan, the prince of demons." MATTHEW 12:24

When we look at today's verse, we might think, *Those Pharisees! They don't understand that Jesus' healing power comes from God the Father, not from Satan.* We're quick to judge them because we know the end of the story.

But are we really all that different from the Pharisees?

In modern medicine, we often give credit to doctors or researchers for their breakthroughs in healing. We award the Nobel Prize for physiology or medicine, but we don't give awards for healing to the Great Physician. Shouldn't the credit for all those award-winning insights or discoveries really go to God?

In some cases, in their acceptance speeches, the winners of the Nobel Prize thank God for his guidance in their research and discoveries. However, by the time the ceremony is over, the only name the public remembers is the name of the person who received the award, not the name of God.

Even in experimental scientific studies, we don't account for God's hand in healing. When we study new drugs or treatments, we compare them to a placebo, which should have no scientific effect on the illness or disease. For a drug to receive approval from the Food and Drug Administration, it must be statistically better than a placebo. That makes sense. An effective treatment should be better than something that is supposed to do nothing.

But what if a placebo isn't actually doing nothing? What if, in some cases, the placebo is actually the means by which God does his healing? Every year, there are thousands of drugs and treatments studied by scientists or doctors that don't do any better than the placebo. And study after study reveals that placebos can have measurable cure rates. In other words, doing something that should have no scientific reason to affect a cure often does.

I believe this is evidence that we are like the Pharisees. We don't give credit to God for the cure when he is ultimately the source of all healing.

TODAY'S RX

Give credit where credit is due. Don't overlook the hand of God in your healing.

Lord, please forgive me for when I've doubted you or turned a blind eye to you. You are the healer of all. Even when I am struggling or in pain, help me to always acknowledge your faithfulness.

ONLY GOD'S PROMISES

Reassure me of your promise, made to those who fear you. . . . Remember your promise to me; it is my only hope. PSALM 119:38, 49

Remember the TV quiz show *Who Wants to Be a Millionaire?* The game offered contestants three lifelines if they didn't know the answer to a question. The first lifeline was to phone a friend, the second was to poll the audience, and the third option was to have the producers narrow the possible answers down to two, creating a fifty-fifty chance. If I were playing, I'd want God to be my "phone a friend" lifeline! I would gladly give up the other two options if I could phone God anytime I had a question.

I know that's how Allen must have felt. When I walked into his hospital room, he turned and said, "Dr. Anderson, the oncologist told me that I have a fifty-fifty chance of survival if I do chemo. But here's the thing. I had a friend who had the same kind of cancer, and he did the chemo and then got very sick and died anyway. I'm not sure I want to go through what he did. Do you think I could get a second or third opinion and go with the majority vote?"

The oncologist had given him a fifty-fifty chance, and now Allen wanted to poll an audience of other oncologists to see what the majority would say. I guess that made me the "phone a friend" option. Allen was using all of his lifelines, but his concern was more important than any game show question. The answer he chose could determine the outcome of his life.

"Allen, I think you're smart to ask all these questions and get as much information as you can. We can get a second opinion and a third if that's helpful. The Bible says that with many counselors there is much wisdom. But let me just say that we don't know anything for certain. Even something that sounds as mathematical as a fifty-fifty chance is only a guess. The numbers come from large population studies, and even there we see notable variations. I recommend that we look at the odds optimistically and pray that God will intervene and heal you 100 percent, not 50 percent."

Though medical science can make mathematical predictions, our hope isn't in science; it's in the God of hope.

TODAY'S RX

God alone knows best, and his promises bring hope.

God, what a comfort it is knowing I'm saved by your grace. Because of your Son, my debt is paid in full—not half or any other amount. You have preserved my life and given me hope.

OCTOBER CHECKUP

October brings the smell of crisp apples and the color of pumpkins and falling leaves. As the air takes on a chill, we pull on our favorite sweaters and boots. There's no better time for a walk to enjoy the tapestry of trees transitioning from summer to winter in hues of burnt gold, rustic brown, and bright orange.

October is a great month for tea, a good book, and the first crackling fire of the season. It's also a great month for "kindness capers."

Over the next few months, you'll be busy with the holidays. So take a few moments in October to share gifts of kindness with those who are least suspecting. Maybe it's paying it forward at a drive-through restaurant, offering a single mom a night of babysitting, or covering for a coworker who seems especially stressed. Maybe you and the kids can make sandwiches and take them to the homeless in the park while passing out scarves and mittens. They'll need them as temperatures drop.

In the Gospels, we read about how Jesus came to reconcile us to God. He didn't wait until we had cleaned ourselves up and deserved to be reconciled. He gave us a gift we didn't deserve. How can you do the same for someone else this month? Is there someone you can forgive who doesn't deserve it? Is there someone who is hard to love that you can love this month? Is there someone who made poor choices and now finds himself or herself in difficult circumstances with a need you can meet?

Set a goal for yourself. How many kindness capers can you think up? Make a list. How many can you complete from your list? Can you have a kindness competition with someone else to see who can out-give the other?

Our family has many October birthdays. By the end of the month, we've had enough cake and ice cream to last us through the winter! Celebrating each birthday as the culmination of the preceding year, and looking ahead to the hope it brings for the upcoming year, gives us time to reflect on and commemorate the person and to thank the Lord for all his blessings.

October may feel chilly, but it doesn't have to be cold. I can think of no better way to warm someone's heart than with an act of kindness or appreciation.

October Booster Shot: As the cooler air drives us inside, we tend to sit more and eat more carbohydrates, leading to an increased risk of obesity, hypertension, and diabetes. So get outside and walk. Exercise will help to prevent many chronic illnesses.

INCREDIBLE SACRIFICES

God also bound himself with an oath, so that those who received the promise could be perfectly sure that he would never change his mind. So God has given both his promise and his oath. These two things are unchangeable because it is impossible for God to lie. Therefore, we who have fled to him for refuge can have great confidence as we hold to the hope that lies before us. Hebrews 6:17-18

"I'm wondering if I can get along with just one kidney," Steve said.

"Why are you asking?"

"My sister has renal failure, and she has to go on dialysis until she can get a kidney transplant. I'd like to give her one of mine. I've prayed about it, and I think it's the right thing to do."

Steve had obviously thought long and hard about this decision and had prayed for wisdom, but I warned him that donating a kidney is a serious and complex business.

"First we would need to see if you two are a match. If so, we can explore other questions, such as whether your current kidney function is healthy enough. We need to make sure you can live a long and healthy life with just one kidney."

"Let's do it!" Steve said.

The test results showed that Steve was a perfect match for his sister. In addition, his kidney function was healthy; he could make the donation without compromising his own health.

"I know you love your sister very much, and this is an admirable thing you're doing, but you have to remember that this sacrifice of love is forever. There's no turning back once you decide to move forward."

"I've never been more certain about anything," Steve said without hesitation. "I just want my sister to have her old life back."

Giving a kidney to someone in need is a sacrificial act of love, but it pales in comparison to the sacrifice that Jesus made on the cross. He willingly gave up his life, not to preserve our old lives, but so that we could have *new* life in him.

TODAY'S RX

When we lovingly sacrifice for others, we do what Jesus first did for us.

Father, help me to give to others as you have given to me. Help me not to cling to worldly goods, but to share them with others in need. I desire to have a sacrificial spirit like yours.

HE ALWAYS ANSWERS

I am praying to you because I know you will answer, O God. Bend down and listen as I pray. PSALM 17:6

"When you told me I had ALS, you said my prognosis was about two years. Is that still what you think?" Albert asked.

"Only God knows the hour, but based on those who've been in similar circumstances, I think that's about right."

Albert was a large, burly man who spoke with a deep-toned voice. Today that voice was filled with resignation. His petite wife sat quietly at his side, taking it all in. Of all the diagnoses I give my patients, ALS, or Lou Gehrig's disease, is one of the worst. I know how many challenges the couple will face in the next few months.

"Now Albert, that's just what the textbooks say. But God is still God, and it doesn't mean we can't pray for a miracle."

"My wife and I pray every day that when I wake up in the morning, I won't have this cross to bear. But so far, God has answered differently."

Albert was right. It wasn't that God didn't answer their prayers; it was just that he hadn't answered them the way they had hoped.

I've begun to understand that, even when God's answers are not what we hoped for, there *is* a reward that comes later. Jesus himself experienced this right before he went to the cross. He asked his Father in heaven to remove the cup of suffering from him if it was aligned with his will. The answer Jesus got was not the one he hoped for. But he followed his Father's plan anyway. He knew the reward that would come at the end of his mission.

When you ask God for something, do you get disappointed or even angry when the outcome is not what you wanted or expected? Do you sometimes misinterpret God's answer as not answering?

Albert's journey was hard, but he understood that God always answered his prayers, even when the answers weren't what he had hoped for. And this knowledge transformed his prayers. Over time, his prayers were transformed as he learned to pray for God's will first and foremost.

Albert was eventually healed of ALS but not here on earth. The reward for his faithfulness came when he entered eternity.

TODAY'S RX

God always hears and answers our prayers. And God always keeps his promises.

God, thank you for bending down and listening to my prayers. You hear my praises and my cries, and you answer faithfully all I ask. Help me to be patient and steadfast in my faith as I wait on you.

MAKING STRAIGHT THAT WHICH HAS BEEN BENT

One Sabbath day as Jesus was teaching in a synagogue, He saw a woman who had been crippled by an evil spirit. She had been bent double for eighteen years and was unable to stand up straight. When Jesus saw her, he called her over and said, "Dear woman, you are healed of your sickness!" Then he touched her, and instantly she could stand straight. How she praised God! LUKE 13:10-13

The woman described in today's verses likely had kyphosis of the spine. In Luke's day, that condition was impossible to cure. Even today, the treatment would be long and laborious for someone who had been stricken for eighteen years. It would require years of orthopedic surgeries and physical therapy working in tandem.

In reading Luke's account of this woman, I realize how terribly she must have suffered. She likely endured debilitating pain as well as breathing and digestive difficulties. Even the act of retrieving water for her basic daily needs would have been a tremendous struggle. The fact that she was still up and about, attending synagogue after eighteen years of suffering from this condition, was a testament to her persistence in the battle for daily survival.

When Jesus saw this woman in such suffering, he had to have felt the same compassion toward her that he exhibited toward so many others who were shunned, outcast, and hurting.

So he healed her.

For the first time in eighteen years, the woman stood up straight, and the first person she saw was Jesus, her healer. Imagine how her eyes must have sparkled and her face glowed as she could finally see the faces of other people rather than always looking at their sandals. When she strolled into the market the next day, few would have recognized her.

Jesus not only has power over our physical health, but he can also straighten out our bent and crooked lives—our marriages, our finances, our jobs. If we're downcast because of guilt, shame, or depression, he can give us a new outlook on life. Jesus straightens the bent and helps us lift our eyes to the heavens, as we once again walk with confidence, knowing that he has not only healed us, but he has also forgiven all our sins.

TODAY'S RX

Give God the bent things in your life. He wants to heal your pain and your shame and allow you to walk upright.

Lord, please remove the sin and shame that weighs me down and keeps me from looking up to you. I long to stand straight, to be free, and to walk with confidence and joy.

THIRSTING FOR MORE OF HIM

LORD, how great is your mercy; let me be revived by following your regulations.
PSALM 119:156

"I don't know what's happening to me," Annette said. "I just don't feel like myself. I'm craving sweets all the time, but I'm losing weight. And I'm so thirsty that I'm always drinking something, which means I constantly have to go to the bathroom—even in the middle of the night!"

"Sounds like it could be your sugar," I said.

"That doesn't surprise me one bit. Half of my family is diabetic, and several are on hemodialysis with end-stage renal disease."

"Let's do some blood work and see what we can learn."

When the results came back the next day, Annette's hemoglobin A1C, which measured the glucose in her blood over the past two to three months was almost twice the normal level. Other tests confirmed that she was a type 2 diabetic. This was actually encouraging, because diet and exercise can positively affect the treatment. Annette's weight loss needed to continue but in a controlled manner, rather than as a result of hyperglycemia.

"We'll start you on a strict program to see if we can get things under control quickly. We also need to have some long-term goals in mind. Let's pray that God will give you the strength and stamina to continue. Remember, this is going to be a marathon rather than a sprint."

Annette's faith was bold. "I know that if I work the plan," she said, "God will have mercy on me. He'll protect me from having to do dialysis and prevent me from being afraid."

As Annette got her health under control, her physical thirstiness decreased. But her thirst for God grew stronger.

TODAY'S RX

God can and will protect you, even when you're facing serious health challenges.

God, give me the stamina to continue this road to recovery. Despite how I feel physically, I know the plans and treatments are for my benefit. Thank you for providing for me during this time and for helping me through.

A FAITH HARVEST

"You don't have enough faith," Jesus told them. "I tell you the truth, if you had faith even as small as a mustard seed, you could say to this mountain, 'Move from here to there,' and it would move. Nothing would be impossible." MATTHEW 17:20

When I was a young boy, my dad and granddaddy planted a garden every spring. As soon as I could toddle after them, I was enlisted to help. In the summer and early fall, we ate fresh vegetables from those gardens, and during the rest of the year, we ate the surplus harvest that we had canned.

One of my first jobs in the garden was planting the seeds. There was a rhythm to it that I quickly learned. Corn seeds were planted every eight to twelve inches. Butter beans could be planted much closer together. But when it came time to plant the mustard seeds, I wasn't allowed to do it. They were too small for me to handle. They'd either disappear in the pudgy folds of my hand, or they would spill out too fast and be wasted. So Dad and Granddaddy were always the ones to plant this small but very important seed.

Because I wasn't allowed to handle them, mustard seeds took on special significance for me. So imagine my interest when I heard that Jesus described the mustard seed as a measure of faith. Most sermons I've heard on the topic emphasize that we only need a tiny amount of faith to do big things. But my understanding is quite different because of my experience in the garden.

When I read today's verse, I ask myself if I am ready and able to handle even that small amount of faith. Am I a good steward, planting the right amount at the right time in the right place?

If properly planted, a small amount of mustard seed produces a lot of greens. Can our faith bloom and grow in the same way? Does our faith grow to provide not only for the season in which we harvest it, but also for a surplus that will provide sustenance during even the longest and coldest winter when nothing grows?

When we harvest a great bounty of faith that was once as small as a mustard seed, I like to imagine God grinning like my granddaddy did when he anticipated a feast of mustard greens for dinner.

TODAY'S RX

Mighty faith comes from a mighty small seed.

Father, your Word reminds me time and again of how you can do a lot with just a little. Help me to remember that when I'm feeling useless or purposeless. I know you can do limitless works through me.

RELAXING IN THE ARMS OF THE SHEPHERD

Save your people! Bless Israel, your special possession. Lead them like a shepherd, and carry them in your arms forever. Psalm 28:9

When our children were little, Karen and I decided it would be a good idea for them to experience a taste of farm life. So we bought a few goats and sheep for our little Tennessee farm.

The goats multiplied so fast that it wasn't long before we had more four-legged kids than two-legged kids! The sheep, on the other hand, were a different story. They never reproduced, and there were never any lambs.

There were other differences between the animals. The sheep were content to stay in one place. They would eat all of the grass in that area, but they refused to venture beyond where they felt comfortable. I had to lead them to greener pastures, or they would have eaten every blade in that one area.

The goats, on the other hand, were regular escape artists. One day, I found all five of them stuck on a bank near the river. I had to lift each one up and out to safety. They relaxed in my arms as I carried them home.

We are a lot like sheep and goats; we need God's guidance and encouragement to stay in the right pasture. But whether we are a sheep or a goat, there are times in life when we don't understand where God is leading us or why. As today's verse says, the Good Shepherd has a plan to save us, bless us, lead us, and carry us in his arms forever.

TODAY'S RX

Today, relax in the arms of the Good Shepherd.

Jesus, thank you for being my Goof Shepherd. You guide me away from danger and lead me to green pastures, caring for my every need along the way. Help me to obey your calling and follow after you.

POINTING TO PROMISES

Do not throw away this confident trust in the Lord. Remember the great reward it brings you! Patient endurance is what you need now, so that you will continue to do God's will. Then you will receive all that he has promised. HEBREWS 10:35-36

Among my son David's friends, Ben stood out from the crowd. He had bright red hair, piercing blue eyes, and a smile as welcoming as it was infectious. Like most young men during their high school years, Ben was eager to get out of the house and change the world. And it turned out that he would do it in a most extraordinary way.

I'll never forget the day when Ben and his parents received the news: "You have cancer of the kidney. But with surgery, we believe you can be cured."

That's when things changed. The young men's Bible study that both David and Ben attended was fairly typical, with a little teaching of God's Word wedged in between a lot of pranks and joking around. Ben's diagnosis changed these young men. Though they still had fun, the teaching time became more vital as they studied God's eternal promises. These young men, forged in fire, began to sharpen each other in the heat of battle.

Ben, of course, was right out front. Leading by example, he used each day to share the love of Christ with others. The center of his witness was always the promises of Jesus. As a result, many lives were changed, and many people joined him in the battle.

When the surgical reports gave the all-clear, we rejoiced with Ben.

Four years later, the cancer returned. Though some may have doubted God's goodness, Ben remained confident. Once again, he chose prayer and love as his weapons, inviting everyone who crossed his path to come along on a great journey of faith.

When others faced problems, Ben was the first one to offer encouragement. "Focus on the things you can control, and don't get overwhelmed by the things you can't," he said. Day by day, breath by breath, Ben focused on the promises of Jesus, especially those promises of a full and complete healing.

This young man with fiery hair and a fire in his soul continued leading others to the Cross until his final breath, when Jesus fulfilled his promise to heal Ben completely and permanently.

TODAY'S RX

Never stop loving, and never stop pointing people to Jesus. His promises will always be fulfilled.

Lord, help me to be patient and trusting at all times, knowing you are in control. In my darkest moments, revive my spirit and allow me to share with others all that you've done for me.

THE FIRST STEP IS ADMITTING YOU HAVE A PROBLEM

He will die for lack of self-control; he will be lost because of his great foolishness.
PROVERBS 5:23

Bryan believed he should at least be able to have a little taste of his birthday cake, but one little taste led to a much larger portion of the forbidden, fruit-filled cake.

At three hundred pounds and growing, Bryan was unable to control his appetite. Having cake in the house only fueled his obsession. Knowing the cake was available, he continued to go back for more until he had eaten the whole thing and lay on the floor, unconscious.

His mother found him and immediately tested his blood sugar. It was so high that it didn't register a number—it just read "high." By the time he got to the hospital, he had a reading of 900—a potentially life-threatening blood sugar level.

"I didn't even buy him a birthday cake," she said, as she waited anxiously in the emergency room. "He went out and bought his own and kept it hidden from us."

"I know he has trouble controlling his appetite, but this could have killed him," I said as gently as I could.

"I know. I know. We're going to have a heart-to-heart with him when he gets out of the ICU."

The next morning, I overheard her pleading for her son's life.

"Bryan, you have to get this under control! You could have died, and I can't take that. Your behavior is going to kill both of us. Please stop."

"I'm sorry, Mom. I know. I'll get help with this food addiction. I promise."

I recommended that he meet with a psychologist before being discharged. When I went in to check on him, I could tell he was taking the situation seriously.

"I don't want to be a food addict for the rest of my life. Will you pray for me? Will you pray that I overcome this compulsion?" he asked.

I assured him that I would continue to pray for him, but I encouraged him also to look to the Lord each day for strength. When we are weak, our God is strong.

TODAY'S RX

There are many forms of addiction. If your life is out of control, acknowledge your problem to someone else; then seek help from God and a professional who can advise you on how best to overcome it.

God, I lack control in a number of areas, and I need you to help me. Please lead me away from unhealthy habits, and direct me to your Word, where I know I will receive counsel.

BLESSED WITH IMMUNITY

They will not work in vain, and their children will not be doomed to misfortune. For they are people blessed by the LORD, and their children, too, will be blessed. I will answer them before they even call to me. While they are still talking about their needs, I will go ahead and answer their prayers! ISAIAH 65:23-24

As she bounced her squirming baby in her lap, the new mother seemed concerned. "I brought him in to get his vaccinations, but I'm not sure I want to now. I keep hearing talk in the media and from celebrities saying that immunizations aren't safe. Some say they don't work or that they might cause autism."

"I know you're concerned. But a lot of doctors and scientists have studied this issue. They've tried to connect vaccinations to all sorts of side effects—but the evidence just isn't there for a connection between the two. The vaccinations won't have any long-term adverse effects on your baby."

"Are there short-term effects?" she asked.

"Well, he might have a little soreness in his leg from where the shot is given or a low-grade fever for a day or two, but the benefits far outweigh the side effects. Without the vaccinations, the consequences could be far worse. He'd be at risk for measles, mumps, rubella, Hepatitis B, diphtheria, pertussis, meningitis, and tetanus. Those could be deadly."

"I don't want *that*."

"Because of vaccinations, the World Health Organization has practically eliminated smallpox and reduced other diseases to only periodic outbreaks. Modern medicine is one avenue through which God has protected our children, even before we were aware of the dangerous diseases lurking outside our doors."

"I just want to do what's right for my son," she said.

"Here's how I like to think of it. With our immune system, God has already given us the greatest defense against disease we could possibly have. Vaccination programs are used to activate what God has already given us."

"That makes sense. Let's go ahead with the vaccinations."

"The only thing that could protect him better is God himself."

TODAY'S RX

An ounce of prevention is worth a pound of cure. Get your kids vaccinated, and get your flu shot each year.

Father, help me not to be distracted by what this world says is right or wrong, but to determine my course of action by what you promise. Thank you for providing cures to so many illnesses and preventative vaccines to keep illnesses away.

RUNNING A NEW RACE

And Jesus said to the man, "Stand up and go. Your faith has healed you." LUKE 17:19

I was in the ER one rainy night when the EMS radio crackled.

"MVA.[9] Single motorcycle in ravine just north of Ashland City on Coyote Curve."

When the ambulance pulled in, the motorcyclist was on a spine board, unable to move his lower extremities.

Jacob was an avid athlete who had run track when he was in high school. After he graduated, he got a job as a mechanic and married his high school sweetheart. She was a nurse, and they were hoping to buy a house and start a family. Instead of getting a second car, Jacob had gotten a used motorcycle to save money.

Tests revealed a T7/T8 spinal fracture. Coupled with the paralysis, it meant that Jacob was in bad shape. He was airlifted to a trauma center for further intervention.

Six months later, Jacob rolled into my office in a wheelchair. "I need your help filling out travel papers," he said. He wanted to fly out of the country for an experimental treatment in Mexico. "There's a doctor there who can do stem cell treatment for paralyzed patients, and I want to give it a try."

I was aware of the controversy surrounding stem cell treatment, but this doctor used a new technique drawing stem cells from the patient's own body, though the procedure had not yet been approved in the United States.

"Jacob, I can't stop you from going and trying this or any other procedure, but I want you to know that I haven't lost faith that God can do all things for those who place their trust in him. If it is his will, I believe you will walk again one day."

Another six months passed, and Jacob was still in the wheelchair, but now he could move his toes and control his bladder. Also, his pain had lessened.

At his next appointment, Jacob reminded me of our earlier conversation. "You know, Dr. Anderson, you're right. I believe God will allow me to walk. He's given me a new outlook on life through all of this. In fact, he's already helped me to run. Though I can't physically walk, my spiritual walk is more like a race that I intend to run for the rest of my life."

TODAY'S RX

Run the race that God sets before you. With his help, you will finish strong.

Lord, keep me from becoming discouraged by the obstacles I face. Lift my spirits so that I may continue running the race before me, doing it all to the glory of your name.

THE BRAVE BOY BORN TO HELP OTHERS

Wait patiently for the LORD. Be brave and courageous. Yes, wait patiently for the LORD.
PSALM 27:14

Karen was twenty weeks pregnant when we found out that our unborn son, David, would be born with a bilateral cleft lip and palate. The face ultrasound was new—only having been used for a few months at the time—otherwise we wouldn't have known that early.

We didn't have a lot of information, so our minds were filled with questions. What caused this? What else might be wrong with him? When can we fix it? Who will fix it? Where will the surgery have to be done? We prayed each day that God would direct our paths and bring the puzzle pieces together in due time.

When David was born, we were blessed with a screaming, bouncing baby boy who was healthy except for the cleft lip and palate.

Karen had done part of her master's work in nutrition on special feeding problems in newborns, so she was prepared. I had done extra rotations in plastic surgery as a family practice resident, so I knew who to call. God had prepared us years before by answering many of our questions before we even asked.

The corrective treatments required patience. The plastic surgeon told us to be prepared for eighteen years' worth of treatments and surgery for David. His cleft lip and palate had a tremendous impact on him but not in the way we were expecting.

Last year, David graduated from Samford University with a degree in nursing. He's hoping to go back for more study so he can become a nurse anesthetist. He told us, "After thirty-five surgical procedures, the person who always gave me the most hope and comfort was the anesthetist who put me to sleep and woke me up. I want to be that person for other people, to help them be brave and courageous when they are facing those same fears."

TODAY'S RX

Bravery develops with time and experience of God's faithfulness.

Help me to see the bigger picture behind my illness, God. Use this often-painful experience to shape my life going forward, so I may see the good that will come from it and glorify you.

THE APPOINTED TIME

When he came to the village of Nazareth, his boyhood home, he went as usual to the synagogue on the Sabbath and stood up to read the Scriptures. The scroll of Isaiah the prophet was handed to him. He unrolled the scroll and found the place where this was written: "The Spirit of the LORD is upon me, for he has anointed me to bring Good News to the poor. He has sent me to proclaim that captives will be released, that the blind will see, that the oppressed will be set free, and that the time of the LORD's favor has come." He rolled up the scroll, handed it back to the attendant, and sat down. All eyes in the synagogue looked at him intently. Then he began to speak to them. "The Scripture you've just heard has been fulfilled this very day!" LUKE 4:16-21

In my practice, the appointment book is full every single day. But my staff always finds a way to squeeze in someone who is acutely ill. Often it means I'll be a few minutes late to the rest of my appointments. But acute illness is always a priority, regardless of the schedule. Typically, I feel as if I'm doing a good job if my schedule is off by only ten or fifteen minutes. But I can feel the tension rising in the waiting room on days when I'm further behind.

We all have appointments to keep, and we try to take these predetermined meetings seriously. We show up on time, and we come prepared. But there are days when the oil change appointment takes longer than expected and we're late getting home for the cable guy. We can't always predict how things will go.

When Jesus arrived at the synagogue in Nazareth, he was keeping an appointment that had been on the books for hundreds of years. Before Isaiah's words were ever written, God knew the exact moment when his Son would announce to the people of his hometown that he was the Messiah.

And just as Jesus had an appointed time at the synagogue, so we all have an appointed time when we will meet him face-to-face. He won't have to squeeze us in, and no one will be fifteen minutes late.

TODAY'S RX

Live your life prepared for the most important appointment you'll ever have.

Jesus, thank you for coming to this earth and sharing your ministry. I look forward to the day when I can walk with you and talk with you and be part of your visible Kingdom.

CLEANING UP A SMOKY MESS

Please help us against our enemies, for all human help is useless. With God's help we will do mighty things, for he will trample down our foes. PSALM 108:12-13

"Dr. Anderson, I'm dying. I just know it. Can you help me?" Clyde said.

I had known Clyde for a long time. He was a tough guy, and he had raised his family the same way. I knew he must be scared because he'd come to see me straight from the fields—he still had wet mud on his boots and overalls.

"Now hold on, Clyde," I said. "Let's tackle this together."

Clyde had been a farmer all his life and a smoker nearly as long. I'd occasionally see him driving his tractor in the fields, and it was hard to tell whether the rising smoke was from the tractor or from his ever-present cigarette.

"Tell me why you came in today."

"This morning I started coughing like I usually do, but this time I coughed up a cup of blood."

"I know that must be frightening for you. But let's turn your fear over to God and pray. We'll ask him to help us through the medical maze that lies ahead."

After we prayed, I arranged for him to have some tests and meet with a specialist.

When the CT scan results came back, they confirmed Clyde's fear—there was a mass on the right lower lobe of his lung. The other scans were clear, and there were no metastatic lesions, which was the first of many answered prayers.

The pulmonary and thoracic surgeons agreed that a lobectomy would be the best chance for cure. The following week, Clyde had his surgery, and everything went perfectly. That was the second answered prayer.

Clyde's recovery proceeded on schedule, and he was back in the saddle by spring planting. This time, it was only diesel smoke wafting in the air. I counted that as a third answered prayer.

When Clyde came in for his next checkup, he said, "Last year's mess with that lung cancer was hard, but God did so many good things through it. I don't smoke anymore, and my faith has never been stronger."

I was glad that Clyde was able to see his recovery as the miracle it was. And it was wonderful to see him become a new man in Christ.

TODAY'S RX

Do you need to clean up the mud in your life? Jesus has the living water to do the job.

Father, strengthen my faith throughout this time in my life. Help me to see the good you're doing. Thank you for all the blessings you've bestowed on me.

TRUST GOD FOR THE TRIP

Do not dread the disease that stalks in darkness, nor the disaster that strikes at midday. Though a thousand fall at your side, though ten thousand are dying around you, these evils will not touch you. PSALM 91:6-7

Each week, the news is filled with stories of countless people who are dying from either disaster or disease.

A breathtaking number of people die in earthquakes, tsunamis, hurricanes, tornados, fires, and mudslides every year. The diseases we hear about are equally frightening. As we're finishing up this devotional, the Zika virus has grabbed worldwide attention. A few years before that, it was the Ebola crisis that seemed as if it would never end—until it suddenly disappeared from the front page. Before Ebola, there was a never-before-seen strain of flu. Ten years before that, we were all afraid of getting SARS. And remember the bird flu?

For those who lost loved ones to those diseases, those tragedies were truly sad days. But millions more people changed their plans because they were worried that one of those dangers might affect them. Fortunately, most of the worries were unfounded.

I was chaperoning a choir trip to Chicago about the time that SARS was affecting China. A friend who was with me on the trip was in the process of adopting a little girl from China. He was making plans to pick her up when the news broke that China was threatening to close its borders to contain the outbreak.

It was a scary time as he tried to figure out the best course of action. We prayed today's verse, and as we prayed, his resolve to go was strengthened. He and his wife left earlier than they'd planned to pick up their daughter, but God protected their family. The borders were never closed, and the whole family returned home safely and healthily.

TODAY'S RX

Despite all the fearful reports in the media, the Bible tells us to fear not. Trust the Lord to protect you.

Lord, please be with all those who are hurting right now due to a disease or a disaster. Keep them safe and provide for their needs. Thank you for keeping your hand of protection over me.

HEARING WORDS THAT HEAL

He sent out his word and healed them, snatching them from the door of death.
Psalm 107:20

Many patients assume that a doctor's primary job is to give out medication. They'd be surprised to know that our treatments are more likely to be spoken than dispensed. Most of my day is spent gathering, evaluating, and disseminating information, not pills. The number one thing that most doctors do is give advice.

Unfortunately, most people ignore their doctor's advice. It is fairly consistent across the board for nine out of ten patients not to comply with their doctor's recommendations. In fact, it's so rare for patients to heed my advice that I'm often surprised when they do.

When patients come in after making a big change and I ask why they lost weight or quit smoking, I'm always pleasantly surprised when they say, "You told me to because you said it would improve my health."

As doctors, we know what to say and how to say it, but the receiver has to be ready to hear it and act on it before a positive outcome can take place. I wish I knew how to make my words stick and get patients to act on them so they could live healthier lives.

The same is true of God's words. A preacher can preach to us on Sunday, and we can read our Bibles Monday through Saturday and in that time hear a lot of wise words. But if we don't heed God's wisdom by doing what he says, it is as if we never heard it in the first place. When we come to God for wisdom, we need to make sure that our ears, hearts, and minds are open and ready to take in whatever he says. More than that, we also have to be willing to act on what he says. A failure to do both ensures that we will never truly be healed from what ails us.

TODAY'S RX

Stop, listen, and then act on the wise words of God.

Father, help me to obey your Word and implement your instructions in my life. I want to please you with all I do and say. I know that when I'm living in you, I'm living life to the full.

MOUNTAINTOP EXPERIENCE IN THE VALLEY

Send out your light and your truth; let them guide me. Let them lead me to your holy mountain, to the place where you live. There I will go to the altar of God, to God—the source of all my joy. I will praise you with my harp, O God, my God! Psalm 43:3-4

Nancy was a busy mother of four, and she seemed stuck in her hectic lifestyle.

"Every day, it's the same thing," she said. "I get up and rush to fix breakfast for my husband and kids. It's always a pain to get them out the door in the morning, and then I have to drop kids at three different schools and fight traffic to get them all there on time. About the time I drop the last one off, the baby starts to cry, and she cries the whole way home. Then *I* start to cry. What I need is a vacation!"

After Nancy and I talked, I realized that she wasn't depressed; she was just exhausted.

"I know you feel like you're in the valley right now, and you'd rather be on the mountaintop, but the valley is where things grow."

We discussed some things she could do, such as taking a nap in the afternoon while the baby slept, eating healthier, and taking a walk outdoors before the kids came home from school.

"I can do those things," Nancy agreed, "but I don't know if they'll help."

"When you take a few minutes to stop, reflect, and rest, it can change your perspective," I said, "even if your circumstances don't change. Taking a few minutes to look back at where you've been and refocus on where you want to go can give you a fresh vantage point on your life."

"You can't take a vacation right now, but you can get the same change in perspective if you will carve out some personal time from the crazy pace you're running."

Today's verse tells us that God's light and truth will guide us to the holy mountain where he lives. It's easy to think of that as a physical place, but the psalmist reminds us that the source isn't a place; it's a person. God is the source of all joy. And when we see him, we will want to praise him.

TODAY'S RX

Don't get stuck in a rut; make time to rest in God, the source of all joy.

Lord, help me to take the time to reflect on my healing process. Allow me to see where I've been and where I'm going. Remind me of your faithfulness throughout this journey.

JOB-RELATED BENEFITS OF TAKING CHRIST TO WORK

They began their circuit of the villages, preaching the Good News and healing the sick.
LUKE 9:6

When I moved to Cheatham County, I was the third doctor in the county. Though I knew that at least one of the other two doctors was a believer, I also knew that he believed it was best to separate his faith from his work. That made me the only openly Christian doctor practicing in that rural community.

For me, the decision to be both a Christian and a Christian doctor was an easy one. Though it seemed that some people were able to put their faith and their work into separate boxes, God had always jumbled my boxes together. There was no way I could function as a doctor without God's backing or leading.

So often in today's world, we live our Christian lives apart from everything else we do. We don't want to be perceived as ignorant and politically incorrect or narrow-minded. But in my experience, following Jesus is the most politically correct and open-minded thing we could ever do. Jesus taught us to love one another. And he taught us to win others to faith through our love for them and each other. My faith doesn't make me intolerant, it makes me more loving. I have never met a patient for whom I didn't wish the best, regardless of what his or her beliefs were.

As Christians, our position is one of serving and pointing the way to God. Just as the gospel and healing went hand in hand in today's verse—in fact, in the whole New Testament—I've learned they go hand in hand in my office too. Years of practicing medicine as an openly Christian doctor have given me the opportunity to share my faith in ways that encourage others who are experiencing the greatest hurts this broken world has to offer. I've received countless invitations to be with families and be a part of their conversations during their most trying hours. Being asked to pray with and for a patient in one of those situations is one of the greatest gifts of living an openly Christian lifestyle at work.

TODAY'S RX

Love others so much today that tomorrow they will invite you into their lives and share their hurts.

Father, help me to proclaim your name through all I do and say. May I point others to your love by serving them well and helping them through their hurts.

THE MIRACULOUS TURNAROUND

Through Christ you have come to trust in God. And you have placed your faith and hope in God because he raised Christ from the dead and gave him great glory. 1 Peter 1:21

"Ma'am, your son is very, very sick. Do you know what happened?"

"I don't know," Barb said through her tears. "He's been struggling to fit in at school this year. We just moved, hoping that would help. His old friends just hung out together and got high. I always told him that nothing good would come from that."

She started to cry harder.

"Colin came home last night from his AA meeting, and he seemed on top of the world. He played with his little sister, and we told him how proud we were of him. He was doing better and getting his life back on track. Around nine, he went upstairs to his room. I knew he was tired, and I didn't think anything about it until this morning when my husband tried to wake him up. Then he started CPR while I called 911 . . . is he going to be okay?"

"It's too early to tell," I said. "His oxygen saturation levels were dangerously low. We've got him intubated, and there's a machine helping him breathe, so right now his blood pressure and his pulse are good. We need to transfer him to downtown Nashville to the ICU—"

"I just want him to be okay," Barb sobbed as she watched the EMTs wheel Colin out to the ambulance.

"Could we stop right now and pray for your son and your family?" I asked.

Barb nodded.

After I prayed, asking God to surround and protect Colin, Barb and her husband left to follow the ambulance. But things didn't look good for Colin.

The next day, I dreaded getting the report from the ICU. But when the call came, the pulmonologist sounded giddy. "There was a miracle in bed 15!"

"Colin, the young man with the overdose?"

"Yes! He woke up this morning and smiled at me."

"What?"

"We took him off life support, and he's doing great. He should be out of the hospital and back home by the end of the week."

Without a doubt, I knew that Colin's life had been snatched out of the jaws of death and that God alone deserved the glory.

TODAY'S RX

God has the power, and the will, to snatch us from the very jaws of death.

God, you are mighty to save. Thank you for the miracles you perform. Even when I am disobedient, you show your grace and favor to me. I am forever grateful.

THE HANDS OF MY FATHER

Yet I still belong to you; you hold my right hand. PSALM 73:23

Growing up on the farm, I often went fishing with my dad. As a little boy, I held my father's hand as we crossed over Mulberry Creek to get to one of our favorite fishing holes. His grip gave me confidence that I was safe and cared for. But as I grew older, I no longer took his hand when he held it out. I thought it looked like a sign of weakness for a "big boy" to hold his father's hand.

"I can do it on my own," I said, and my father reluctantly pulled back.

After graduating from high school, I headed off to college. For the first time, I was on my own physically. But I felt alone spiritually. I had decided I didn't believe in God anymore after a family tragedy. During this time, I was unmoored. I was vulnerable to whatever way the wind tossed me. There was no anchor grounding me when storms blew through my life.

But a few years later I felt lost and no longer wanted to be on my own anymore. I once again raised my hands to God. He reached out with his mighty grip, grasped my weak and trembling hand, and held it firm and safe in his—just like my father had done when I was a small boy.

Like the Good Shepherd he is, over the years our Savior has used his hand to gently guide and nudge me to greener pastures. Looking back now, I can see that even when I was an atheist and I told God to let go because I didn't want to walk with him anymore, his grip on me never changed. Years of walking with our Lord has taught me that my heavenly Father will never let go of me.

TODAY'S RX

Jesus is waiting for you. Put your hand in his, and he will never let go.

Jesus, what a comfort it is to know that I am secure in you. You hold my life in your hands and keep me from faltering. Walk with me as I cross this bridge to healing.

NOT OUR WILL, BUT GOD'S

Dear friends, if we don't feel guilty, we can come to God with bold confidence. And we will receive from him whatever we ask because we obey him and do the things that please him. 1 JOHN 3:21-22

I examined Scott's CT scan results one more time before opening the exam room door. The report showed renal cell carcinoma—one of the most ominous and aggressive cancers known to man. The only hope for a cure was complete surgical removal of the kidney.

I broke the news to him as gently as I could, and then together we discussed the treatment plan. "Your right kidney needs to come out as soon as we can get your surgery scheduled. As long as it hasn't spread, I would expect you to live a long and full life with your remaining kidney." Scott took the news as bravely as any man could. Then he asked me to pray with him.

A few weeks later, Scott had the surgery. Afterward, the oncology urologist called me with the verdict. It was mixed news. The next day while on rounds, I stopped by Scott's room to deliver the report. "Great news," I said. "The surgeon didn't see any metastatic disease. However, he did see a cyst on the left kidney that warrants watching."

I watched as Scott slowly took in the news. If there was cancer on his left kidney, he would have to have it removed as well. He knew that he couldn't live without any kidneys, and the chances of getting a donor kidney weren't very good.

He slowly nodded his head and then looked at me and said, "Do you remember when we prayed before my surgery? What did you say at the end of your prayer?"

I remembered because it's something I say at the end of all my prayers: "Lord, not our will, but yours be done."

"Then we'll leave it to him," Scott said. I'll come in for my visits and get my tests done, but from now on it's in God's hands."

Scott found comfort and confidence in trusting God's will. As I write this, it has been six months, and the cyst has remained stable. Scott shows no signs of cancer, and he shows no signs of worry. He is leaving the end result to God.

TODAY'S RX

Are you worrying about something? Stop and tell God that you trust his will for you.

God, ease my mind of worry today, and let me find rest in you.
Your promises are what I cling to in times of confusion and
doubt. Help me to trust in your timing for my life.

PASTOR WILLY'S LAST BREATH

Christ has rescued us from the curse pronounced by the law. When he was hung on the cross, he took upon himself the curse for our wrongdoing. For it is written in the Scriptures, "Cursed is everyone who is hung on a tree." Through Christ Jesus, God has blessed the Gentiles with the same blessing he promised to Abraham, so that we who are believers might receive the promised Holy Spirit through faith. GALATIANS 3:13-14

When I admitted Pastor Willy into the hospital, I knew that when he left, it would be to the other side of the veil. After making my morning rounds, I stopped in to see him.

"Good morning, Pastor. Do you mind if I pull up a chair?"

"C'mon in, Doc," he said.

As always, Pastor Willy had stories to share. We discussed some of the things he'd witnessed in his life and the sermons he'd preached. He had started preaching when he was eighteen years old and just out of high school. And he hadn't stopped preaching until the previous Sunday, at the ripe age of one hundred.

As he reflected on his century of life and some of the highlights of his ministry, he said, "Dr. Anderson, I have seen a lot of amazing sights in my years. And man has done a lot to help this world. But I've also witnessed the curse we live under. I have suffered many a trial and tribulation, and this morning I am ready to go home. That's what Jesus promised. He promised to take me home."

I marveled at his faith. His life was an example of a race well run. "Pastor, though I don't think you have much more time left, I don't know when your last breath will be any more than I know when *my* last breath will be. But I do know that your last breath here will be your first in glory." I paused for a moment and then added, "I wish I could join you when you go. If you will save me a seat near the throne, I would greatly appreciate it."

Jesus promises redemption and relief from our suffering through our faith in his saving grace. Ask him to give you his peace until the moment you take your last breath—just as he did for Pastor Willy.

TODAY'S RX

Today, give thanks to God for every breath he has given you.

Lord, thank you for my breath. You've blessed me beyond words, and I'm grateful.

THE KIDNEY PAIN OF HUMILIATION

The Lord will deliver me from every evil attack and will bring me safely into his heavenly Kingdom. All glory to God forever and ever! Amen. 2 TIMOTHY 4:18

I had lost somewhere between twenty and twenty-five pounds, and I was in the best shape of my life—or so I thought.

Three months earlier, in an attempt to lose weight, I had researched the medical literature and found a high-protein diet that had been successful for many. As an experiment, I thought I would give it a try. I didn't always have time to eat healthy, and I thought perhaps the diet would help me lose unwanted pounds.

Karen, however, was completely against the idea.

"You're just being overly protective," I said.

"Let me remind you, I have a master's in clinical nutrition," she countered.

As part of the diet plan, I was supposed to drink large amounts of water. But because I was always on the go and didn't want to have to stop to go, I forgot about drinking the water.

I didn't realize until it was too late that water was a crucial part of the diet—to flush out excess protein and other poisons from my system. The day I first realized I had a problem was the day I had a sudden pain in my left flank. Then I noticed blood in my urine. I had a kidney stone!

Though it was a simple diagnosis, the pain was not easy to endure. Within an hour of arriving at work, I found myself in the ER receiving IV fluids and pain medication. Karen met me there, and she didn't have to say a word. I knew that "I told you so" look.

When the second stone came, I was home alone, and the pain almost did me in. It was so intense that I cried out to God, "Take away the pain, Lord, or take me with you!"

Suddenly, the pain resolved, and I was able to drive myself to the ER. A seven-millimeter stone was passed with lithotripsy later that week, and I quickly recovered.

God did not take me with him that day, but he did take away my pain. And I learned to listen to my wife when it comes to matters of nutrition.

TODAY'S RX

Men, listen to your wives. There's a reason God created them to help us!

Thank you for the people you've put in my life, Lord, who've helped me in many ways. I wouldn't be where I am today without them, and I praise you for designing those friendships.

REST IN THE LORD

Praise the LORD who has given rest to his people Israel, just as he promised. Not one word has failed of all the wonderful promises he gave through his servant Moses.
1 Kings 8:56

Our world is becoming more complicated and stressful. I often tell my patients that humans weren't created for a rat race. We need more rest. What if we went to sleep when the sun set and woke up when the sun rose? That's more rest than we typically allow ourselves to enjoy.

My day begins at five o'clock each morning. The great thing about waking up that early is that I get to enjoy a twenty-minute hot shower and then a twenty-minute commute to work. I drive east, watching the sun rise as I travel. My mornings start with a sense of calm and awe for the Creator and the plans he has for my life that day.

I once heard a preacher say that God rested on the last day—after his work—but our week begins with a day of rest. In fact, the first day that Adam and Eve knew was a day of rest. That wasn't by accident. God created us to begin our days rested and refreshed.

God also wants us to rest in him and his words. Take time before you start your day and your week to be still in God's presence. Rest in his promises, even if it means going to bed a little earlier so you can get up a little earlier. This simple discipline will pay off with many returns throughout your day.

TODAY'S RX

Tonight, go to bed a little earlier so tomorrow you will be rested and can spend more time showering in God's promises. Repeat daily.

Jesus, you say in Matthew 11:28, "Come to me, all of you who are weary and carry heavy burdens, and I will give you rest." Thank you for that promise. I choose to rest in you today.

BREATHING EAGLE AIR

You know how I carried you on eagles' wings and brought you to myself. Exodus 19:4

Gene didn't seem to have much left physically or emotionally. He had end-stage chronic obstructive pulmonary disease, with less than 20 percent lung capacity, and he was limping through the last leg of his race here on earth. It was hard for him to breathe, and his quality of life was greatly impaired.

When I saw him, he was straggling down the hall to the exam room, dragging his oxygen tank. From the way his body slumped, he looked downtrodden and depressed. He also looked more tired than usual.

"Everything okay, Gene? You look tired."

"Yeah, I'm exhausted."

"Well, I looked at your numbers. Your oxygen saturation is 93 percent when you're on it. That's better than it was the last time we checked."

"I know." He paused for a moment, then said, "You know, my wife died last year. And all my kids have moved away. The only pleasure I had left was smoking, and then you told me to quit. I just don't know what to do anymore. I don't feel like going on; all the joy has left my life. Have you ever felt that way?"

I put my hand on his shoulder, "Look, Gene, I know this next question isn't directly related to your checkup, but have you tried praying lately?"

"No, not really."

"Do you have a relationship with God?"

"It's been a long time since I went to church. But maybe I could go this weekend."

We talked a little more, and I encouraged him to give it a try.

At his next appointment, two months later, Gene entered the exam room with his head up. He was still very ill, but he had a bit of a pep in his step.

"How are you doing?' I asked.

"The pastor at my church told me that Jesus would lift me up on eagles' wings if I would let him. So I did."

"That's great!" I said.

What Gene said next made me smile and remember today's verse. "You know, Doc, when you're flying with eagles; it's a lot easier to breathe!"

TODAY'S RX

When you cannot take another step, allow Jesus to carry you on eagles' wings. He will renew your life and give you air to breathe.

Father, refresh my spirit today, and give me a renewed sense of vigor.
I desire to hold my head up high and enjoy this life you've given me.

LISTEN, TRUST, AND OBEY

Lord, your discipline is good, for it leads to life and health. You restore my health and allow me to live! Isaiah 38:16

I'm sure my patients think I sound like a broken record! I'm always telling them what they should eat and drink (or what they shouldn't eat and drink). Patients who listen show signs of improved health. Those who don't? Well, often they don't fare as well.

Your doctor's job is to listen to you and your needs. Then he or she should help you map out a strategy for good health. Your job is to listen to what the doctor says, provide input into the strategy, and then follow the plan as best you can.

Today's verse shows that the Lord's discipline is good and leads to good outcomes. Of course! That's a strategy crafted by the Great Physician himself. He cares about every aspect of our lives and health.

In the desert, God not only directed the Israelites' path, but he also directed them to healthy food and drink. When they didn't have food, he sent manna. When the water was unfit to drink, he purified it. But to benefit from his advice, the people had to listen and obey.

I have patients who claim to hear what I say, but they don't always do what I tell them. I keep repeating the same things to them, however, because I desire to see them healthy.

TODAY'S RX

Listen to your doctor and do your best to do what he or she says. When the Israelites listened and obeyed, great things happened. The same will be true for your health.

Lord, help me to trust you throughout my healing process and listen to my doctors' advice. Thank you for putting well-trained physicians in my life and for providing for me along the way.

UNEXPECTED ANSWERS

We are confident that he hears us whenever we ask for anything that pleases him. And since we know he hears us when we make our requests, we also know that he will give us what we ask for. 1 JOHN 5:14-15

What happens when things don't go your way? Maybe you've asked God for something, and all you've heard is silence? Or, perhaps God answered your prayer but not the way you thought he would. What do you do then? Do you lose faith? Do you begin to doubt God?

Clancy came to see me because of a small ulcer on his tongue that wouldn't heal. It had been annoying him for more than two months. While in my office, he also asked me to feel a nodule on the back of his neck.

"I think we're going to need to send you to the head and neck surgeon for a biopsy," I said. For years, I had been trying to talk him out of chewing tobacco. I was afraid that his symptoms were a sign that the tobacco had finally caught up with him.

I made a referral and set up an appointment, and I could tell that Clancy was worried. Before he left he said, "Dr. Anderson, will you pray with me that this isn't cancer?"

Unfortunately, my suspicions were right. The next time I saw Clancy, he had a tracheotomy and most of the right side of his neck had been removed in a radical neck dissection. This wasn't the answer we'd prayed for; but it had saved his life. Though he had cancer and a pretty nasty surgery, Clancy said that he felt God's presence throughout his journey. God had saved his life and comforted him when he needed it most.

It would be easy to say that God didn't answer Clancy's prayer. But what if God had a higher purpose for Clancy's life?

Five years after his surgery, Clancy was not only alive and thriving, he was also a crusader, teaching young people about the dangers of tobacco. He had the real-life scars to illustrate the pain and suffering that can occur when you use chewing tobacco.

In God's infinite wisdom, he was able to take Clancy's past and turn it into a lifesaving ministry to those who would learn from his mistakes.

TODAY'S RX

When we pray, the road to God's answer might be rocky, but the destination is worth it.

God, you have always been faithful to intervene at just the right moment, removing me from harm and showing me the path to take. Thank you for helping me through many trials and showing me your ever-deepening love.

SEEK GOD, NOT YOUR EXPECTATIONS

But Naaman became angry and stalked away. "I thought he would certainly come out to meet me!" he said. "I expected him to wave his hand over the leprosy and call on the name of the LORD his God and heal me!" 2 Kings 5:11

So often when we seek healing we think we have all the answers as to where we should look. I have patients who consult with specialists, some at internationally recognized medical centers that specialize in their particular condition. Some comb the Internet in search of an unknown cure. Others have sought help from vitamins, cleanses, or a faith healer.

Despite trying everything, their condition continues to worsen. They're not seeing the healing they envisioned. After consulting with specialists, they return to me with the news that nothing can be done. I know how discouraging this is.

Naaman was so discouraged that he was angry about his situation. He expected a miraculous healing, but because his pride got in the way, he hadn't listened to the simple instructions he'd been given!

If you or someone you love seems to be in a no-win health situation, pray about whether or not the healing you're seeking is what God wants you to seek. It may be that in that moment, he has something more important for you than physical healing.

TODAY'S RX

Seek Jesus as Lord, trusting him to heal what most needs healing.

Jesus, you heal more than just physical ailments; you heal the heart. Thank you for showing me your grace as you've walked beside me through this season.

CARRIED BY THE SPIRIT

Don't you realize that I could ask my Father for thousands of angels to protect us, and he would send them instantly? MATTHEW 26:53

"Hello, June. I'm Dr. Reggie."

In the rehabilitation unit that I oversee, patients tell us their stories, and we often get to share in their experiences of God. That was my privilege the day I stopped to talk to June, a new patient to our unit, who had come in the previous day with a hip fracture.

"I heard you had a little fall. Can you tell me what happened?"

"My husband died a number of years ago, and I've lived alone ever since. I've gotten out of bed thousands of times in the middle of the night to go to the bathroom or get a drink of water. The other night, I remember getting up around 1:30, but I'm not sure what happened. When I woke up again, I was lying on the floor, and my clock read 3:36. I tried to stand, but the pain in my right leg was too much. I was so frightened that I just remained on the cold floor and prayed and prayed until I saw the first rays of the sun through my window. The next thing I knew, it was daylight and my son Mike was knocking on my door."

"So, he's the one who found you on the floor?"

"No, he found me in bed. That's the strange thing—for some unexplained reason, when Mike knocked on the door, I woke up, and I was in my bed! I'm sure the Lord sent an angel to pick me up off the floor. How else could I have gotten there?"

"Yes, June, God does send his angels to keep watch over us," I reassured her. "And now that you're here, he's sent these nice young ladies and strong men to help you recover. When it's time for you to walk, they will be with you step-by-step."

"Doctor, I really appreciate all of your help and the help of all these nice people, but I know who really saved me that night—it was my Lord. And he continues to hold my hand every day."

TODAY'S RX

You are never truly alone. But if you or someone you know lives alone, consider a medical alert system.

God, please be with the elderly today, watching over them and protecting them from falls and injuries. Comfort them when they are lonely, and reassure them of your presence.

DIRECTIONS FOR LIFE

If you refuse to serve the LORD, *then choose today whom you will serve. Would you prefer the gods your ancestors served beyond the Euphrates? Or will it be the gods of the Amorites in whose land you now live? But as for me and my family, we will serve the Lord.* JOSHUA 24:15

Ever since Karen and I got married, the last sentence of today's verse has been framed and prominently displayed on the wall of our home. We felt it was important to have this declaration and promise as the foundation for our life together, for our family, and for all those who enter our home.

When we start any journey, we need to know where we are going. If we take a step without having a destination, or at least a road map, there's a good chance we will end up lost and adrift. This is also true with our health. If we don't know where we're headed, we could end up stumbling through life, eating what we want, rarely exercising, and picking up other unhealthy habits.

To be healthy, you must have an intentional plan for your life. If you want to change something about your health, you need direction. Do you want to lose weight? Do you want to be able to climb stairs without getting winded or run a 10K? Do you want to get rid of the pain in your knees or get rid of a sinus infection?

It's only by knowing where you're going and what the outcome or destination will be that you can make progress toward your goal. That's why the first thing I do with my patients is take their medical history and discuss their symptoms. The history of where they've been helps me know where they are going.

After I make a diagnosis, the most important part of the visit occurs. Does the patient want to get better? If so, we put together a treatment plan—a direction for the patient to follow. We also know the desired destination or outcome before we even start. We may want to lower blood sugar levels or blood pressure numbers. We may want a cough to subside or a headache to go away so the patient can sleep.

If you choose to follow the Lord, you need to know where you're headed. We know that eternal life will be the final outcome.

TODAY'S RX

Few choices have a known and perfect outcome. But following Jesus is one.

Lord, I declare for myself and my family that we will serve you. Help us to faithfully follow after you in this journey of healing and beyond. May we always stand on Christ, the solid Rock.

HEALING PARTY

Jesus returned to the Sea of Galilee and climbed a hill and sat down. A vast crowd brought to him people who were lame, blind, crippled, those who couldn't speak, and many others. They laid them before Jesus, and he healed them all. The crowd was amazed! Those who hadn't been able to speak were talking, the crippled were made well, the lame were walking, and the blind could see again! And they praised the God of Israel. MATTHEW 15:29-31

On one of my trips to Ecuador, we converted the town hall, which was actually a mud hut, into a clinic for the week. My exam room was a small corner of the hut where patients came to see the American doctor.

In broken Spanish, I asked them what they needed. All day long, as soon as I finished with one patient, another showed up. Some conditions were easily treated, but unfortunately, many were not. As a doctor, I've never felt so inadequate and ill-prepared. Crowds of people, all with pressing needs, surrounded us, but because we lacked the necessary resources, we couldn't cure them. Often those we could help received only temporary relief from their suffering. It was frustrating and overwhelming to see so many in need and realize I could do so little for them.

Perhaps that's why I was so thankful that we could pray with them. Despite our lack of resources, we knew that God doesn't lack for anything. We could trust in him to heal those we couldn't. And we saw some miraculous and inexplicable cures.

When I read today's verses, I think about those frustrating moments in Ecuador when I wanted to do so much more than I could. The verse reminds me that Jesus not only cured diseases, but he also healed every part of the person—mind, body, and soul. No wonder the crowd was amazed!

When I think of the sick Ecuadorians we were unable to help, I take comfort in knowing that one day they will be fully healed and filled with joy, not because of anything we did, but because of everything Jesus did.

TODAY'S RX

Picture yourself dancing and singing praises on the day you are finally and completely healed!

Jesus, your power has no limits. You brought healing to the masses by simply speaking a word. I realize that what I lack, you fulfill, and I praise you for that. I wait with anticipation for the day when I'm fully healed by you.

MIDNIGHT IN THE ER

Weeping may last through the night, but joy comes with the morning . . . You have turned my mourning into joyful dancing. You have taken away my clothes of mourning and clothed me with joy, that I might sing praises to you and not be silent. O LORD my God, I will give you thanks forever! PSALM 30:5, 11-12

Graveyard shifts in the emergency room can bring out the worst cases. It seems that patients with strokes and heart attacks arrive at the same time as victims of horrific car accidents. Crying babies can be heard above all the usual noises, and the line for X-rays can get lengthy with all the broken bones. During the overnight shift, weariness sets in for both the sick and those who treat them.

"Will this pain ever end?"

"Will this night ever be over?"

"How long will our weeping last?"

Waiting for answers while the night grows longer can cause both patients and providers to lose patience. But as a doctor, I know that when dawn bursts over the eastern sky, our cortisol levels start to rise as well. We experience a kind of rush of adrenaline. With this boost of God-given energy from the body, we can often experience a lift in our moods. We begin the new day with hope.

During those rosy-pink hours of early daylight, doctors often find that they are able to wean patients off of artificial systems and oxygen tubes that have kept them alive. They have made it through their dark night, and during the first hours of light, they begin their journey back to independence.

TODAY'S RX

No matter how dark the night or how loud the cries, morning releases mourning and restores the soul to new life.

God, thank you for piercing the darkness with your light. You reenergize me daily with your hope. This world does its best to cloud my vision, but you lift the fog and show me your great love.

NOVEMBER CHECKUP

By November 1, most stores will already have Christmas decorations hung and holiday merchandise on sale. During the next few weeks, it will be tempting to focus on what needs to be purchased rather than on the bounty we already have. To combat the pull of materialism this month, start a blessings journal. Each day, write down five things you're thankful for—things that God has given you that make your life better. Ask your family and close friends to do the same. Maybe it's a relationship, something you already own, or a favorable test result. It could be as simple as appreciating that you still have all your teeth each time you brush, or as big as being thankful that you and your family are together for one more holiday season. On Thanksgiving, share with everyone a few things you're thankful for. Nothing can enhance your mood quite as quickly or as well as being thankful.

Our forefathers took time during this month to sit with friends and neighbors to enjoy the bounty of the autumnal harvest for which they were thankful. The table would have been stocked with fresh fruits and vegetables that they had grown over the summer. With the winter rapidly approaching, it was probably the last chance they had to eat fresh food.

Consider how different that display is from the food we will prepare this month. Our potatoes and squash will be covered with butter and cheese. Pumpkin and sweet potatoes won't be eaten as raw vegetables; they will be mixed with sugar and baked into a pie. The early settlers used salt and vinegar to preserve the bountiful harvest so it could be eaten throughout the long winter. Now, many of our food sources are processed and preserved with chemicals that remove many of the vitamins and minerals that made the food healthy. In addition, we often replace natural ingredients with artificial ingredients or additional fats, sugars, and salt.

This time of year, it is very common to diagnose gallbladder disease. The high-caloric Thanksgiving meal tends to exacerbate gallbladder attacks. To keep everyone healthy, substitute fresh or frozen fruits and vegetables for your processed or prepared menu items throughout the month. And remember, you don't have to fill your plate or clean it. The only thing stuffed at Thanksgiving should be the turkey!

At halftime during the football games, take a short walk outside or play a game of touch football. To get the most enjoyment out of the holidays, do all things in moderation—except for gratitude, which should be done in abundance.

November Booster Shot: Take a moment this month to thank God and your family and friends for the many blessings they have bestowed upon you. As we thank God for our physical food at the table, we should also thank him for the spiritual nourishment he has given us throughout the year.

SEEK WISE COUNSEL

Come and listen to my counsel. I'll share my heart with you and make you wise.
Proverbs 1:23

I could see that Lisa Anne was doing her best to console her crying newborn baby, but she wasn't having much success.

"I'm a single mom and pretty much all alone except for my baby. Can you help me?" she asked, handing me the crying bundle. "I'm not sure I'm doing it right. I'm not even sure I know how to be a mother!"

I'm always honored when I'm invited to be a caregiver, especially in situations like this. It was obvious that Lisa Anne was intimidated by caring for her new baby.

"Tell me your concerns," I said. "I'll do whatever I can to help you."

She began to pour out all her questions and concerns, beginning with when she left the hospital with her baby. It was easy to see that her fear of the future had a choke hold on her heart. She wanted to be the best mom she could be, but with a lack of good parenting role models in her life, she didn't know how.

I listened intently and wrote down every question she asked—recording notes for her to take with her, containing detailed instructions on everything from feeding schedules to immunizations. Then I examined her bundle of joy—a healthy, squirming baby boy.

Over the next few years, Lisa Anne regularly brought her son in for well-baby checkups. She made sure he got his shots and made sure I answered all her questions. I tried not to overwhelm her with too much information as I guided her through each stage of her baby's growth.

As quickly as her son grew in size, Lisa Anne grew in confidence as a mother. She continued to seek out wise counsel both for herself and for her baby until she was so confident in her skills as a mother that she was advising other young moms on the things she'd learned.

TODAY'S RX

Be willing to share your fears with a trusted friend, professional, or family member. They will learn what is important to you, and their advice will help you become wise.

Father, you are the Wonderful Counselor. You see me when I am overwhelmed, listen to my needs, and calm my fears. Thank you for putting trusted people in my life who care about me and help me in times of need.

CHASING AWAY THE DARKNESS

The creation looks forward to the day when it will join God's children in glorious freedom from death and decay. ROMANS 8:21

Driving to work in the morning, I look toward the eastern sky. As the sun stretches and yawns, it chases darkness into the shadows. The sky's canvas in front of me is constantly moving and changing as the first pink and golden tendrils of day light up the horizon.

The colors never rest. Like a mood lamp slowly changing colors, the sunrise moves through cranberry, pinks, and golden brushes before choosing the brilliant yellow that will hang throughout the day.

I marvel at how it looks new minute by minute and day by day. No artist or digital camera could replicate the masterpiece that lives and breathes each morning before my eyes.

Some say that creation speaks God's glory. I believe it shouts. But too often we're blind and deaf. We focus not on the burgeoning life before us, but on our weakness and inevitable decay. Though we are citizens of a dark, broken world, the beauty of creation reminds us that it won't be that way for long.

As each new day shines the light of heaven into the dark shadowy crevices of this world, the sunrise reminds us that the powers of darkness cannot survive in the heat and brilliant light of day.

As God's children, we were made for the light, not the darkness. That's why we respond with joy to the sunrise. It is but a glimpse of what we will experience when all darkness is defeated. The sunrise is merely a reminder that one day soon we will see another Son rise. And that Son will never set.

Take courage; it won't be long. The glorious return that the morning sky foretells is imminent.

TODAY'S RX

Turn your eyes toward the risen Son, who will chase away all darkness, disease, and decay.

Jesus, I never have to worry about losing sight of you; you are everywhere—in the beauty of a sunrise, in the calling of the birds, in the dew on the grass. Fill me with your light today so that my heart may be full and I can sing your praises. Thank you for my many blessings.

REGARDLESS OF THE THREAT, GOD CAN OVERCOME

At that time some Pharisees said to him, "Get away from here if you want to live! Herod Antipas wants to kill you!" Jesus replied, "Go tell that fox that I will keep on casting out demons and healing people today and tomorrow; and the third day I will accomplish my purpose." LUKE 13:31-32

When the Pharisees threatened to kill Jesus if he wouldn't stop healing the sick and demon possessed, Jesus didn't stop. He had come to do his Father's work, and nothing would deter him. In my medical practice, I've never been threatened by religious leaders, but at times I have been threatened by a patient.

At our local jail, when an inmate is sick or injured, a jailer will accompany the prisoner to the emergency room for treatment.

During my first year of practice, a man who was jailed for domestic abuse became ill with severe nausea, vomiting, and dehydration. Preliminary testing confirmed my hunch that he was suffering withdrawal from an abused substance—in this case PCP, which was one of the most dangerous illegal drugs at the time.

We decided to keep him overnight, so the jailer spent the night with him in the hospital room, and a second guard would relieve him at the next shift change.

When the patient was so sick that he slept most of the night, the first guard decided to leave before the second jailer had arrived. The patient was still asleep when he left.

Minutes later, a nurse on a routine check found the inmate standing on the windowsill pounding on the locked window. He was wide-eyed and shouting profanities. I saw the nurse backing out of the room and went to see what I could do.

PCP can sometimes linger and cause wild behavior and hallucinations. As I slowly entered the room and sat down, the man remained on the ledge, spewing vulgarities at me.

"Can you get down, please?" I said. "There's really no place for you to go."

"If you make me get down, I'll cut you," he said.

Not wanting to agitate him further, I sat and quietly prayed. It seemed to work. The longer I sat praying under my breath and refusing to leave, the calmer the inmate became.

Eventually, the new jailer arrived, and a nurse was able to administer a sedative.

TODAY'S RX

When chaos reigns around you, remain still and know that God will calm the storm.

Lord, be with me in fearful moments. Permeate the air with your peace and cast out all evil. I know you can overcome whatever threatens me, and I thank you for watching over me.

THE BLESSINGS OF KNOWING YOUR KINFOLK

Now that you belong to Christ, you are the true children of Abraham. You are his heirs, and God's promise to Abraham belongs to you. GALATIANS 3:29

"Marry out of state," Grandma Anderson used to tell her kids and grandkids. She was a farmer's wife, not a geneticist, but she knew that growing up in the South we had to be careful to trace our lineage so we didn't end up marrying our cousins. "Marry out of state," was her way of telling us to broaden the gene pool.

Being kinfolk helped bind our large Southern family together. Even if we didn't see our relatives often, we were still close. We watched out for each other. Though generations of my family were spread across two states, we regularly got together for holidays. In the summer, I worked on my grandfather's farm alongside relatives, though I wasn't always sure of their relation. I just knew we were family.

Knowing your kin is not only helpful for feeling connected, but it can also be helpful to your doctor. Some diseases, such as diabetes, hypertension, heart disease, strokes, and cancer, run in families. Knowing the diseases that are a part of your family history can help a doctor to look for and more quickly recognize diseases in you. Often, the earlier a disease is diagnosed, the more options there are for treatment.

The same is true of your spiritual lineage. As Christ followers, we are heirs to the promises that God gives us in his Word. And as brothers and sisters in Christ, we have bonds of faith.

As today's verse acknowledges, knowing where you're from can tell you a lot about the direction you're heading.

TODAY'S RX

Create a diary of your family's health history. It can help your doctor to make an early diagnosis. Create a list of spiritual kin, as well. Brothers and sisters in Christ can give early warnings about sin or support you in prayer.

God, help me to take my physical and spiritual health seriously. Give me the wisdom I need to eat well, exercise, and take preventative measures against what may lie ahead. Help me, too, to be prayerful and in fellowship with my brothers and sisters in Christ.

A CRITICAL SABBATH HEALING

One Sabbath day Jesus went to eat dinner in the home of a leader of the Pharisees, and the people were watching him closely. There was a man there whose arms and legs were swollen. Jesus asked the Pharisees and experts in religious law, "Is it permitted in the law to heal people on the Sabbath day, or not?" When they refused to answer, Jesus touched the sick man and healed him and sent him away LUKE 14:1-4

From Luke's description of the man with swollen limbs, it's likely he had edema (sometimes called dropsy), which happens when fluid builds up, especially in the legs and feet.

Though edema can be a side effect of some modern medications, at the time of Jesus it was likely caused by either congestive heart failure, kidney failure, or an even more serious condition. In a modern setting, a patient with these symptoms would be admitted to the hospital immediately, possibly even to the ICU, for proper diagnosis and treatment. Treatment would include bed rest, salt restriction, and diuresis to remove the stress of the extra fluid on the heart and lungs.

In today's verse, Luke notes that it was the Sabbath. Breaking the Sabbath—even to heal someone—while in the home of a leader of the Pharisees would go against prevailing Jewish beliefs. But Jesus didn't worry about cultural norms and man-made rules. When he asked whether it was okay to heal on the Sabbath, he wasn't asking for permission; he was asking the Pharisees what they believed.

When the Pharisees didn't answer his question, Jesus didn't hesitate to act. He knew that without help, the man could die at any moment. So Jesus intervened, even if it meant breaking the Pharisees' rules. He knew that his Father's will superseded anything that man could contrive.

God loved this man enough that Jesus healed him, even on the Sabbath. He loves you just as much and can heal you just as quickly, regardless of any man-made obstacles that are put in the way.

TODAY'S RX

Have faith that Jesus sees your needs. If God so chooses, no man-made obstacle will stand in the way of your healing.

Jesus, thank you for acting out of love rather than following a set of rules. Help me to have that same compassion for the people you put in my life. I desire to see them through your eyes.

COME DIRTY AND GET CLEAN

I will save them from their sinful apostasy. I will cleanse them. Then they will truly be my people, and I will be their God. EZEKIEL 37:23

Nick had once owned his own business and had been a well-respected member of the community. But as I watched the prison guard escort him down the hall, what defined his life now was an orange jumpsuit. Once Nick was settled in the exam room, the guard walked out and closed the door.

"I can't take it!" Nick said. This is my third DUI, and they sentenced me to eleven months and twenty-nine days. That's a year in jail, and it will ruin me! What am I going to do? I've already lost my business, and now my wife is leaving with the kids."

"I can help you medically, Nick, but only God can restore what's broken in you. I know he can restore your health and life while you're in jail. If you let him, he can work a miracle."

Nick settled back in his chair and seemed to think about what I had said.

"St. Paul spent time in prison," I said. "In fact, God spoke to him there many, many times. I'm going to pray that God speaks to you, as well."

What in your life is keeping you in prison? What idols distract you from the love of God? Whether it's a relationship, an illness, an addiction, or a preoccupation with the wrong things, God wants to cleanse your lost and broken soul and restore you to wholeness.

A year later, Nick came to see me in my office—not as a new patient, but as a new man. He had a spring in his step and a lift in his voice as he told me how God had not only forgiven him, but had also restored him to his family.

"I began reading the Bible again," he said. "And you were right. That jail time saved my life."

I asked Nick about his plans for the future.

"I'm already working," he said with a grin. "I'm a drug and alcohol counselor at a rehab facility. I get paid to bring the hope of new life through Jesus Christ to those who need a fresh start."

TODAY'S RX

It's easy to become a prisoner to the idols in our lives. Ask God to cleanse you and restore your love for him.

God, I pray that you would remove any unhealthy habits that have become a stronghold on my life. Take away the distractions and idols that keep me from finding my identity in you. I desire to start fresh and be made whole.

CRYING OUT

I cried out to the LORD in my great trouble, and he answered me. I called to you from the land of the dead, and LORD, you heard me! JONAH 2:2

"I lost both my parents this year!" Faye said, tears gathering at the corners of her eyes. "I don't have anyone left."

I had known Faye's parents well. They had been faithful followers of Jesus and had left a rich legacy in the community.

"Tell me why you're feeling this way," I said.

"Well, I'm the oldest, so I have to take care of everything. First, I had to settle Dad's estate, and now I'm in the middle of doing my mom's. I was the one who had to pay for both funerals, and since I'm the only one of my siblings who lives in town, I'm the one who goes to the cemetery to put flowers out."

"Does that help you feel better?"

"No, I just sit there and cry. Sometimes I stay there for hours. I miss them so much. I know my kids need me here, but I have nothing left to give anyone. I can barely get out of bed and get dressed, much less worry about getting the kids ready. I don't know what to do. I can't keep living like this." She buried her face in her hands and began to sob.

Like many who have suffered a major loss, Faye was clinically depressed. "Let's start with some medications to improve your sleep and increase your serotonin levels. Then I'm going to make an appointment for you to see a friend of mine who can help you organize your thoughts." I hoped that a Christian counselor would be someone to whom she could talk.

A few months later, Faye came in to see me.

"I don't go to the cemetery as often as I used to. Now when I go, my husband comes with me. He reminds me of what great parents and Christians they were, and that makes it easier. I don't know where I'd be if you hadn't sent me to counseling."

We should always cry out to Jesus, but there are days when we need to cry with other people.

TODAY'S RX

If you are mourning a loss, find a good Christian counselor or a pastor who can help you.

Father, I know you give and take away. Help me to celebrate the gift when given and mourn the loss when taken away. May I share my joys and sorrows with others so I may not lose sight of your purpose in my life.

GOD COMMANDS REST

They must realize that the Sabbath is the LORD's gift to you. That is why he gives you a two-day supply on the sixth day, so there will be enough for two days. On the Sabbath day you must each stay in your place. Do not go out to pick up food on the seventh day. EXODUS 16:29

Karen and I often visited my parents when they lived in Alabama. Dad occasionally wanted my help with a small project or two, but most of our visits were spent sitting, talking, and eating. Our favorite afternoon activity—napping—usually followed a big Southern meal.

One steamy Sunday, we were relaxing in the front room, and the TV was on. I don't remember the show, but it might have been Mutual of Omaha's *Wild Kingdom*.

The screen filled with lions roaming the hot plains of Africa. While the narrator described the pride and how they lived in the stifling heat, we were enjoying the modern convenience of air conditioning. Dad seemed to be enjoying it the most, occasionally snoring to let us know he was still breathing.

As the program continued, the narrator explained that one way the lions dealt with the heat was by sleeping twenty hours a day. Just then, my father, the king of our pride, roused just enough to mumble, "Well, I must be related to the lions." Then, just as quickly, he slipped back into slumberland.

Every good thing comes from God—even naps. If our Lord, the lion of the tribe of Judah, commands us to rest, I believe, for our good health, we should.

TODAY'S RX

Don't feel guilty when you need sleep. God commands us to rest. You don't have to belong to a pride to be proud of taking a nap.

Father, help me to lay down the demands of the day and seek proper rest. I realize I cannot do the work you call me to when weariness fogs my vision. Thank you for giving me the gift of sleep.

LETTING GO AND LETTING GOD

Do not judge others, and you will not be judged. Do not condemn others, or it will all come back against you. Forgive others, and you will be forgiven. Give, and you will receive. Your gift will return to you in full—pressed down, shaken together to make room for more, running over, and poured into your lap. The amount you give will determine the amount you get back. LUKE 6:37-38

"After that kid got my daughter pregnant, he ran off with another woman. He left Maria with no child support. I just want to wring his neck. Or worse!"

Ralph was understandably upset, and I knew the family was facing a lot of pressure because of the recent circumstances.

"Where's Maria now?"

"She and the baby moved in with us. We were looking forward to retirement, and now we're raising our granddaughter. The baby is up all night crying, so Maria's up all night crying. Then my wife gets up to help, and she's crying too. That's why I'd like to make that boy cry! I need you to give me something to help me sleep."

"Look, Ralph, I know how you feel. But the best way to move forward is not to be so preoccupied with this boy. You need to forgive him—even if you don't feel like it. Otherwise, the hatred you feel will keep smoldering in your heart and will flare up when you least expect it. That's not healthy. So, I have a prescription for you, but it's not what you think. Your prescription is to pray that God will help you forgive this young man who hurt your daughter."

Ralph didn't like what I had to say, but he agreed that my advice was better medicine than a sleeping pill.

When Ralph brought Maria and the baby in for a newborn checkup, I watched as he oohed and aahed over his granddaughter. When Maria stepped out for a moment, Ralph said, "I started out hating that boy, and I still don't like what he did. But I told him I forgave him, and he started to cry. Now at least I can talk to him and give him room to grow."

"Good for you, Ralph!" I said.

"Nope, good for God. He's the one working on me. And now the boy is trying to reconcile with Maria."

TODAY'S RX

Forgive your grudges, and allow the love of God to fill the void.

Jesus, thank you for modeling forgiveness for me. You bore no grudges when you were nailed to the cross, but gladly carried my sin so that my life could be restored. Help me to remember that always and to be quick to forgive.

A SECOND CHANCE FOR MARTY

When people do not accept divine guidance, they run wild. But whoever obeys the law is joyful. PROVERBS 29:18

Marty was a shadow of his old self. His weight loss over just the past few months was dramatic and ominous. But he seemed to have no idea how serious his situation was.

"I know you keep telling me to quit smoking," he said, "but I'm just not ready to clean up my act and fly straight. I've been smoking since I was fourteen, and it's the only thing I enjoy doing."

"Marty, this is serious. You need to get a chest X-ray."

He looked at me, surprised. "What for?"

A few days later, he was back in my office for the bad news. The chest X-ray confirmed my suspicion. He had a 3 x 3 cm tumor on the lower lobe of his right lung.

"Do you think it's cancer?" Marty asked. He was much more solemn than he'd been earlier in the week.

"I'm afraid it has the appearance of cancer, but we won't know for sure until we do a biopsy."

When the biopsy revealed adenocarcinoma of the lung, we scheduled Marty for surgery.

I saw him before he went under, and he stopped me and said, "Doc, will you pray for me? I've never been one to follow God's direction in my life, but I want to change that now." We prayed together, and Marty said he was ready for whatever happened.

The results we received the next day were encouraging. The skillful surgeon had been able to remove the tumor, and by all indications, Marty was completely healed. I shared the good news with him, and we rejoiced together.

Six months later, Marty was back in my office, and I asked him the same question I always asked him: "How much do you smoke, Marty?"

This time his answer was very different from before. "Because of the grace God showed me, I have changed a lot of my ways. I cleaned up my act, and I'm doing my best to fly straight." He looked at me and smiled. "After forty years, I have quit smoking. God gave me a second chance at life, and I figured I would honor him by trying to take care of the body he has healed."

TODAY'S RX

It's never too late to start on the right path.

Lord, thank you for showing me your mercy. You forget my sins and right my path, bringing me joy.

THE REBUKE OF LIFE

"I brought [my son] to your disciples, but they couldn't heal him." Jesus said, "You faithless and corrupt people! How long must I be with you? How long must I put up with you? Bring the boy here to me." MATTHEW 17:16-17

Obviously, God wanted this young boy to be healed because Jesus healed him. But that wasn't the original plan. The disciples were supposed to be part of the healing process. But as the father of the boy said, the disciples couldn't do it.

When Jesus heard the news, he rebuked the disciples for not having enough faith to heal the boy. Perhaps this was the lesson they needed to learn because in other parts of the New Testament we see that the disciples went on to heal many people.

As a resident in training, I received a similar rebuke from my instructor. A patient had come into our clinic with what seemed like a summer cold. He was coughing and producing white, foamy sputum. I didn't see any signs of an infection, so I assumed it was a cold.

Because it was my first week in the clinic, I was asked to present my patient's case to the attending physician. I told him about my exam and my conclusion. The attending physician asked a few probing questions, such as, Can he walk up a flight of steps? Does it get worse when he lies flat? What do his neck veins look like? Does he have a heart murmur?

As I answered those questions and more, I suddenly had a sick feeling in my stomach. I realized that the patient had more than a summer cold. He was in heart failure! And I had missed it!

To this day, I remember my attending physician's rebuke. As a result, from that day forward, I've always considered the most life-threatening conditions before concluding it might be something less serious. It was a good lesson, and it was done in such a way that I never forgot it.

My guess is that the disciples remembered their rebuke from Jesus long after he was gone. He taught them that faith was a critical part of healing. From then on, they seemed to have the faith necessary to heal those whom God wanted healed.

TODAY'S RX

Rebukes are sometimes God's way of instructing us. But learning to have faith can save us or someone else from physical or spiritual death.

I long to have faith that is rooted deeply in you, Father. Nourish me and help me to stand firm in your ways. Allow me to flourish and bring your Good News to others who are looking for hope.

WHEN THE WALLS CAME TUMBLING DOWN

A person without self-control is like a city with broken-down walls. PROVERBS 25:28

Thirteen-year-old Haley was exquisitely beautiful at a time when many middle school girls are awkward. She had unblemished porcelain skin and thick, dark curly hair. When she entered a room, people were stunned by her beauty. At the county fair, she won Fairest of the Fair. Wherever she went, everyone noticed her. Whatever the "it" factor was, she had it. In spades.

Then things began to change. When she turned fourteen, she came to see me for a sore throat, and I noticed a hint of cigarette smoke in her hair. A few months later, she blemished her otherwise snow-white skin with the first of many tattoos.

One day, when she was sixteen, I pointed to a homemade tattoo emblazoned on her upper arm and asked, "Whose initials are those?"

"Oh that's for Dougy-D."

I knew the young man she was talking about, and he wasn't exactly a role model. He was ten years older than she was, and he'd been in and out of the ER with injuries from fighting and drug use. I warned her that the cracks in her self-control and judgment could lead her where she didn't want to go. But she paid no attention.

A few months passed, and I saw her again. This time I noticed fresh marks on her arm—not from new tattoos, but from IV drug use. Again, she dismissed me.

Like today's verse warns, the walls of this beautiful girl's character had been dismantled one brick at a time until the barbarians at the gate had run roughshod through her fair city. Her pristine beauty was gone, replaced with dark eyeliner and darker circles under her eyes.

Nothing that anyone said could prevent her further destruction. She continued her risky behavior and eventually dropped out of school. With no structure and no self-control, it wasn't surprising when the next time she showed up in the ER, she was dead on arrival from a drug overdose.

Untended cracks in a wall become great divides until the wall crumbles under disrepair. Haley was a tragic example of how self-centered choices hurt not only ourselves, but everyone around us. Only through self-control and accountability can we shore up the walls of defense against the enemy's fiery darts.

TODAY'S RX

Preserve the walls around your heart and mind so you won't be tempted to let them decay.

Guard my heart and mind, Lord. Keep me away from temptation. Help me to plant myself firmly in your Word, so that I can be faithfully grounded in you.

WISE ADVICE FOR A HEALTHY LIFE

Those who trust their own insight are foolish, but anyone who walks in wisdom is safe.
PROVERBS 28:26

"My wife made me come in. She's the one who thinks I need a checkup. I haven't been to a doctor in more than twenty years, and I'm doing just fine. Nothing hurts, and I pretty much do whatever I want."

Elmer's body told a different story from the one he was voicing to me. He was fifty-three but looked sixty-five. He was fifty pounds overweight, and his blood pressure was elevated.

"Let's get a medical history on you and run some tests, and then we'll see," I said. "Does anyone in your family have a history of diabetes, heart disease, or cancer?"

"Yeah, Daddy died of a heart attack when he was fifty-two, and my brother died last year of a heart attack. I think he was fifty-three. My momma had diabetes, but that was only 'cause she was fat like me."

I could tell I had my work cut out for me. Elmer seemed blissfully unaware of the connection between the premature deaths of his close family members and his own prospects for long-term survival. And he was oblivious to his own body's warning signs.

His tests for diabetes and cholesterol both came back abnormally high.

"Elmer, you're not doing as well as you think you are," I said, showing him the results. "You're behind in your health care, and if you don't change, you'll likely die before you're fifty-five. You have a lot of work to do. The good news is that, if you listen to me and work hard, you can fix a lot of this."

"You've got my full attention, Doc. I've got kids that I want to see get married, and I want to be a grandfather one day."

I prescribed medication for his blood pressure, his diabetes, and his cholesterol. We talked about how he needed to quit smoking and stop eating so much processed food. Elmer was obviously surprised by everything I said.

"Am I doing anything right?" he asked.

"Yes. You listened to your wife when she sent you in for a checkup. Be sure to thank her when you get home."

TODAY'S RX

Seek wise counsel and follow the advice you're given if you want to live a healthier life.

Help me to be obedient in all aspects of my life, Lord, by listening to my doctor's advice, along with what your Word tells me. I desire to be healthy in body, mind, and spirit.

THE ROAD TO RECOVERY

Letting your sinful nature control your mind leads to death. But letting the Spirit control your mind leads to life and peace. ROMANS 8:6

During my college years, I became an atheist and embraced the prevailing thought of the day—that science alone could explain everything. I didn't believe there was a God or an afterlife because there was no way to prove it.

I was also very angry. My best friends had died a tragic death in the most unimaginable and cruelest way possible. I didn't see any point or purpose to life, and I chose to live as if there were no tomorrow. My sinful desires controlled my mind and body. I drank too much and didn't take care of myself physically.

But one day, I met death eyeball to eyeball as I stared into the face of the cadaver I'd been assigned in my medical school lab. Somehow, seeing my own mortality reflected back to me made my spirit come alive. Weeks later, I repented of my atheistic beliefs and fully accepted Christ as my Savior.

It was only then that I realized how spiritually dead I had been. It was as if my soul had been wandering around in a dry desert, longing for living water. When Jesus rescued me, I hadn't had any spiritual food or water for many years. I was anemic, anorexic, and bulimic when it came to spiritual sustenance.

Jesus took over my dying case and became my treating Great Physician. Under his care, my spirit began to recover. He gave me new life as well as an understanding of and a longing for eternity with him in heaven.

Though I'm still in spiritual recovery, and will be as long as I am here on earth, my soul has been revived and refreshed and is a thousand times more alive in Jesus than it ever was before.

TODAY'S RX

It is better to be a recovering sinner than afloat on a raft of rebellion and lost in an ocean of sin.

Father, I acknowledge my need for you, day in and day out. Sustain me through tough seasons, keep my fire lit, and increase my desire for you.

AN AMERICAN HERO

You need not be afraid of sudden disaster or the destruction that comes upon the wicked, for the LORD is your security. He will keep your foot from being caught in a trap.
PROVERBS 3:25-26

Jack was the all-American boy next door. He was captain of the high school football team and well regarded in our town. He had it all and then some.

No one was surprised when he joined the military to fight for our freedom. His blue eyes sparkled with anticipation of helping his country and touring the world in the hope of spreading freedom.

The whole town sent him off with well wishes and prayers for Godspeed to return him home soon, safe, and sound. No one said it out loud, but they all thought that God would certainly protect such a fine young man going overseas for such a gallant cause.

A few months after Jack deployed overseas, a call came to his home alerting his family that Jack's unit had come under attack, and his vehicle had been hit by a roadside bomb. Word spread fast, and the town pulled together to pray for their hero while awaiting further news.

In the end, Jack made it out, but his entire body was covered in third-degree burns, except for his legs—they were missing. The force of the explosion should have killed him instantly, but God had different plans for this hero. Not only did he survive, but he also recovered. Then one day, he walked into my office.

I recently watched the movie *American Sniper*, and I couldn't help reflecting on how war and the threat of destruction affects our soldiers to the very core of their being. So many of America's finest have returned home with scars—and often the worst scars are ones we can't see.

But when Jack walked into my office, his clear blue eyes still had the old sparkle. And his question was the same one he'd asked before he left: "How can I help someone less fortunate?"

The town knew that God had been a part of Jack's life early and often, but now God was with him continuously. Jack is not just our hometown hero; he's an American hero as well. Though war took his legs and left him with scars, it could not diminish his desire to serve others.

TODAY'S RX

Fear not. Trust God to lead the way.

God, thank you for our servicemen and women who give so much of themselves for our country's freedom. You've blessed them with a sacrificial spirit much like your own, and I pray that I may honor these people and show them the dignity and respect they deserve.

DROWNING IN TEARS AND COMPASSION

My life is an example to many, because you have been my strength and protection. That is why I can never stop praising you; I declare your glory all day long. PSALM 71:7-8

Kurtis and I had been in the same practice years ago. Recently, he and his wife came over for dinner, and we shared memories of the days we'd worked together in the ER.

"You taught me a lot of things when I was working with you," Kurtis said. "But do you know what the most important thing was that you taught me?"

As I tried to think back through twenty years of cases, Kurtis said, "I'll give you a hint. It happened the day that baby drowned."

There had been several children who had drowned over the years I'd practiced medicine in that rural ER, but I distinctly remembered the one he was referring to. A baby, in full cardiac arrest, had been brought in after being rescued from a pond. But despite our best efforts, the Lord had taken this precious baby back into his bosom that day.

"I'm stumped," I said. "Everything we tried that day was pretty much standard procedure. I can't think of anything new or unusual."

"It's what happened after the baby died that stuck with me," Kurtis said. "What you showed me had nothing to do with medicine and everything to do with practicing medicine."

"What do you mean?"

"You sat down with those young parents, held their hands, and looked them right in their tear-filled eyes. Then you explained that God had their baby. I remember the wife sobbing on your shoulder, and the father crying into his hands. You reached out to touch him and gave him physical comfort. When their crying slowed, you reminded them that this wasn't anyone's fault. Then you asked them to pray with you. I'll always remember the part of your prayer where you said that each day from that day forward would bring all of us closer to the day of reunion with our loved ones who had gone on before us."

I had no idea that I'd made such an impression on Kurtis. I could only give God the glory for being present at that moment and prompting my actions. As today's verse says, he is our strength and protection.

TODAY'S RX

Live out your faith even in the most difficult situations; you never know who might be watching you.

Father, may my faith radiate through my words and actions.
May I be a source of comfort to those in need, embracing
them in your truth and enfolding them in your love.

STUBBORN SHEEP AND OUR FAITHFUL SHEPHERD

Once you were like sheep who wandered away. But now you have turned to your Shepherd, the Guardian of your souls. 1 PETER 2:25

When our children were young, we had a menagerie of animals: two dogs, six cats, three horses, twenty-six goats, and two sheep. The goats frequently wandered off, but they were smart and usually came home when they knew we had food or treats.

The sheep were less prone to wander than the goats, but they were dumb animals. When they got lost in the fields, they didn't care what we were offering; they weren't interested. They didn't listen when we called, and they wouldn't come home on their own. One of the kids would have to go lead the stray sheep back home.

The sheep were often so much work that the kids would give up on them and prefer to play with the more obedient goats. I understood that feeling. I also found myself wishing we had not gotten all those animals.

So often in the Bible we're compared to sheep, which I now know isn't a flattering comparison. However, I'm glad that God is our Shepherd and that he continues to gently guide and protect us even when we wander. He is so determined to bring us back home that he was even willing to sacrifice his Son for our stupidity and sin.

Are there places in your life where you're wandering from the Good Shepherd? Do you ever act like a sheep lost in the field, far away from the safety, security, and nourishment of the barn? I know I have.

When God starts to nudge us back home, it's important for us to realize that his staff and rod are there to catch us and protect us, not to punish us for our disobedience. Like my kids trying to lead the sheep home, God is trying to lead his kids home. Fortunately, God doesn't give up as easily as my kids did!

TODAY'S RX

As sheep, we are prone to wander. That's why we must always listen for our Shepherd's voice.

Thank you for gently leading me in the direction you desire for me, Lord. As I wander away, you step in and guide me back to the fold. I will praise you all the days of my life for your faithful pursuit of me.

RICH AND NOT POWERFUL

Once a religious leader asked Jesus this question: "Good Teacher, what should I do to inherit eternal life?" . . . "You know the commandments: 'You must not commit adultery. You must not murder. You must not steal. You must not testify falsely. Honor your father and mother.'" The man replied, "I've obeyed all these commandments since I was young." When Jesus heard his answer, he said, "There is still one thing you haven't done. Sell all your possessions and give the money to the poor, and you will have treasure in heaven. Then come, follow me." But when the man heard this he became very sad, for he was very rich. Luke 18:18-23

Adam's mother, Marjorie, inherited a fortune and continued to increase her wealth throughout her lifetime. She had a modern Midas touch, and she was also generous in her support of several local charities and her church.

As she grew older, the family began to notice that she no longer gave money to organizations she had supported for years. When she also became withdrawn, refusing to go out with the family, they asked me to see her.

My first surprise was her appearance—once very regal but now unkempt. I administered a short exam to test her mental state, and she failed. A neurologist and a psychiatrist later confirmed a diagnosis of Alzheimer's disease, and placement in a suitable care facility became the next step.

When the family had settled on the safest and healthiest place for her to live, admission required a power of attorney—but no one had been appointed. As a result, Marjorie was stuck in limbo because she couldn't make her own decisions, and no one had been designated to make them on her behalf.

In her dementia, she attached herself in a very miserable way to her possessions and wealth, constantly accusing her children of trying to steal from her. When the court finally appointed Adam as her trustee and gave him power of attorney, Marjorie was legally forced to remove her grip on her money and possessions—and her health improved dramatically.

Medication and therapy helped to slow the dementia, and the nursing home chaplain was able to guide Marjorie out of her paranoid shell and back to the old, generous person she'd once been.

TODAY'S RX

Don't let your riches possess you. Be rich in God's love, and use your material wealth to bless others.

Father, help me to remember that everything I have on this earth is because of you. May I be generous with what you've blessed me with and give to those in need. After all, you gave your all for me.

A BREATH OF PRAISE

Make thankfulness your sacrifice to God, and keep the vows you made to the Most High. Then call on me when you are in trouble, and I will rescue you, and you will give me glory. PSALM 50:14-15

Lillian's presence was magnetic; she had a way of drawing people in with her joy and laughter. But a terrible thing happened when she contracted HIV after her husband had an affair.

HIV is a terrible disease that has killed thousands of people and weakened many more through complications. I would have thought that Lillian would be angry and bitter, but she wasn't. Even when she was at her weakest and couldn't laugh or talk, she could still smile—and she did.

When she came in to see me one day, I could see that the disease was slowly draining the life out of her.

"I don't know why I'm on this journey," she said. "But I believe God has a purpose for my life. I know my time on earth is going to be shorter than I expected, but I plan to use every breath for my Lord."

She paused to catch her breath, and it was obvious to me that she had pneumonia. I admitted her to the ICU and placed her on a ventilator to help prevent complete respiratory failure.

Through it all, Lillian remained awake but sedated. I stopped by each day to see if she needed anything. She couldn't speak, but she would clasp her hands together in prayer, so we prayed together. I knew she was silently praising and thanking God.

Today's verses tell us to make thankfulness our sacrifice. If we call on God when things look bleak, he will rescue us. Lillian was such a great example of that because she truly sacrificed each breath to pray. It was a lot to endure, but she fought bravely—and God rescued her.

About a week into her hospital stay, Lillian turned a corner and started to regain her physical strength. By the time she was ready to go home, she told me, "Without all of the prayers, I never would have made it." Even in her darkest moments, Lillian was giving the glory to God.

TODAY'S RX

Make thankfulness your sacrifice. Give God all the glory and praise. Then, when you call on him, he will rescue you.

Lord, even when I'm hurting and do not feel very thankful in the moment, help me to have a heart that thanks you and praises you. I may not understand why this hurt has happened, but I know you are in complete control and that you care for me.

DEFEATING DARKNESS

Jesus said, "All right, receive your sight! Your faith has healed you." LUKE 18:42

I want you to try something. If you have an inside room that is totally dark, go into that room and sit still for ten minutes. While you're there, think about the gift of sight and how most of us take it for granted. Go ahead and do it now. I'll wait here until you get back.

Our ability to see is a marvelous gift, and we often don't realize how important it is until it's gone.

One summer while on a solo camping trip, I went spelunking in a cave. I was about seventy-five yards in when I dropped my flashlight. When it hit the ground, the light flickered out. Suddenly, I was standing in pitch darkness, and it was immediately clear to me why you're never supposed to go exploring alone. I couldn't see a thing, and I didn't know what to do. There was no way I could make my way out of the cave alone without a light source. I began to panic.

I didn't realize it at the time, but being trapped alone in the darkness of a cave was symbolic of my life as an atheist. I thought I could handle everything, until suddenly I couldn't. That's when I realized I was trapped, alone, and blind.

As I stumbled around in the dark, my foot hit something, and I backed up. It was the flashlight! When I kicked it, it turned on, casting its beam on the far wall of the cave. In that instant, the darkness had no choice but to retreat into the crevices and the shadows. The light was victorious.

Though I didn't see the connection right then, I later understood that Jesus, the Light of the World, could defeat the darkness in my life. My joy was made complete when he shone his light and love into the previously darkened corners of my life.

Go back into your dark room again, and think about the darkness. How does it feel to be alone and blind? When you're ready, flip on the light, or light a candle and see how quickly the light defeats the darkness. Now imagine what God's light can do for the darkness in your life.

TODAY'S RX

Things may be dark for a while, but God's light always overcomes the darkness.

Jesus, you are the Light of the World. Thank you for shining your light on me.

STRENGTH IN THE SPIRIT

Dear friend, I hope all is well with you and that you are as healthy in body as you are strong in spirit. 3 John 1:2

When I look into the eyes of my patients, feel the firmness of their handshakes, and listen to them talk, it's obvious which ones are strong in spirit. And they are the ones who give me great hope. From experience, I know that patients who are strong in spirit will face with resilience and resolve anything that comes their way.

When the apostle John wrote his third recorded letter, he recognized the connection between body and spirit. In his greeting, he mentions his hope that his friend's body will reflect the strength and health that John already knows is in his spirit.

There's a lesson here for all of us. Just as we should not neglect our physical health, neither should we neglect our spirits. We exercise and eat right to take care of our bodies. And to have healthy spirits, we need spiritual exercises and nutrition such as prayer, reading Scripture, and fellowshiping with other believers.

Despite the many adversities my patients face, those who are strong in spirit often overcome their health problems and go on to live into their nineties or even longer. Is it because they are healthier in body or spirit? No one knows for sure, but my guess is that the answer is both.

TODAY'S RX

When making healthy choices for your body, remember to also make healthy choices for your soul and spirit.

Lord, I know that my spiritual health often dictates my physical and emotional well-being. I ask that you help me to remain firm in my Bible reading and prayer, knowing you will preserve me in spirit and body.

THE BLESSINGS OF CONTENTMENT

From his abundance we have all received one gracious blessing after another.
John 1:16

Bernie, my first patient of the morning, took one look at me and said, "You look tired."

He was right. I knew I did. It was a Monday morning, and I had just finished a weekend shift in the ER.

"For an old watermelon farmer, I'm doing fine," I said.

Bernie laughed.

Every day I feel blessed beyond measure. Growing up, I had much less materially than I do now. But even back then, I remembered being content and happy with what God had given me.

Though my fatigue was showing that morning, it didn't keep me from counting all the ways God has blessed this poor country boy from Alabama. For example, I love serving underprivileged country folks just like the ones I grew up with. God has given me an amazing wife and four wonderful children, and we all have more than enough clothes and food and a comfortable home. The kids are all healthy and doing well, and we have friends at both church and school.

"Enough about me, how are you and your kids doing?" I asked Bernie.

I listened as Bernie told me about his family. We were both blessed not only to have our families and our jobs, but also to have grown up in America, where we can take advantage of the opportunities that this country offers. No matter what troubles we face, our blessings certainly outweigh them.

Our contentment shouldn't be determined by the idols we have created. It should come from our appreciation of what God has done for us. Even on a Monday morning when I am tired from working all weekend, I can still say that God has blessed me, and I am content.

TODAY'S RX

If you search for contentment, you may never find it. But if you count your blessings, you surely will.

Father, help me to remember and be thankful for all the blessings you have bestowed on me. Even in the difficult times, may I never forget all you have done for me.

REMEMBER ME AND SHOW ME FAVOR

Remember me, LORD, when you show favor to your people; come near and rescue me. Let me share in the prosperity of your chosen ones. Let me rejoice in the joy of your people; let me praise you with those who are your heritage. PSALM 106:4-5

A big city hospital can be a scary place for some of my patients, and sometimes it can be overwhelming for me too.

One day, I called the regional hospital on behalf of Diana, who had presented in our ER with heart attack symptoms and needed to be seen by a cardiologist. The staff said they were full, but they would do what they could.

By the time I reached the hospital, Diana had been moved to the last room at the end of a very long hallway, in a far corner of the hospital. It was a miserable experience walking through endless cold and sterile hallways looking for her room.

When I arrived, it felt isolated and dark with only a single small window, but I knew it was the only available room.

"I'm so glad to see you!" Diana said. "You're the first familiar face I've seen here!"

I knew what she meant; she was the first familiar face I'd seen, as well.

Diana looked frightened as I sat down beside her bed. "Don't worry. I know this place is big and can seem scary. But God is with you, and he allowed me to be here to help you navigate through the confusing maze of hallways and all the paperwork."

She smiled.

"The specialists here are top-notch," I said. "And the cardiologist will be here in a short while." As a country doctor, my presence at the bigger hospital was often more about making the patients comfortable than for medical purposes.

Diana and I chatted until the cardiologist arrived. He ordered some tests, and we learned that Diana had a cardiac arrhythmia. In the cardiology lab, they were able to quickly diagnose and fix the abnormality in her heart's electrical system.

In medicine, we all do what we can to make our patients feel better. The cardiologist was there to steady her heartbeat, and I was there to steady her nerves.

TODAY'S RX

Don't be afraid. Wherever you are, the Lord is with you, and you are not alone. He will never leave you.

Lord, help me to be still and trust in you when the path ahead is frightening. I know you're beside me, lighting the way.

PERSISTENCE IS NOT A PROBLEM

Everyone who asks, receives. Everyone who seeks, finds. And to everyone who knocks, the door will be opened. MATTHEW 7:8

"I've got a problem, and I was wondering if you could help me," Drew said. "It seems kind of silly, but my wife—"

"Your problem is your wife?" I asked.

"No," Drew said, laughing. "My wife thinks I may have a problem, but I'm not so sure. I'm here because she made me come, and I'm hoping you'll tell me it's not a big deal."

"Sure. What's up?"

"I have a spot on my back, near my right shoulder. My wife pointed it out a few months ago. I thought it had always been there, but she said it hadn't. Now she thinks it's growing, but I think it's pretty much the same size—of course, I can't see it that well because it's on my back. It's not painful or anything, but she won't let it rest until I hear from you that it's nothing to worry about."

"All right, let me take a look," I said.

I noticed the spot immediately. It had signs of melanoma—irregular borders, with different shades of brown and black.

"Well, Drew, I think your wife is right to worry about it. I know you're a farmer, and farmers can get a lot of sun even when they're not trying. I think it would be wise for you to have a biopsy done."

I sent him to a dermatology department that specialized in melanoma. The report confirmed my initial diagnosis. Drew and his wife both came in to get the results. "We're going to storm the gates of heaven with our prayers," she said, after hearing the news. She also wanted a list of the best oncological surgeons. "I'm going to call around and get as many answers as I can, and we'll just keep praying until God makes each step clear."

"Drew, it looks like your wife is looking out for you. Not only was she persistent about getting you in here, but I have a feeling she'll be even more persistent in her prayers for you."

TODAY'S RX

Is there something irregular in your life? Don't wait until it causes you pain; pray about it now. When it comes to prayer, persistence is not a problem.

God, help me to pray frequently and fervently, lifting my worries to you, knowing that you will hear me and answer me. Thank you for listening and keeping me under your watchful care.

THE FIRST STEP IS THE MOST IMPORTANT ONE

Jesus immediately reached out and grabbed him. "You have so little faith," Jesus said. "Why did you doubt me?" MATTHEW 14:31

When I ponder Peter's act of faith in stepping out of the boat to walk on the water toward Jesus, I don't think about his walk or his fall. I think about that first step. What kind of courage did it take for him to hoist himself over the side of the boat and onto the water? I've often tried to imagine what he was thinking as his foot touched the waves. Frankly, I'm impressed that he did it; I would have been cowering in the back of the boat!

Sometimes, the first step is the hardest. Many of my patients come to me with an addiction to alcohol, tobacco, or even food. They want to quit the behaviors that are killing them, but they feel powerless. To overcome any kind of addiction, you can't keep doing what you've always done. You have to take a first step toward the life you want. That first step is often to admit that you have a problem and you're powerless over it. You need to ask for someone's help—maybe a friend, a pastor, or a doctor. God can work through many people to show his love for you.

Do you feel paralyzed by inaction? Are there places you want to go in your life, but you're not sure how to get started in that direction?

The first step is to take that first step.

Whether you sink or swim, you have to get out of the boat and begin moving toward your destination. Fortunately, we know that Jesus is with us every step of the way. If you look, you will see him coming toward you. If you fall, it is his arms that will reach out to catch you. The faith to take the first step is all you need to propel you in the right direction.

Take that first step toward healthy living, and have the confidence that even if you get a little wet, Jesus will be your life jacket.

TODAY'S RX

If you're afraid to step out, at least talk to God about your fear. He can give you the courage you need to move forward.

Jesus, I want to take that first step toward a healthier lifestyle. Help me to stand firm in my commitment and have faith in my ability to persevere. Be with me every step of the way.

NO DOUBT

Jesus said to the disciples, "Have faith in God. I tell you the truth, you can say to this mountain, 'May you be lifted up and thrown into the sea,' and it will happen. But you must really believe it will happen and have no doubt in your heart. I tell you, you can pray for anything, and if you believe that you've received it, it will be yours."
MARK 11:22-24

Martin had a bulging disc, and his neurologist recommended back surgery as soon as possible to stabilize it. But Martin wasn't sure about the surgery. He wanted to wait and pray about it first.

A few weeks later, he showed up in my office, "Hey, Dr. Anderson, I just got back from a prayer service. I want you to check me out to see how well it worked."

"I'd be happy to," I said, unsure of what to expect.

Martin had struggled for many years with severe arthritis and pain in his lower back. During that time, I'd ordered a series of tests, including an MRI, a nerve conduction study, and a neurosurgery evaluation. He had also seen several specialists. They all agreed that back surgery was his only option.

"Stand up and show me how you're moving," I said. He got off the exam table a little spryer than I remembered from the last time. "Now lie back down, please." After he was back on the table, I asked him to do a straight leg raise. Martin was much more mobile, and he had full range of motion without as much pain as he'd had before.

"Well, I don't think I need surgery. What do you think?"

"I could not agree more."

In England, back surgery is often delayed for six months or more. Maybe we Americans should be more patient as we wait upon the Lord. If we rush into things, we may miss the great work the Lord has in store for us.

Jesus told the disciples that they could pray for anything, and if they believed, they would receive it. Martin believed that God would heal him, and he received the healing he prayed for.

TODAY'S RX

Today, pick something to pray about, and pray in faith, without doubting. God is faithful to hear you and to answer in accordance with his will.

Father, I pray for you to work a miracle in my life and rid me of this pain. Revive me. Refresh me with your Holy Spirit. Allow me to experience life without this thorn in my side.

NO PRAISE WAS SPARED, ONLY THEIR LIVES

Yes, the LORD is for me; he will help me. PSALM 118:7

Though it had been snowy the night before, Lynne and Larry decided it wasn't anything their front-wheel-drive sedan couldn't handle. So they got in the car and left at the same time they always did. They were talking and laughing when they rounded a bend on the highway and saw a jackknifed eighteen-wheeler blocking the road in front of them.

Larry slammed on the brakes, but the car slid straight toward the cab of the truck. There was nothing they could do to stop. Though their car may have been able to handle the weather, it was no match for the massive semi. Their little sedan was crushed.

Those at the scene said that Lynne's and Larry's heads were less than four inches from the tires that had run over the demolished car. They were still seated, side by side, holding hands and praying—trapped, but by God's grace still alive. Rescuers used the Jaws of Life to cut them out of the wreckage, and they were amazed that the couple still had all their limbs.

Lynne and Larry spent two weeks in the trauma unit at Vanderbilt, and everyone who heard their story was astounded at how they'd survived. It didn't take a miracle—it took a succession of miracles for them to make it out alive.

I had read about the wreck in the local paper, and I'd heard reports on the couple from friends and family, so when their names were on my appointment schedule one morning, I knew who they were, but I didn't know what to expect. I was sure they'd gotten treatment for all their physical injuries, but I worried about their emotional and spiritual condition. Major trauma can cause more "head" injuries than a concussion, not to mention what such a harrowing experience can do to a person's heart.

To my surprise, they both entered the office upright, though walking with the aid of walkers. More important, they were upright in their spirits, singing praises to God. Hearing firsthand the story of their miraculous survival and how God had carried them through gave my own faith a shot in the arm.

TODAY'S RX

If your life has passed in front of you and you lived to tell about it, give all the glory to God.

To you be the honor and glory, God. I praise you with all my heart.

SAYING GOOD-BYE TO THE OLD

This means that anyone who belongs to Christ has become a new person. The old life is gone; a new life has begun! 2 CORINTHIANS 5:17

In the depths of my rebellion against God, I went on a camping trip alone. I arrived at the campsite an atheist, but two days later, I left a changed man. Out in the woods, Jesus met me in a vivid dream, and that encounter changed my life.

When I arrived at the clearing that afternoon, I unpacked my gear and started a small fire, where I reclined and read for a while. Suddenly and without warning, I fell asleep and dreamed of heaven. In the dream, I was enveloped by vibrant colors and sounds, and I breathed in the scents of lilac and citrus. It was a dream so incredible that it seemed more real than real life. But heaven was so much better than a dream. I never wanted to leave! Though I had no idea what questions I should ask, Jesus spoke to my confusion and hurts. When I woke up next to the fire, only embers remained, but there was a new fire in my heart.

The next day, I walked down the mountain toward a shimmering waterfall, and I reflected on the person I had been and who I now was in Christ. As a symbol of my new commitment, I baptized myself in the stream. As the cool mountain water drenched my forehead, I felt my old, tarnished self washing away. I was a new creation; the old was gone. The person I used to be had died in the woods next to that fire. I would never be able to resuscitate that deceased part of me, nor would I ever want to.

When we become a new creation in Christ, it is important to reflect for a moment on what has been washed away. By acknowledging the old, we make way for the new. Only after we seeing the reflection of our previous filth in the pool can the waters of change cleanse us. Pausing to see that old reflection allows us to say good-bye to our old selves and vow that we'll only move forward with the Lord.

TODAY'S RX

Becoming a butterfly is a journey, and the first part of flying free is to discard the chrysalis that once confined us.

Wash over me, Lord. Cleanse me of my sin, and revitalize my spirit. I desire to be made new.

WAITING FOR HIS MASTER

Since the world began, no ear has heard and no eye has seen a God like you, who works for those who wait for him! Isaiah 64:4

I entered the sunroom as the first rays of dawning light were shining through the nursing home windows. Throughout the day, the temperature in that sunny room would continue to rise by several degrees as light spilled through the glass and reflected off the walls, producing a radiant glow.

Marvin, an elderly man with a few remaining wisps of white hair, sat in the sunniest part of the room with his face lifted toward the rising sun. He looked up expectantly, as if anticipating a glimpse of something. But if Marvin saw anything out those windows, it was something the rest of us couldn't see because Marvin had lost his eyesight many years ago.

Before he arrived at the home, he'd been a preacher for nearly eighty years. His ophthalmologist had tried valiantly for many years to stem the tide of darkness that gradually washed away Marvin's sight, but nothing could stop the deterioration.

During his first few years in the nursing home, he would smile when I greeted him. But now, even shouting, "Good morning, Marvin!" wouldn't get a response, because the years had taken his hearing, as well. Now, he just sat by the window in silence, like a loyal dog waiting for his master to return.

I touched his shoulder, and he clasped my hand and gave me an affirmative squeeze. This was our sign that all was still well with the world.

To those who didn't know Marvin, his world may have seemed dark, quiet, and meaningless. But I knew that his heart and mind were alive with thoughts of what would come next. He'd never missed a Sunday as a preacher, and during those years he taught about the promises of God. Though he could no longer communicate with others, I knew he was rehearsing God's promises in his very active mind. Marvin greeted the sunrise every morning. Though he couldn't see it, he could feel it. To him, it was a reminder that God's promises are new every day, as he waited expectantly for his Master to call him home.

TODAY'S RX

Attune your spiritual eyes and ears to see and hear what God is doing all around us.

God, help me not to take my health for granted, but to be grateful for all I have. I desire to be in tune with you always, listening for your call and feeling the warmth of your presence.

NOT IF, BUT WHEN JESUS HEALS

"What do you mean, 'If I can'?" Jesus asked. "Anything is possible if a person believes." The father instantly cried out, "I do believe, but help me overcome my unbelief!"
MARK 9:23-24

If is one of the biggest little words I know. So much can ride on a question that begins with this tiny word.

What would happen if you ate this or that food or if you exercised more? Maybe you've asked *if* questions about your disease. You want to know if one drug is better than another or if you should try surgery.

Medical professionals aren't exempt from asking *if* questions of their own. We wonder if our patients would be more compliant if we prescribed drugs to be taken once a day rather than four times a day. We wonder if more education will help our diabetic patients keep their sugars under control or if our obese patients would lose weight if they consulted a nutritionist.

But the saddest *if* questions we ask are the *what if* questions. What if our patient hadn't smoked a pack of cigarettes every day for twenty years? What if the woman with ovarian cancer had gone to the doctor sooner? What if the patient had properly cared for the wound on his foot?

We could take the *what if* questions all the way back to the first couple in the Garden of Eden.

"What if Adam and Eve had not eaten the forbidden fruit? Would we still have sickness and disease?" But for all these *what if* questions, we will never have an answer this side of the veil.

In today's verse, Jesus tests the man's faith by repeating back to him his question: *"If I can?"* The father replies with perhaps the most honest answer ever. "I *believe*, but I need help for those time when it's hard."

As a doctor, I know that a treatment is more likely to work if the patient believes it will. I suspect the same is true with our faith. The more we believe, the more we see Jesus' healing works in our lives and in the lives of others. But we're not stuck with a lack of faith. If we're honest with Jesus, even about our unbelief, he can bolster our faith in an instant and heal our diseases.

TODAY'S RX

Cry out to God for help in overcoming your unbelief. He is faithful and able.

Lord, in my most desperate and trying moments, when the world has me down and all options have failed, please help me to overcome my unbelief. I know you are able, and I trust you for complete restoration and healing.

DECEMBER CHECKUP

It's December. Do you hear the bells of Christmas? Stop and listen to the tinkling sounds and gongs of the hand bell choir at your local church. Or cheer for the exuberant preschoolers who shout Christmas carols enthusiastically at a local school. Pause long enough to drop a gift in the Salvation Army's red buckets, and shake the hands of the volunteers who faithfully collect funds for the needy.

Everywhere you go in December, there are reminders of Christmas but not always of Christ, whose birthday is the reason we celebrate. Don't let all the commercialization, glitz, and glamor of the season distract you from unwrapping and getting to know the greatest gift you will ever receive—our Lord and Savior, Jesus Christ.

The Creator of the universe came down to earth to live, walk, talk, and sing among us. His birthday present was his presence here on earth. This year, worry less about exchanging presents and more about being present. Put down the technology, and laugh with those around you. Forget the stress of capturing the perfect moment on your phone. Instead, concentrate on seeing it with your eyes and feeling it with your heart.

When attending holiday parties, be present in the moment. Look people in the eye and have real conversations. When people tell you they're "fine," tell them you want to know how they're really doing. When someone asks how you are, don't just tell them you're busy; tell them what is really going on in your life. Take time to reconnect with old friends whom you haven't seen lately. Call relatives in distant places and tell them you're thinking of them. Instead of sending so many mass-produced Christmas cards, handwrite a few to those who matter most to you.

Start a new holiday tradition. Go back through this book and select an "ornament" that represents what you've done each month. Hang something on the tree that reminds you of your internal reflections from January. Attach a photo of a new relationship made in February or of one of your October kindness capers. Pick a symbol of fire for July and water for August. As you go through each month, reflect on all the ways you've healed and grown.

As you're out and about this holiday season—listening, looking, smelling, feeling, and being present—know that each toll of the holiday bell is an invitation to open your heart to others and to God. Nothing will change your life more than a little open-heart spiritual surgery. God the Father opened up his heart and invited us in. This Christmas, return the favor with an invitation for him to come into your heart.

December Booster Shot: Just as you winterize your car, boat, or home, take a few minutes each day to winterize your body. Wear warm clothing. Check the weather forecast for snow and ice before venturing out, and tread carefully as you walk or drive. We tend to stay inside and huddle together during December, which allows bacteria to breed and germs to spread. Watch for signs of respiratory infections and seek medical care early.

BE PRESENT

Encourage each other and build each other up, just as you are already doing.
1 THESSALONIANS 5:11

As a doctor, I am sometimes called upon to deliver bad news. Occasionally, these discussions involve preparing a patient for the end of life. These conversations are never easy, and I take time to walk my patients down this dark and lonely road.

What I've found is that these moments call for a flashlight—a spiritual flashlight. I want my patients to know what the next life offers and that they can have it. I want them to see death as a glass half-full and to be optimistic and encouraged, even as their time on earth draws to a close.

I often tell my patients that I wish I could join them on this journey to our heavenly home, and I mean it. I truly want to be with the Lord, and I'm a little envious that they are in line ahead of me. Even those who are on their deathbeds and are no longer speaking will smile and give my hand a slight squeeze when I say those things.

As parents, I know we often tell our children when they're hurting that we would gladly substitute ourselves for them if we could. Each of my children has heard both Karen and me say this. It somehow gives them the courage to endure the pain.

I don't think it's unusual that the best military leaders in history were always the ones who led in the battle. They willingly put themselves in harm's way alongside their soldiers. Troops follow this kind of a leader anywhere—even into death.

As you walk with people facing death, it can be hard to know what to say to them. My advice? Just let them know you're with them.

TODAY'S RX

In the worst of circumstances, there are no adequate words. Just be present.

Lord, help me to be present with those I love this holiday season. Do not allow me to be distracted by the world, but help me cling to what matters most—the celebration of your coming into this world.

LISTENING: HOW TO STAY OUT OF TROUBLE

Watch your tongue and keep your mouth shut, and you will stay out of trouble.
PROVERBS 21:23

When my classmates and I made rounds in medical school, no one wanted to be asked a question he or she couldn't answer—or worse, ask a question for which he or she should have known the answer. Either situation signaled to the attending physician that we hadn't studied enough. It was like an open invitation for more questions we couldn't answer. Our attending physician usually had a bunch of trick questions up his sleeve, and he couldn't wait to pull them out if he thought we were unprepared.

Over time, I found that the best strategy was to look engaged and interested but remain silent. If I did that, I could usually make it through rounds without drawing attention from the attending physician. By listening more than talking, I also picked up pearls of wisdom that helped me later on. What I thought was a strategy to avoid unwanted attention turned out to be a prudent way to learn.

One day, we had a Christian professor visit who imparted the most important lesson we would ever learn in medical school: Be quiet and listen carefully to your patients. "If you'll just listen," he said, "they will tell you the diagnosis."

To this day, I believe he was trying to teach us the same valuable lesson that today's verse teaches. We need to stay calm and quiet. We need to listen before we speak.

After practicing medicine for so many years, I've learned that patients hang on every word a doctor says. Often they repeat back to me something I've said, but they say it with even more clarity and intensity. That makes it critically important for me to be careful and thoughtful with my speech.

Though I first learned the lesson in medical school, it doesn't just apply to medicine. The wisdom of "listen first" applies to marriage, parenting, and other relationships. If we listen first, we will speak softly, calmly, and with the backing of wisdom.

TODAY'S RX

The next time you're in a conversation, look the other person in the eye and listen first to what he or she has to say. When you speak, it will be with the wisdom of understanding.

Help me to remain quiet and have a listening ear, Father. I desire to understand those I'm in fellowship with and not speak over them or instruct them. Thank you for imparting your wisdom to me.

HEALING FLOWS FROM GOD

Fruit trees of all kinds will grow along both sides of the river. The leaves of these trees will never turn brown and fall, and there will always be fruit on their branches. There will be a new crop every month, for they are watered by the river flowing from the Temple. The fruit will be for food and the leaves for healing. EZEKIEL 47:12

Ezekiel was an Old Testament prophet who had an apocalyptic vision of the Temple, God's dwelling place, which he metaphorically revealed to be the source of divine, life-giving water.

This reminds me of the Amazon River and the surrounding rain forests. Did you know that many of our favorite foods, such as oranges, lemons, grapefruits, figs, bananas, pineapples, coconuts, and mangoes are found in the rain forest? Though in the West we eat only about two hundred different kinds of fruit, natives of the area have access to a much broader diet, including nearly two thousand varieties of fruit.

Rain forest plants are also rich in medicinal properties. Nearly one out of every four ingredients in our modern medicines comes from the flora grown there. Furthermore, two thousand plants found in the rain forest have proven anticancer properties. It's as if the rain forest is nature's pharmacy, providing us with healthy foods and healing medicine.

It's exciting when scientists discover new technological breakthroughs in food and medicine. But we must remember that some of the greatest modern miracles were discovered in trees and shrubs that God gave us thousands of years ago. Healing can come to us in many forms. Sometimes it comes miraculously. Other times it comes through medicine, and still other times it happens through healthy eating choices.

As today's verse mentions, a river flowed from the Temple with healing waters, which nourished the trees on both sides. The trees were also a source of food and medicine. Ezekiel poetically reminds us that no matter how we're healed, healing always flows from God.

TODAY'S RX

The healing properties of food aren't found in a vending machine. If you can grow it or pick it, you'll be much closer to the way God intended you to eat.

Lord, I desire to fill my body with the healthy, nourishing foods you intended for me to eat—not the sugary, processed foods that lack nutritional value. Help me to make wise choices this Christmas season to keep my body running well.

KNOWING THIS ISN'T OUR HOME

They have defeated him by the blood of the Lamb and by their testimony. And they did not love their lives so much that they were afraid to die. REVELATION 12:11

For a variety of reasons, many people are afraid of death. Parents worry about who will take care of their children if they are no longer around to care for them. Seniors worry about dying alone. Some people fear a painful or protracted death. For others, the fear isn't of dying, but what happens after they die. They're not sure what, if anything, comes next.

After I became a Christ follower, I no longer feared death. I was on a solo camping trip when I had an encounter with the risen Jesus; and in a dream, I caught a glimpse of heaven that forever changed my views about death. In this dream, I saw that what follows this life for believers is better than anything we can imagine. As a result, I long to go to heaven, and that knowledge has removed all fear of death.

Both personally and as a doctor, I have been able to look death squarely in the eye and know beyond a shadow of a doubt that Christ has conquered death for me. For all who believe in Jesus, death has been defeated and is a mere shadow we pass through on our journey to our forever home.

I first sat at the bedside of a dying patient when I was in medical school. Since then, I have sat with many patients who have died of causes ranging from cancer to car accidents, from diseases to suicides. The one thing that consistently stands out to me is that my patients who have faith in Jesus are different from those who don't. Those who were believers were happy and joyous the moment that heaven welcomed them home.

We fear the unknown, and for many, death is the great unknown. That's why the testimony of the saints who have gone on before us to great victory is so important to grasp. If we understand that our ultimate transition from earth to heaven is a step into a real and forever life, then our fears will fade.

TODAY'S RX

If you're afraid of what will happen after you die, today is the day to secure your future home.

Jesus, I know I have no reason to fear death when the glory of your presence awaits me. Thank you for providing a way for me to spend eternity with you.

THE ROAD LESS TRAVELED CAN STILL GET YOU THERE

God remembered Rachel's plight and answered her prayers by enabling her to have children. She became pregnant and gave birth to a son. "God has removed my disgrace," she said. GENESIS 30:22-23

Alexis was afraid that her second marriage would end for the same reason as her first—her husband wanted children, and her body was unable to carry a baby to full term.

Alexis had miscarried three times that she knew about, but she suspected it had been even more. Her second husband understood her plight and stood by her during what they thought would be a surgery to correct the problem.

Unfortunately, soon after the surgery, Alexis started to bleed and went to the ER for a blood transfusion. The hospital admitted her overnight, but by the morning her situation had become life-threatening. The OB/GYN who saw her the next morning gave her the bad news: she needed to undergo an immediate hysterectomy to save her life. She had the surgery that afternoon.

When I saw Alexis the next morning, she was devastated.

"I know in my heart that I'm supposed to be a mom," she said. "I trusted God, and look what happened." She began to cry as the questions burst forth from her pain. "How can so many women get pregnant and then have an abortion, when I'll never be able to conceive again?"

"I'm so sorry, Alexis," I said, patting her hand. "I know God has a plan for you; I just wish I knew what it was."

"I know you're right," she said.

"Have you considered adoption?" I asked. "I've had lots of patients and friends who've grown their families that way. I could refer you to an agency if you're willing to consider it. They could give you more information and answer your questions."

Alexis said she would talk to her husband, but she was worried because her first husband hadn't been open to the idea.

A few weeks later, Alexis called and asked me to help her fill out the paperwork they needed to provide to the adoption agency.

Less than a month after they turned in the paperwork, they got a call from the agency, and Alexis left this message on my voicemail: "Thank you! My husband and I are headed to Florida to pick up our new baby daughter!"

TODAY'S RX

When the road seems blocked, God may have a different path for you to travel.

Father, thank you for knowing the desires of my heart. You've known them all along, and I praise you for providing the means you see fit for answering my prayers.

LAST HOPE

Jesus said, "Someone deliberately touched me, for I felt healing power go out from me."
LUKE 8:46

Elaine sat quietly in the corner of the waiting room. When her name was called, she got up slowly from her chair and made her way down the hall to the exam room.

"I don't know what to do," she said. "I'm swelling all over. It's worse in my legs, and I'm losing my strength. I'm always short of breath, and I don't think I can take another step."

We helped her into the room, and I began my exam.

"I've seen at least ten doctors before I came to see you, and they all just shook their heads. They couldn't give me an answer. You're my last hope."

She had visited a number of specialists, and most of the doctors on her list were much more qualified than I was. If they hadn't turned up anything specific, how could she expect me to have an answer? I was just a country doctor.

But I was also a believer. "Let's pray that God will show us what's wrong," I suggested. "Perhaps he can use one of the tests I'll run to give us some answers."

After we prayed together, I said, "I'll track down the test results from the other doctors you've visited, and I'll order some additional ones. Once we have all the results, we'll see what God can tell us."

During the week, while I pondered Elaine's condition, I thought about the bleeding woman who had reached out to touch the robe of Jesus. I'm sure she had sought help from other healers and that none had been able to help her. As she approached Jesus, he was her last hope.

A week later, with the test results in hand, I had an idea of what was causing Elaine's symptoms. She had nephritic syndrome, which her nephrologist later determined was due to abnormal protein flowing through her blood. After another week, we were able to confirm a diagnosis of amyloidosis—a condition that causes protein to build up in other tissues and organs. Once we identified the cause, we were able to determine the treatment. Elaine needed a bone marrow transplant.

A few months later, Elaine walked into my office and smiled. She was back to her normal self.

TODAY'S RX

When seeking treatment, be persistent, and never give up. Lean on the Lord in faith, and trust his wisdom.

Lord, give me the patience to endure what I'm facing and the reassurance that you have all the answers. I trust in you to direct my path to healing.

KICKING THE HABIT

No discipline is enjoyable while it is happening—it's painful! But afterward there will be a peaceful harvest of right living for those who are trained in this way.
HEBREWS 12:11

As the medical director at our critical access hospital, my job is to oversee patient rehabilitation. Most are there to get physical therapy for something they've broken—and for the geriatric set, that's usually a fracture in the hip joint.

Judy was no stranger to the hospital, but this was the first time she'd been admitted into the rehab unit after breaking her hip. Usually she came in for exacerbation of her chronic obstructive pulmonary disease. She would stay a day or two until she could breathe better, and then she'd go back home and resume her smoking habit.

Her stay in the rehab unit would be much longer and much harder than she was used to. It was also a nonsmoking facility with strict rules. All of this seemed to catch Judy by surprise. She wasn't ready for the pain of rehab, much less ready to give up her cigarettes.

I was paged to her room one morning when she tried to light a cigarette.

"I'm going crazy not being able to smoke," she said when I reminded her of the rules, "and the pain of rehab is also getting to me. I'm not sure I want to do this."

I decided to take a different tack. "Did you know that the phrase 'no pain, no gain' has biblical roots?"

She looked at me like I was crazy.

I told her about today's verse from Hebrews. "God knows that sometimes we must struggle to reach our goals. It's not always easy, but it's worth it. While you're here to rehab your hip, it's a great time to kick your cigarette habit. Why don't you think about it?"

When I left her room, she was as stubborn as ever, but at least she had handed me her remaining cigarettes.

Nine months later when I saw that Judy was my next appointment, I walked down the hall to escort her to my office. But before I could get to her, she jumped up from her chair and held out her hand to shake mine. "Dr. Anderson, I kicked it to the curb!" she said, showing off her functioning hip with a low kick. "I'm no longer a smoker!"

TODAY'S RX

What you're going through may be difficult, but the reward at the end is worth it.

God, thank you for providing road blocks to divert me from harmful behavior. You created me for more than what I've limited myself to, and I pray that with your help I can begin making great strides toward an abundant life of faith.

A MOTHER'S LAST WISHES

Whether we are here in this body or away from this body, our goal is to please him.
2 CORINTHIANS 5:9

Ann was ninety-five years young and had been in very good health all her life. Whenever she stopped in, we often talked more about our shared faith than we did her health. More than anything, she wanted to live her life in a way that pleased God.

As she got along in years, she often spoke about how ready she was for this life to end so she could begin her forever life with Jesus. Her husband had died five years earlier, and she wanted to see him again. Her living will ruled out any heroic measures during her final days. Her family, however, was divided about her wishes. Two of her children didn't want to let her go without every possible medical intervention taken. The other two wanted to honor their mother's wishes to go quietly when her time came. As often happens, the family was unable to come to a consensus.

A few months later, Ann had a stroke in the middle of the night. When she was found the next morning, they sent her to the ER. As soon as I entered the room to examine her, I could hear the familiar end-of-life breathing pattern called Cheyne-Stokes. Ann was unresponsive, and I knew the end was near.

When her children came to see her, they predictably responded according to their own desires. After discussing a few options at their request, I said, "Now is the time for you to come together as a family. Please look at her living will, and see her last wishes."

People who have lived a long and good life, and who have a relationship with Jesus, often can't wait to run toward eternity. But that can be hard for their family members to understand. For many years this wasn't even a topic of discussion because we didn't have the medical means to prolong life as we do now. Even so, I've observed that many seniors who live into their nineties don't want to be kept alive artificially. They're ready to go.

Ann's family finally agreed to let her go without taking extraordinary measures to keep her alive. With her family surrounding her, we stood on heaven's front porch to wish her good-bye as she stepped across.

TODAY'S RX

If your end-of-life preferences have not been formalized, consider a living will to make your desires known.

Father, I long to please you with my life. May all my choices be an effort to honor you, praise you, and know you more deeply. Thank you for being in relationship with me.

THE GIFT THE WORLD CANNOT GIVE

I am leaving you with a gift—peace of mind and heart. And the peace I give is a gift the world cannot give. So don't be troubled or afraid. JOHN 14:27

Susan sat in my office in a bundle of nerves and tears. I'd known her for a number of years and was aware that she struggled with anxiety. She was normally able to handle her fears with medication and counseling, but her husband had recently been diagnosed with renal cell carcinoma, and it had caught her off guard. Though Marcus had undergone successful surgery to remove the cancer, Susan's anxiety hadn't abated.

"Is Marcus going to be okay?" she asked with a quivering lip.

"All indications are that he's going to be fine," I said.

"Are you sure?"

"From the report the surgeon sent me, he thinks he got it all."

"I know that's what he said, but I'm still worried. What about the sepsis?"

Marcus had twice come to the ER with postoperative fevers. Each time, to be cautious, they had admitted him, completed a sepsis workup, and sent him home with medications.

"The antibiotics should take care of that," I reassured her.

"But could he die from the sepsis, even though the cancer surgery was successful?"

"What are you truly afraid of?" I asked.

Susan chewed her fingernails and stared off into space for a moment. With fresh tears running down her cheeks, she whispered, "I don't want him to die."

"God is the only one who knows all the details, Susan. He's in charge of every breath we take. At some point, we're all going to die. But when he calls us home, we will live with him forever in heaven."

"I know," she said as she tried to stop the tears.

"I spoke with Marcus right after his surgery, before we got the pathology report back." I said. "He expressed some of the same fears that you're describing now. But he told me he was totally at peace with whatever God chose to happen."

Susan looked at me, surprised. "He said that?" I nodded, and she wiped her eyes. "Well then, so am I."

God calmed her heart and gave her peace of mind—which only he can truly provide.

TODAY'S RX

Be open to God's will for your life. He will calm your fears and allow you to live in peace.

God, only the peace that you supply is sufficient to calm my fears. Please remove any anxious thoughts from my mind, and replace them with promises of your provision and love.

WHO ELSE?

That evening many demon-possessed people were brought to Jesus. He cast out the evil spirits with a simple command, and he healed all the sick. This fulfilled the word of the Lord through the prophet Isaiah, who said, "He took our sicknesses and removed our diseases." MATTHEW 8:16-17

This story of Jesus taking our physical illness and removing our diseases is just a foreshadowing of greater things to come. On the cross, not only did Jesus take our sicknesses, he also took all of the sins of the world—past, present, and future. His death made us clean and spiritually healthy once again.

No matter how hard we try, and even with all of the tools of modern medicine, doctors cannot heal everyone. Even diseases that have cure rates nearing 100 percent still have an isolated case or two that doesn't respond to treatment. But with Jesus, his cure rate is always 100 percent.

When we look to Jesus for healing, we need to understand that his healing isn't limited to just our earthly world. Sometimes, to see his healing hands at work, we need to look beyond this world and realize that he may heal something greater than just our mortal bodies. He may choose not to heal us here on earth; he may want us to wait until he heals us permanently, for all of eternity.

Who else but Jesus could take our illnesses and heal them by the touch of his hand? Who else but Jesus and his death on the cross could heal our mortality?

The answers we receive to our prayers and requests for healing may be different from what we are asking, but that doesn't mean God hasn't heard or that he has denied us healing. Healing can occur on both sides of the veil that separates this world from the next. Complete healing of our mortal bodies will only happen on the other side of the veil.

TODAY'S RX

Look expectantly for God's healing, wherever it may happen.

Father, give me the courage to accept your plan for me, even when it deviates from what I ask. Embolden my faith so that I may trust you with all my heart through whatever lies ahead.

JESUS HAS COMMAND OVER DISEASE AND TIME

Suddenly, a man with leprosy approached him and knelt before him. "Lord," the man said, "if you are willing, you can heal me and make me clean." Jesus reached out and touched him. "I am willing," he said. "Be healed!" And instantly the leprosy disappeared. MATTHEW 8:2-3

As soon as Eve took the first bite from the forbidden fruit, she blamed the serpent. Adam also took a bite, and he blamed Eve. Today, we live in a broken world where we often want to blame others for our problems. When we think we've been wronged, whether by our parents, our boss, or our politicians, we want retribution and repair. And we want it done yesterday!

When something goes awry and doesn't turn out the way you think it should, do you look for someone or something else to blame?

When we look for the causes of sin and disease, it's often easy to point to things that someone else should have done differently. But we're all guilty and responsible for our separation from God and for spoiling the perfect world he designed for us. When we fell away from God through our disobedience, sin and disease entered the world.

Jesus came to restore that broken relationship. As part of that restoration, he sometimes heals people who are sick. In today's verse, we see a leper who could have blamed others for the disease that had likely left him scarred and missing fingers or toes. Instead, he reached out to Jesus, believing that he alone could heal him.

To fix this man's medical problems would have taken years of modern medical treatment, but Jesus not only healed the leper completely, he healed him instantly. When Jesus performed this miracle, he repaired what was broken in this man's life. In doing so, he took control not only of the disease, but also of time. It was a perfect example of Jesus' authority and sovereignty over the world.

TODAY'S RX

The next time you're tempted to blame someone else or demand that what's broken be fixed immediately, let go of your expectations and allow God to heal what is broken. And let him do it in his perfect timing.

Lord, help me to be honest and humble. I know my sin is a result of my own actions and no one else's; and I know that my saving grace is from you and no one else. May I grow to resemble you more closely every day of my life.

BEHIND THE SMILE

The LORD your God is living among you. He is a mighty savior. He will take delight in you with gladness. With his love, he will calm all your fears. He will rejoice over you with joyful songs. ZEPHANIAH 3:17

"Dr. Anderson, I have a question for you," Virginia said. "Why do you smile all the time? You're surrounded all day by sick and dying patients."

Virginia had been very observant of the moods of the caregivers who had come in and out of her hospital room that day. She was in an especially reflective state of mind because we had just diagnosed her with metastatic pancreatic cancer. She knew that her time on earth was coming to an end.

"I smile because I believe there is a very thin veil that separates us from where we are right now to where we are meant to be in heaven. Heaven isn't something we run to, it walks alongside us. When I have the honor of being at a patient's bedside when that veil is pulled back, I get a small sneak-peek into heaven. That experience fills my soul with gladness."

"I know you have only a few minutes before you have to attend to other patients," Virginia said, "but would you pray with me, and *for* me, this morning? I would be honored if you would."

"I always have time to pray," I said as I took her hand.

"Lord, we know that the timing of Virginia's journey is in your hands. Help her know how close you are and that her journey home is not a long one. Reassure her that we, as your servants, will do everything we can to make the time she has left on earth as free of pain as possible. Encourage her to know that we will be by her side as she is delivered into your hands."

Three days later, I was back in Virginia's very crowded room. Her loved ones had come to help deliver her into the next world. Right before the veil parted, Virginia looked up and to the right in what I call "the gaze of glory." She had a glow on her face when she took her last breath. Everyone in the room could feel the Lord's presence as she passed, and we all smiled.

TODAY'S RX

It's possible to smile at death when we know that heaven's foyer is on the other side of the veil.

Jesus, Prince of Peace, you are the calmer of the seas. You bring perfect peace to the hearts of all who have faith in you. I thank you for the peace you've given me.

A SOLID ROCK

Trust in the LORD always, for the LORD God is the eternal Rock. ISAIAH 26:4

"My emotions are all over the place," Jillian said. "One minute I'm crying because I feel sad, and the next moment I'm angry. But that's not all. It's the dead of winter, and I'm having hot flashes that are so bad I'm sweating while everyone around me is freezing. I feel like I'm in a raging river being tossed around while my family is standing on the banks wondering what's wrong with me."

Jillian was fifty-two, and her menses were as irregular as her emotional state.

"You're going through menopause," I said. "Your ovaries are shutting down. They gave you four great children, but now they're getting confused. They don't know which hormones to produce and how much to release at a time. That's why you get surges that make you feel as if you're not on solid ground—because, hormonally speaking, you're not."

"What can I do about it? I can't live like this. Should I go on hormone replacement therapy?"

"There are many options, and just as many opinions, in medicine today. In the past, we put everyone on replacement treatment, but now we tailor treatment to your individual needs. The studies are still coming in about the risk/benefit ratio for hormones. I agree that we need to focus on how to minimize and manage the symptoms you're experiencing."

I talked with Jillian about several options. I wanted to make sure she understood the importance of good nutrition, exercise, and other techniques, such as relaxation treatments. We also discussed medications that were available to help her with the emotional ups and downs she was experiencing.

"How long does menopause last?" she asked.

"The average is about two years, and then things should settle down."

"I feel like I just need a solid bit of ground to stand on until then," Jillian said.

You may not be going through menopause, but perhaps something else is rocking your world and making you feel as if you're being tossed around. Today's verse promises us that God is our Rock. If we build our life on him, we may take a battering during a storm, but the strong winds of adversity won't be able to knock us down.

TODAY'S RX

Trust God. He is our eternal Rock.

When my life is spinning out of control, I know I can go to you for refuge, Lord. You are my steady ground. Thank you for remaining constant when all else is in flux.

SACK RACE TO HEAVEN

I press on to reach the end of the race and receive the heavenly prize for which God, through Christ Jesus, is calling us. PHILIPPIANS 3:14

"How long do I have before this cancer takes me home?" Allen asked me one December.

"Only the Lord knows our days, but the cancer you have is advanced, and surgery isn't an option at this point. Typically, most patients at this stage have fewer than six months."

"I have a few things I need to do before I go," Allen said, "and I'm going to do my best to press forward. Please don't tell anyone else my prognosis."

Allen's family was aware that he had cancer, but they had no idea how little time he had left. When anyone asked him about it, Allen simply replied, "Jesus and I have this thing beat!"

Allen wanted to live long enough to be at his son's wedding, but by the time the family sent out the announcements, Allen had already lived six months longer than expected—and the wedding was still six months away.

"I'm still running the race," he told me at his next appointment, "but it feels like a three-legged sack race. My son is getting married in June. I think I can make it. What do you think?"

"You've already lived longer than all the studies I've read, so we'll just trust God with this," I said.

"It's a good thing that Jesus is my partner in this sack race!" Allen said. "We've got it beat!"

A few weeks before the wedding, Allen was having trouble swallowing. I arranged for him to have a feeding tube inserted into his abdomen to help with his nutrition.

"Let's fight the good fight," Allen said.

By the time of the wedding, Allen was in a wheelchair. But the bride was beautiful, and the groom was beaming with pride. When I saw Allen the next week, he said, "I'm ready now. Everything on my list is checked off. Jesus and I, we got this thing beat."

Two months later, Allen finished the race, still holding tight to the promises of his heavenly sack race partner.

TODAY'S RX

With Jesus as your partner in the race of life, you will be victorious every time.

Jesus, help me to have a positive outlook as I fight the good fight and keep my eyes on the finish line. You are the fuel I need to keep going, the partner to root me on. Thank you for being beside me always.

THE PARALYSIS OF MODERN MEDICINE

Immediately, as everyone watched, the man jumped up, picked up his mat, and went home praising God. Everyone was gripped with great wonder and awe, and they praised God, exclaiming, "We have seen amazing things today!" LUKE 5:25-26

When patients show up in the emergency room complaining that they are unable to walk, our protocol is to admit them into the hospital.

Over the next few days, we'll run a battery of tests, including an MRI, a nerve conduction study, and a neurovascular workup. The physical therapist is consulted, and depending on the diagnosis, a usually long and laborious course of treatment follows. However, modern medicine is limited in what it can do. In some cases, the patient could be disabled for life. New treatments from stem cells that are created from the patient's own blood may offer increased mobility, but the focus on stem cells is so new that it's far from a sure thing.

But with Jesus, all things are certain. The outcome is known before the patient even arrives. Like everyone in the crowd who witnessed the events in today's verses, I am gripped with great wonder and awe for the lame who are immediately healed, can walk, and even jump for joy.

There's no doubt that as a doctor, Luke had seen and treated many patients who were lame. But neither he nor I have seen a man go from lame to dancing in an instant. This miracle once again proves that Jesus is in control of time and the physical world in which we live. It would take modern medicine months, if not years, for patients to achieve even a partial recovery. But Jesus heals instantly and completely.

Are you limping through life? Is it hard to put one foot in front of the other? Do you take one step forward and two steps back? Pick up your mat and set it at the feet of Jesus. Ask for his guidance. His loving arms and healing hands will embrace you and encourage you to move forward.

TODAY'S RX

The lame jump for joy and praise him. Shouldn't we do the same?

When fear cripples me, Lord, and I cannot move forward, take my hand and help me to put one foot in front of the other. Your gentle guidance is all I need.

A JOURNEY OF FAITH

Through faith in the name of Jesus, this man was healed—and you know how crippled he was before. Faith in Jesus' name has healed him before your very eyes. ACTS 3:16

The man who stood in my office said, "I didn't come to see you because I need a doctor; I came to see you because I need something else."

"Tell me more."

"I was born with a heart defect," he said. "I had my first surgery before I was a year old. The cardiologist has continued to monitor my situation, and he says I need one more surgery. I hope this one will be my last. I have it set up with the hospital in Nashville for next week."

"Okay, but how can I help you?"

"I didn't even know who you were until about a month ago when a friend of mine gave me a copy of *Appointments with Heaven*. I got to know you through that book." Then he smiled and added, "And I also got to know Jesus. While reading your story, I rekindled my faith in him. I was drawn closer to Jesus, and my love for him grew. Now I'm having this heart surgery, and I realize there's a chance I might not wake up from it. But I know that Jesus is with me. Your book helped relieve me of so much fear. I'm no longer afraid of dying, and I look forward to my life, whether it is here or in heaven."

His words were touching, and I felt a few tears welling up. I was grateful that God had used my story to reach someone who had distanced himself from him. "Thank you for telling me," I said.

"I came to see you because I wanted you to pray for me during the surgery and my recovery. I know this might be an odd request, but I just wanted another believer to pray with me."

It was pretty unusual for someone to stop by my office and ask me to pray with them on their first visit, but it was obvious that God had opened this door. "I'd be honored to pray with you," I said. "And I'll pray that everyone you meet will know that it's your faith in Jesus that healed you."

TODAY'S RX

Trust that in your journey with God, he is leading you down the perfect path.

Lord, you've proven faithful to me time and again. Help me to share stories of your faithfulness with others, encouraging them to come to know you and experience your great love.

THE HEALING GIFTS OF THE MAGI

They entered the house and saw the child with his mother, Mary, and they bowed down and worshiped him. Then they opened their treasure chests and gave him gifts of gold, frankincense, and myrrh. MATTHEW 2:11

Ask anyone who is familiar with the Bible to name the gifts that Jesus received from the magi, and they will say gold, frankincense, and myrrh. But ask them *why* the magi brought those particular gifts, and the answer may be less certain. Most people recognize the value of gold, but why frankincense and myrrh?

Myrrh was one of the ingredients that Moses used to make a sacred oil for anointing the Ark of the Covenant, the Tabernacle, and all its utensils. Whatever the oil touched was made holy.

In the ancient Near East, both myrrh and frankincense were used to make perfumes, oils, and ointments. In the Tabernacle, the priests would sprinkle frankincense over their grain offerings to create an aroma pleasing to the Lord.

Just as myrrh makes things holy and frankincense makes an offering pleasing to the Lord, Jesus himself was holy, and he ultimately became a wholly pleasing sacrifice for our sins. Perhaps the gifts he received were a way to foreshadow what was yet to come.

Frankincense and myrrh both have healing properties, as well. Myrrh can affect the hypothalamus and the pituitary. It can help to improve our spirits, diminish our fears, and make us more trusting and less judgmental. Myrrh also has antioxidant properties that can help to relieve stress and mitigate diseases. Frankincense is an antiseptic and disinfectant. It can even be used in some cancer treatments. These are but a few of the properties of medicinal oils made from frankincense and myrrh that we are now scientifically validating.

When these gifts were presented to the baby Jesus, they symbolized the emotional and physical healing that he would bring to the people he encountered during his earthly ministry. Today, we use anointing oils with frankincense and myrrh when we pray for the sick and dying. The oil represents and reminds us of the power that Jesus has over death and disease, as well as the presence of the Holy Spirit, who brings renewed health and vitality to those for whom we pray.

TODAY'S RX

If you're sick, invite your friends to anoint you with oil and pray for your health to be renewed.

Jesus, thank you for being the perfect gift to this world. Help me to remember always that I am healed of my sins through your perfect sacrifice.

A PAIN IN THE BACK

What are worthless and wicked people like? They are constant liars, signaling their deceit with a wink of the eye, a nudge of the foot, or the wiggle of fingers. Their perverted hearts plot evil, and they constantly stir up trouble. But they will be destroyed suddenly, broken in an instant beyond all hope of healing. PROVERBS 6:12-15

Owen was a new patient, and I watched out of the corner of my eye as the nurse took him back to the exam room. There was nothing remarkable about his appearance other than a slight limp. Otherwise, he looked like an average middle-aged man. But when I entered the exam room, I quickly found out how aggressive he was. Without even waiting for a greeting, he stuffed a stack of medical records and X-rays into my hands from the last four or five doctors he'd seen.

"As you can see, I've been to all these specialists, and I've had three back surgeries. But none of them worked, and I'm still hurting."

As I did my exam, I noticed that his vitals were a little elevated, and he had a scar from at least one surgery. We discussed treatment options to control his pain with medication. Often, opiates are used in this type of situation, and from his records, it appeared that his prior doctors had prescribed these for his pain.

"I ran out of my last prescription; that's why I'm here to see you today," Owen said.

His story seemed legitimate. I did a urine drug test, which came back negative, confirming that he'd been out of pills at least long enough for the drugs to clear his system.

As I prepared his prescription, I did one last check, and then the truth was revealed. The state recently had started an online program listing all the doctors and pharmacies a patient had visited in the past few months. From the online records, I could see that Owen had never stopped going to his previous doctors. He was getting a full prescription of opiates from each one. A quick check of the pharmacies and emergency rooms he'd visited confirmed our worst fears. Owen was a dealer, selling his pain medication to others. But once he was reported to the district attorney's office, the gig was up. They were happy to take this dealer off the streets.

TODAY'S RX

Be certain to handle your medications responsibly, and properly dispose of unused quantities.

God, when evil seems to pervade all corners of the earth, I take comfort in knowing you are victorious. Thank you for not giving up on your people, but showing us your undying compassion and love instead.

RULES ON THE ROAD TO HEALTH

God detests the prayers of a person who ignores the law. PROVERBS 28:9

I entered the exam room and shook Kevin's hand. "It's good to see you," I said. "It's been a while since you've been in."

"Yeah, I know. I should have come back like you told me. But, you know, life happens, and I was busy."

"Looking at your chart, I see you've been out of medication. You haven't refilled your prescription in months."

"Yeah, I know. When my prescription ran out, I just stopped refilling it."

"Well, what brings you in today?" I asked.

"I'm having a hard time breathing. It seems like I'm always short of breath, even when I'm not exerting myself."

Kevin's complaints were common. Like most people with medical problems, staying healthy required work. In Kevin's case, he had diabetes, hyperlipidemia, and hypertension. To manage his diseases, he needed to do regular blood sugar and blood pressure checks. He needed to take his medications, follow a prescribed diet, and exercise regularly. But following all of those "rules" wasn't enough. He also had to have regular lab work and visits with his doctor to make sure the prescribed treatment was keeping him on the path to physical health. If not, the health rules he lived by would need to be changed.

Unfortunately, Kevin hadn't obeyed any of the rules he'd been given. As I examined him that day, I realized he was having a massive heart attack. He received immediate intervention to save his life and from that point forward had to follow the rules he had previously ignored. He knew that if he wanted to stay alive, he would have to respect these rules and follow them closely.

If you are driving down the highway and disregard the rules of the road, sooner or later you'll have a major crash. Kevin nearly died because he hadn't obeyed the medical advice he'd been given. In our spiritual lives, just like in medicine, noncompliance can lead to death. The laws of the road, the laws of medicine, and the laws of the Bible are there for our own good. Following them leads to health.

TODAY'S RX

Pay attention to the laws of life. They can keep you alive spiritually and physically.

Father, help me to be wise and live in compliance with your laws. I want to experience more of your glory.

THE LAWS I THINK ABOUT MOST

Oh, how I love your instructions! I think about them all day long. Your commands make me wiser than my enemies, for they are my constant guide. Yes, I have more insight than my teachers, for I am always thinking of your laws. I am even wiser than my elders, for I have kept your commandments. PSALM 119:97-100

In college I took a lot of science classes. In chemistry and physics, we learned the laws of nature, such as "a body in motion will remain in motion," or "order gives way to disorder." In biology, we learned the theories that seek to explain the origins of humanity.

Whether it was a law or a theory, the science I studied was supposed to answer questions about the world we live in and how we got here. But often, my studies exposed more questions than they answered.

I went on to medical school with the expectation that I would learn the answers to my questions. At the time, I was an atheist who believed that all of life's mysteries would become known in my study of science and medicine. But the more I studied, the more I realized that no matter how much knowledge I accumulated, there were still questions that the academic disciplines couldn't answer—or couldn't answer convincingly.

That's when my thoughts turned to God.

While sitting in my gross anatomy lab one day, I looked at the human body in front of me, marveling at its beauty and organization. In seeing how the complexity and integration of the various systems were so well conceived and designed, I concluded that an intelligent being must have played a part in our creation.

That's when I became convinced that there was an artist behind the art. And even though the teaching experts explained a lot of what we saw, there was so much more that couldn't be explained. Even at the highest levels of science and medicine, there are still mysteries that point to God, and one of those mysteries is the human capacity to feel, think, act selflessly, and love.

When I left my atheistic thinking behind and began to follow God, the laws of science and the theories of medicine still played a role. But I realized, as today's verses say, that God's laws have more insight than the wisdom of my earthly teachers.

TODAY'S RX

Take a moment today to ponder the beauty of God's laws.

Lord, I praise you for your artistry and craftsmanship. You've made this world so wonderfully complex. Thank you for giving me life.

EXCHANGING "STUFF" FOR THE SUBSTANCE OF GOD

Don't copy the behavior and customs of this world, but let God transform you into a new person by changing the way you think. Then you will learn to know God's will for you, which is good and pleasing and perfect. ROMANS 12:2

We often think of peer pressure as something that happens to our kids, but there are just as many adults who feel pressured to conform to other people's standards. We want the upper-middle-class American Dream of a bigger house, a newer car, and photos from the hottest vacation spots to post on social media. Not only do we want to keep up with the Joneses, we want to surpass them.

Conforming to the ways of others may be as subtle as living in a neighborhood with building codes and mandated color palettes or as monstrous as shared opinions about discrimination or racism. We want to be a part of the "in" group, and we'll do what everyone else is doing to make it happen. Unfortunately, groupthink isn't always the smartest way to think.

God wants us to do our best and enjoy his world. However, if our beliefs and actions are inspired by our desires to keep up with our neighbors rather than honoring God, we might need to rethink our motivation.

God wants us to renew our minds to see and experience the world as he does. When we do, we begin to understand and love others who are different from us. We appreciate diversity in people and nature. The world blossoms and grows more beautiful. We recognize our place as a small part of a much bigger plan.

When God transforms us, our desires will conform to his desires, and our eyes will see the world through the same lens of grace that he uses to see us. Instead of worrying about what the Joneses have, we'll only want more of what God is freely offering.

TODAY'S RX

Be a nonconformist; instead of looking at your neighbors' stuff, spend time with God in nature admiring all that he has created for us.

Lord, I confess that it's easy to focus on what I lack and forget about all I've been blessed with. Help me to not lose sight of the many gifts you've given me, but to appreciate them and use them for your honor.

MUSIC THAT CALMS THE TROUBLED HEART

Let us find a good musician to play the harp whenever the tormenting spirit troubles you. He will play soothing music, and you will soon be well again. 1 Samuel 16:16

Nowhere is the connection between physical, emotional, and spiritual illness more evident than in a psychiatric hospital. While I was the medical director of a mental health facility in Jackson, Tennessee, I saw on a daily basis how even one poor health decision could dramatically affect a person's emotions and spirit. Conversely, I could see how a patient with a positive attitude seemed to improve not only emotionally, but also in spirit and in health. It's as if the physical, emotional, and spiritual strands of our lives weave together to make up the cord of our health.

The power of God's words to heal disease and infirmity is proved over and over again in the Bible. It has also been proven time and again in my own experience. I've watched patients' spirits change dramatically when their family members read Scripture to them. Their screaming seemed to subside as they heard the red-letter words of Jesus. Watching it happen was like watching music soothe a wild beast.

Later in my medical practice, when a belligerent, demented patient confronted me in the emergency room, I reminded myself that it was all connected. Medicine that affects the body also affects a patient's mental and spiritual health. Patients who were mentally unstable often didn't take care of themselves physically. At times, it was very tedious to tease out the difference between symptom and cause.

In those difficult moments, I'd think of Jesus, who healed both mind and body, removing every kind of sickness and disease. Patients brought to his feet were then brought under his healing command. When he simply spoke words of healing, demons and disease would flee the person's body. Even today, his words are the music we use to calm our wild and troubled hearts.

TODAY'S RX

Are you having a hard day? Are your cords fraying under the weight of all you have to bear? If so, turn to Scripture, and allow God's words to be the chords of music that will soothe your ears, heart, and mind.

Jesus, there are so many people who are lost and troubled in this world. They need to know your love and experience your healing touch. Use me as you see fit to shine your light where it needs to be cast.

THE BIRTH OF JOY

Always be joyful. 1 THESSALONIANS 5:16

A mere fifty-seven years and fifteen minutes after I was born, my daughter Kristin gave birth to my first grandchild, Callum. Shortly after his birth, I went to Belfast, Northern Ireland, to meet him and welcome him into the world.

Today's verse reminds us to always be joyful, and at that moment it was easy! I can't begin to describe how happy it made me to cuddle that little bundle of love. When Callum was born, he delighted all of us, and he continues to do so every day.

But what about those moments when things are hard? Was Jesus joyful when he wept for his friend Lazarus? Or how am I supposed to be joyful when I walk from the ER to the waiting room to tell a family that their loved one has died? It's hard to find joy in a room full of grief.

Obviously it's okay to be sad because even Jesus wept. So it must be possible to experience both joy and grief in the same moment. But how?

Though it may not be immediately evident in a hospital waiting room, I think that after some time has passed, it is possible for people to look back and see that grief and joy coexisted in the same moment. When there is a death on earth, there is sadness on this side of the veil as we say good-bye to a loved one. But on the other side, there is great joy as a new soul is born into the delivery room of heaven.

Though we may feel sadness when our friends or family go on before us, there should be great joy in knowing what awaits them on the other side. And when we die, it will be like the ultimate Christmas, because in that moment, we will receive the greatest gift of all—eternal joy with our Father in heaven.

TODAY'S RX

Find joy amid the ashes, and praise God for the promise we have of heaven.

Lord, thank you for the gift of eternal life. May I always have my eyes set on heaven and the glory that awaits me there.

A SACRIFICIAL CHRISTMAS GIFT

The LORD is like a father to his children, tender and compassionate to those who fear him. PSALM 103:13

Daddy was a proud man. He was a teacher and a farmer, and he taught his children how to live upright and work hard. My siblings and I respected him and feared him because of his strength of character. What he said was law, and the law was laid down by biblical principles. "Honor thy father and thy mother" was often repeated in our house. He taught us lessons, not through lectures, but through his deeds.

The Christmas when I was eight started out like any other. My siblings and I waited patiently until the sun came up before racing to the living room, where the Christmas tree stood. As we rounded the corner, we came to a sudden stop.

There were only two presents, but there were three of us. Who was left out?

Turns out it was me! And I had so badly wanted a bike that year.

With a new house, the family budget had been stretched beyond its limits. And though I didn't know it at the time, the new BB gun my parents had gotten me for my birthday in October was supposed to count for both my birthday and Christmas. But in my mind, as an eight-year-old child, I thought Santa had forgotten me.

My sobs awoke my father. When he heard my cries, he was determined to do something about it. This proud man humbled himself to beg and borrow enough money to buy me a bike.

I watched my father exchange his pride for my gift that Christmas. Even at eight, I understood what a selfless gift it was. My adoration for him has flowed ever since. Dad became my hero that day, and though he has since passed on to heaven, he will be my hero forever.

When I think about my earthly father giving up so much, I'm humbled at how much more God the Father sacrificed for us, sending his Son to die so that we could have eternal life.

Not everyone is blessed with an earthly father who would sacrifice the way my father did. But we all have a heavenly Father who willingly sacrificed to give us the best Christmas present we could ever hope to receive.

TODAY'S RX

Adore and worship God this season for the sacrifices he has made for you.

Thank you for sending your Son to earth, Father, to be the sacrifice for my sin. I am forever grateful for this undeserved gift.

CHRISTMAS DAY CAN BE EVERY DAY

On another Sabbath day, a man with a deformed right hand was in the synagogue while Jesus was teaching. The teachers of religious law and the Pharisees watched Jesus closely. If he healed the man's hand, they planned to accuse him of working on the Sabbath. But Jesus knew their thoughts. He said to the man with the deformed hand, "Come and stand in front of everyone." So the man came forward. Then Jesus said to his critics, "I have a question for you. Does the law permit good deeds on the Sabbath, or is it a day for doing evil? Is this a day to save life or to destroy it?" He looked around at them one by one and then said to the man, "Hold out your hand." So the man held out his hand, and it was restored! Luke 6:6-10

When patients come into the emergency room on holidays, they are often surprised to find me working.

"How come you're not at home with your family?"

As I look around at the rooms full of sick and hurting people, I say, "God wanted me to be here with you when you're sick. My family and I will celebrate when I get home."

I didn't realize how unusual this was, until a few years ago when my daughter Kristin called my wife with a question.

"What day is Christmas?"

"December 25," Karen said.

"Is it the same date every year?"

"Yes. Unlike Easter, Christmas is the same date every year."

At the time, Kristen was a young woman in her twenties living in Ireland, and though most people know that Christmas is on December 25, Kristin had rarely celebrated the holiday on the actual day.

As a young country doctor, I often had to work or at least be on call on Christmas Eve and Christmas Day. To avoid my getting called away in the middle of our family celebration, we typically celebrated Christmas on a day when I could schedule another doctor to cover for me. My kids knew that Christmas was in December, but we placed little importance on the exact date. Anytime between December 15 and 30 could be Christmas for us.

On Christmas, we celebrate God's gift to us of his Son. The least we can do is offer ourselves as a gift to someone in need.

TODAY'S RX

On this Christmas Day, do what you can to help someone else.

Lord, thank you for Christmas Day and the joy of this season.
May I always praise the King of kings and be grateful for how
you sent your precious Son, Immanuel, to this earth.

OLD PROMISES OF HEALING IN NEW MODERN WAYS

His people believed his promises. Then they sang his praise. Psalm 106:12

"Dr. Anderson, I know God has promised many things in the Bible, but do you think he can heal me?" Darryl asked.

Stage four colon cancer can be a scary diagnosis. When I was in medical school, and also as a resident, we were told to approach patients with metastatic colon cancer carefully because the diagnosis was the equivalent of a death sentence. We would have a short conversation about treatment protocols, and then the conversation would drift to end-of-life care and the comfort measures the patient wanted.

In those moments, I talked to my patients about what they wanted or did not want in their final moments. I also took the opportunity to discuss their spiritual health. They needed to know that their time on earth was short.

As I considered how to answer Darryl's question, I thought about all those past conversations. With new medical advancements, the diagnosis no longer carries the grave prognosis it once did. That's not to say that everyone will be healed or survive, but great strides in oncology treatment have been made. Many of my patients are still alive and singing God's praises years after their final treatment cycle.

Some call these advances a medical breakthrough, but I prefer to think of them as a medical miracle—one that God has guided. Though these discoveries are made by medical science, I know that God has his hand in every one of them, as he reveals himself and keeps his promises every day. It's exciting to work in a field where I can see such marvelous evidence of God's faithfulness. It's a great reminder of why we need to keep our eyes open to what is happening around us so we can see the fulfillment of God's promises.

"Darryl, I believe that God keeps his promises to heal us. Sometimes it is an inexplicable event that happens here and now. Sometimes it is a miracle of science and medicine that was years in the making. And sometimes it is an indescribable event that happens when we enter our forever home. So, yes, Darryl, I am convinced that God keeps his promises and will heal you."

TODAY'S RX

Open your eyes today to see all of the ways in which God keeps his promises. Then sing praises to him.

Father, I will never cease to be amazed by your faithfulness in keeping your promises. Help me to keep my eyes open to them every day, so that I may witness more of your unfailing love and grow deeper in my faith.

WAITING FOR YOUR TURN

Your promise revives me; it comforts me in all my troubles. PSALM 119:50

Janet had been through a couple of tough years. She'd had surgery for weight loss, and the procedure had gone well, but she started having some complications around the same time her husband, Rick, got sick and died.

Rick and Janet had been active in their church and in the community. It seemed that everyone turned out for his funeral to support Janet. But something was different about her. It was as if Rick had taken the bright light of her personality with him when he left, leaving only a flickering flame.

Janet came to see me several weeks after the funeral. "I don't know how to get out of this nosedive. He was my world, and we did everything together. Now my heart is so heavy that I can hardly fill out the form to see you." I nodded, listening to her as she put words to her pain.

"Are you still gardening?" I asked. I knew their garden had been a source of pride for both of them.

"I don't even go outside. I just stay in my bedroom and keep the shades closed. I've gained twenty pounds in the past two months, and I know I'm eating myself to heaven so I can see Rick again."

"Janet, there are two things I know about you. First, you and Rick had an infinite love for each other. Second, you both loved the Lord even more than each other. Those things are still true. Rick caught an earlier flight to heaven, but I believe that God has also promised you a ticket. When he calls you, and not a day sooner, you'll be ready. Until then, you have to live here."

"On his last day, Rick talked about seeing glimpses of eternity, and he told me what they looked like."

"I believe that Rick gave you those glimpses as a way to sustain you until you can meet him there."

I saw Janet several times over the next two years as the flickering flame was restored to the bright beacon it had once been. One day she said to me, "You have been with me through thick and thin, but the most important thing you ever told me was that when things are the worst, look up. That's what keeps me going."

TODAY'S RX

If your loved ones have gone on before you, glorify God with every day you have left before you join them.

Father, I look forward to the day when I can be reunited with my loved ones who have gone on before me. Keep them in your care, and sustain me here on earth until my time arrives.

A TEMPERATURE OF 103 DEGREES

A raging fever burns within me, and my health is broken. PSALM 38:7

"Nurse, how many patients have we seen today?"

"Forty and counting. The waiting room is standing room only."

"Does everyone in the county have the flu?" I asked. But she had already moved on to the next room.

I was the only doctor available in the entire county that day. The other two were out. One had just finished a twenty-four-hour shift, and the other had the flu.

As I continued to see patient after patient and write the same prescription—Tylenol, fluids, and rest—it occurred to me that everyone seemed to have the exact same temperature: 103 degrees. After seeing a dozen more patients with the same readings, I said, "Is our thermometer broken, or does everyone have a fever of 103?"

"We use more than one thermometer," the nurse said, chuckling.

Still, it bothered me. With this many people presenting the exact same symptoms, my fear was that something other than the flu would slip by undetected.

By late afternoon, I was weary of repeating myself, and we were all tired from the pace we'd been keeping. "Who's next?" I asked the nurse.

"Patient ninety-three. Same complaints: sore throat, fever, temperature of 103."

When I entered the room and saw an older gentleman, I sensed that something different was going on here. Though his symptoms sounded the same, he seemed a little more lethargic than the other patients I'd seen. I did the exam, paying special attention to his head, neck, and throat. When I pulled out the hospital admission forms, the nurse looked at me as if to say, *Why are you admitting him? He has the same symptoms as everyone else!*

"Sir, I'm going to admit you and run some tests. Your neck is stiff. I want to check for meningitis."

Meningitis is a serious and life-threatening disease if not treated with IV antibiotics. At the hospital, the test results validated my instincts: meningitis. The next morning, the man's condition was much improved. Had we sent him home, he might have had a very different outcome. I thanked God for the nudge. Without his help, the diagnosis would have been easy to miss.

TODAY'S RX

Not all fevers are the same, and not all individuals are the same. We need to see others as God sees us—as individuals.

Help me to be alert and aware, Lord, as I go about my day and do my work. Ease my stress, and remind me that you are with me every step of the way.

FADED BODY, STRENGTHENED SOUL

The one thing I ask of the LORD—the thing I seek most—is to live in the house of the LORD all the days of my life, delighting in the LORD's perfections and meditating in his Temple. For he will conceal me there when troubles come; he will hide me in his sanctuary. He will place me out of reach on a high rock. PSALM 27:4-5

Like many young couples, Tony and Amanda enjoyed life—and maybe would admit that they enjoyed it a little too much. They regularly attended parties, and "just say no" was not in their vocabulary.

After years of partying, Amanda decided to cut back and stay home more. But Tony continued to go out with his buddies. Amanda assumed that Tony still used only alcohol and pot, like they had together. She didn't know he had moved on to IV drug use that led to other risky behaviors.

It wasn't until he started losing weight and developed bruise-like lesions on his skin that she suspected something was terribly wrong. When she finally convinced him to seek medical care, he was diagnosed with HIV. But by then, the disease had progressed too far for treatment, and Tony died soon after.

But that wasn't the worst of it for Amanda. One week after Tony's funeral, I gave her the sad news in my office: "You've HIV positive."

Through tears, she said, "Dr. Anderson, what am I going to do? I don't even know where I'm going to live. And what can I do with this death sentence hanging over me?"

"I know this is hard," I said. "But now, more than ever, God wants you to lean on him. We'll make some calls, and I'll help get you connected at the local AIDS clinic. We can reach out to Social Security to see if you can get some financial help as well."

For the next fifteen years, Amanda and I worked together to battle her disease and the complications that followed. Even as her body weakened, I could sense a growing strength in her soul. God had taken care of her, and she knew it.

One day she said to me, "I know that God is my rock. And though my body may wither, my soul will live forever in his sanctuary."

TODAY'S RX

Even as our bodies fade, our souls can soar to new heights.

Lord, I echo today's verse: My greatest desire is to live with you in your house all the days of my life. Thank you for giving me strength when I had none and hope when all else failed. I am grateful for how you've watched out for me.

FEAR NOT!

Jesus responded, "Why are you afraid? You have so little faith!" Matthew 8:26

Scripture repeatedly reminds us to have faith and not to fear.

As a doctor, a lot of my job involves alleviating fear and encouraging faith. When patients are waiting for test results, I tell them not to worry too early. I tell them to wait until we get the results back and know what we're dealing with. When they fear going to the hospital or having surgery, I remind them to trust in the experienced hands of those who will be taking care of them. And with all my patients, I want them to have faith that God is in control.

I understand why my patients fear the unknown and the undiagnosed. When something is amiss with our health, all sorts of thoughts run rampant through our minds. Sometimes the diagnosis is simple and easily treatable. When that happens, a patient's sigh of relief is audible.

"Wow, thanks, I thought it was something more serious!"

Even when the diagnosis is serious or life-threatening, if we put treatment plans in place, the patient has less to fear. Fear grows exponentially when fueled by the unknown.

Maybe that's why Jesus appears so frustrated with his disciples in today's verse. He was sitting right in front of them. What did they have to fear? They had the answer to all of life's questions in their very presence, and they could ask him anything they wanted. Yet they still doubted, and they still had fear.

With two thousand years of hindsight, it's easy to blame the disciples for their lack of faith. But aren't we also guilty of the same thing? We have all the answers that the early disciples had—*and* we have even more knowledge because we can see life through the historical lens of Scripture. We know that Jesus overcame death on the cross! Why should we ever doubt or fear? He is the way, the truth, and the life!

TODAY'S RX

Seeing Jesus' power throughout history should make us faithful and fearless.

Jesus, be with me when my fears are overwhelming. Help my soul to be still. Remind me of your power and victory over evil, and comfort me in your embrace.

GOD'S SUPPLY IS UNLIMITED

When I think of all this, I fall to my knees and pray to the Father, the Creator of everything in heaven and on earth. I pray that from his glorious, unlimited resources he will empower you with inner strength through his Spirit. EPHESIANS 3:14-16

If I could choose only one passage of Scripture to summarize this book, it would be today's verses.

In this world, there are limits to the medical resources we can provide. In this world, there is not enough money to pay for every treatment and test that patients or their doctors want. Your doctor may prescribe a certain procedure only to find out it's not covered, it's classified as elective, or it is considered medically unnecessary. The medical system today limits us to providing only those things that the patient needs, according to the powers that be.

Insurance companies, and sometimes government programs, help to regulate the flow of resources between the wants and the needs. This is the give-and-take reality that confronts so many people who seek treatment for themselves or their loved ones.

Even if we had unlimited financial resources, we still live in a finite world. Steve Jobs had nearly unlimited resources with his material wealth, yet even he wasn't able to buy more time on earth. We all are finite mortals.

When my patients are encumbered by the complexities of the health-care system, I remind them of today's verses. Ultimately, God is our source for all things. His resources are unlimited, and he alone heals. We doctors are just his tools here on earth to help provide temporary cures.

When we look to the infinite, all-powerful, all-knowing God of the universe, we find an endless well of supply. It is from this well that the living waters spring forth to forever heal us.

TODAY'S RX

It only takes a sip of living water for us to never thirst again.

God, there is no one like you. You are infinite, all-powerful, all-knowing, and you love your people with an everlasting love. Thank you for filling my spirit with your living water, reviving me to new life in you.

SCRIPTURE INDEX

Scripture Index

ABOUT THE AUTHOR

REGGIE ANDERSON, MD

Dr. Reggie Anderson was raised in the small, rural town of Plantersville, Alabama, and has come to embody the small-town wisdom and homespun morality that he grew up with. He graduated from the University of Alabama with a BS in chemistry and an English minor. While attending the University of Alabama Medical School, he met his wife, Karen. He completed his residency in family practice at the University of Tennessee in Jackson.

Reggie and Karen have raised four children, three daughters who are married and a son who is currently in nursing school. He and Karen reside on a farm in Kingston Springs, Tennessee, often opening their home as a refuge for those needing shelter following a natural disaster or other crisis.

Recently, Reggie was awarded The Frist Humanitarian Award by the Centennial Medical Center in Nashville. He was chosen from more than nine hundred doctors to be nominated for the national award.

Reggie is a member of the American Academy of Family Physicians and works at the TriStar Medical Group, where he continues to serve the poor and underprivileged in satellite offices in Ashland City and Kingston Springs, Tennessee. He also serves as chief of staff at TriStar Ashland City Medical Center, as well as the medical director of three nursing homes. Learn more about Reggie at www.appointmentswithheaven.com.

JENNIFER SCHUCHMANN

Whether writing or speaking, Jennifer loves the challenge of taking difficult concepts and finding ways to make them easy to understand, practical, and transformational. She excels at organizing masses of raw material into book form, while maintaining the voice and intent of the original communicator. She finds great joy in helping authors with compelling messages tell their stories to new audiences.

Recent books include: *Taylor's Gift* by Todd and Tara Storch, about the story of a couple who donated their daughter's organs after a skiing accident and later met the recipients; *Spirit Rising* by Jim Cymbala, an in-depth look at the Holy Spirit; and *By Faith, Not by Sight* by blind *American Idol* finalist, Scott MacIntyre. A selection of past books includes *One Call Away*, a memoir of Brenda Warner, and *First Things First*, a *New York Times* bestseller by Kurt and Brenda Warner.

Jennifer is the host of *Right Now with Jennifer Schuchmann*, which airs weekly on the NRB Network, Sky Angel satellite, and DIRECTV. She holds an MBA from Emory University, with an emphasis in marketing and communications, and a bachelor's degree in psychology from the University of Memphis. She's been married to David for more than twenty years, and they have a son, Jordan. Learn more about Jennifer at WordsToThinkAbout.com, or follow her on Twitter @schuchmann.

NOTES

1. Adapted from *Appointments with Heaven.*
2. C. S. Lewis, *Mere Christianity* (1952), first HarperCollins paperback ed. (New York: HarperOne, 2001), 136–137.
3. Adapted from *Appointments with Heaven.*
4. Adapted from *Appointments with Heaven.*
5. Adapted from *Appointments with Heaven.*
6. Adapted from *Appointments with Heaven.*
7. Adapted from *Appointments with Heaven.*
8. Adapted from *Appointments with Heaven.*
9. Motor Vehicle Accident

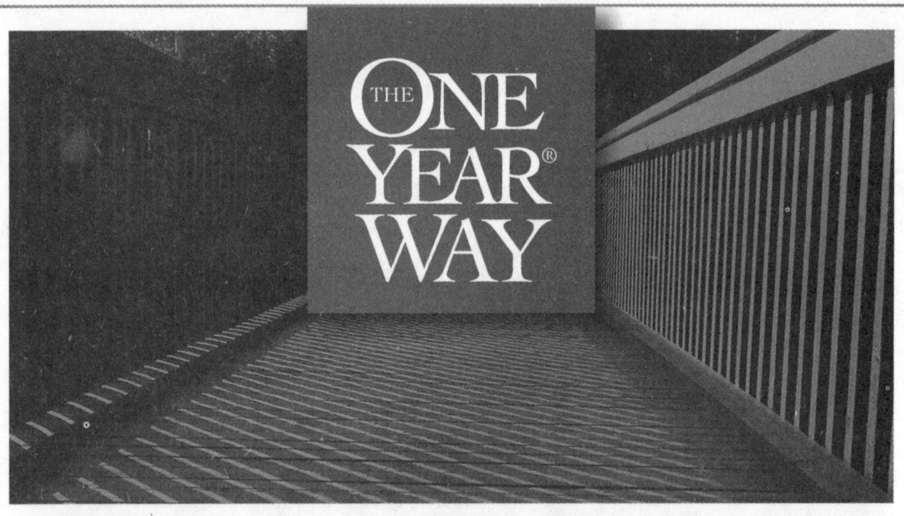
THE ONE YEAR® WAY